Comprehensive Dictionary of Audiology

Illustrated

Brad A. Stach

Chief Executive Officer
Nova Scotia Hearing and Speech Clinic
Halifax, Nova Scotia

Professor
School of Human Communication Disorders
Dalhousie University
Halifax, Nova Scotia

Williams & Wilkins
A WAVERLY COMPANY

THE HEARING
JOURNAL.

Editor: David H. Kirkwood
Production Editor: Wendi L. Neenan
Managing Editor: Kathleen Gaffney
Cover Design: M. Kwesi Brathwaite
Typesetter: Peirce Graphic Services, Inc.,
    Stuart, Florida
Printer & Binder: Edwards Brothers Inc.,
    Ann Arbor, Michigan

Library of Congress Cataloging-in-Publication Data
To purchase additional copies of this book, call our customer service department at **(800) 638-0672** or fax orders to **(800) 447-8438**. For other book services, including chapter reprints and large quantity sales, ask for the Special
Sales department.

Canadian customers should call **(800) 268-4178**, or fax **(905) 470-6780**. For
all other calls originating outside of the United States, please call **(410) 528-
4223** or fax us at **(410) 528-8550**.

Visit *Williams & Wilkins* on the Internet: http://www.wwilkins.com or con-
tact our customer service department at **custserv@wwilkins.com**. Williams &
Wilkins customer service representatives are available from 8:30 am to 6:00 pm,
EST, Monday through Friday, for telephone access.

97 98 99
1 2 3 4 5 6 7 8 9 10

To my mother and father,
Joan A. Stach and Harold L. Stach

PUBLISHER'S FOREWORD

When I joined *The Hearing Journal* several years ago, it soon became obvious that one of our publication's most valuable assets was James H. Delk's *Comprehensive Dictionary of Audiology*. First published by the *Journal* in 1973 and revised three times over the next decade, the Delk Dictionary had established itself as *the* classic reference resource of its kind among not only audiologists, but also hearing instrument specialists, otolaryngologists, and others in the hearing healthcare field.

While there was continuing demand for the dictionary, it was becoming clear that there was a growing need for an entirely new volume reflecting the dynamic changes that had taken place in audiology since the Delk dictionary was last revised in 1983.

To determine the interest in a new dictionary of audiology, our publisher, Williams & Wilkins, conducted a survey of *Hearing Journal* subscribers. Their enthusiastic response encouraged us to proceed with the project.

With Jim Delk having entered well-earned retirement after a 40-year career in hearing health care, our first and most important assignment was to identify someone who had the rare combination of knowledge, skills, and energy required to accomplish the daunting task of compiling a new comprehensive dictionary of audiology. To help us select the right person, we consulted a number of leaders in the field. Time and again, the name of Brad Stach was recommended to us.

It was easy to see why Dr. Stach came so highly recommended. Trained in audiology at Vanderbilt University and at Baylor College of Medicine, where he received his doctorate in 1986 under the direction of Dr. James Jerger, Brad had quickly established himself as a rising star in the profession. Before assuming his present positions as Chief Executive Officer of the Nova Scotia Hearing and Speech Clinic and Professor of Audiology at Dalhousie University, he held a number of other prestigious titles, including Director of Audiology at the California Ear Institute at Stanford University and Director of Audiology and Hearing Research at Georgetown University Medical Center.

Brad also had a proven track record as an author, having written dozens of articles for professional publications and book chapters on a sweeping range of audiologic topics.

Clearly, Brad had all the attributes we were looking for. Therefore, we were delighted when he agreed to become the editor of our new *Comprehensive Dictionary of Audiology*.

As you use this dictionary in your work, I'm sure you will concur with our choice of editor. In compiling this authoritative volume, Dr. Stach has achieved a difficult balance. While he provides complete definitions for all the terminology used in audiology today, he has also succeeded in making the text clear, concise, and eminently usable.

I am confident that Stach's *Comprehensive Dictionary of Audiology* will become an essential part of your professional library.

DAVID H. KIRKWOOD
Editor-in-Chief
The Hearing Journal
Williams & Wilkins

PREFACE

The need for this dictionary was never quite as clear to me as when I began to compile it. A number of sources of words, definitions, acronyms, and the like exist in various textbooks. They typically cover topics specific to the book's theme and highlight pertinent specialized vocabulary. Yet a modern source does not exist that consolidates these diverse efforts and covers the broad spectrum of the profession, practice, and science that we call audiology.

The idea to create this *Comprehensive Dictionary of Audiology* was not mine, I promise. The idea of writing and compiling a dictionary seemed a little like reading a phone book. But the actual process was a fascinating one that quickly proved to me the need for a comprehensive source of terminology for the profession.

The inspiration for this project is a volume often referred to as "the Delk dictionary." In 1973, James H. Delk authored *The Comprehensive Dictionary of Audiology,* a compilation of a *Dictionary of Audiology* series in the publication then entitled *The National Hearing Aid Journal,* which later became *The Hearing Journal.* The 4th edition of the Delk dictionary was published in 1983. The editorial staff at *The Hearing Journal* and Williams & Wilkins believed that it was time to revive the idea of a dictionary devoted to audiology, and it began anew in 1995. I am certain that few people could fully share my appreciation of James Delk's pioneering efforts.

We chose to begin this project from scratch, mostly in deference to the explosion of information and technology that has occurred over the past few years. Our challenge was to be thorough in our coverage of the past, current in our coverage of the present, and cognizant of the manner and speed with which proprietary and obfuscatory terminology comes and goes. To compile the list of terms, I extracted indices, glossaries, tables of contents, and appendices from a number of textbooks and journals. The lists were then consolidated by a colleague into a database that served as the basis of the dictionary. From that point, the task was one of plowing through the alphabet, term by term and letter by letter.

One of the advantages of writing a dictionary is that I was able to design it in a manner that corresponded to the way I might like to use it. More specifically, I was able to avoid those aspects of a dictionary that are less than convenient and useful. There are a number of things that annoy me about dictionaries, especially specialized ones. One is the overuse of cross-referencing. When I am seeking the definition of a term, I am not interested in being referred to two or three other terms to get the answer. Another is the overuse of tables within the body of a dictionary. Multipage tables interfere with efficient access to terminology that has the misfortune to be in alphabetic proximity to them. Another thing I find annoying is the overuse of figure and illustrations. Most of us do not read a dictionary. We get in and get out with the information that we need. Illustrations should serve to educate rather than decorate. To the extent that I could, then, I tried to use cross-referencing, tables, and illustrations judiciously, hopefully in a manner that is congruent with the way in which readers use the dictionary.

One of the goals in creating this dictionary was to make it as authoritative as possible. I consulted a number of sources, many of which are listed in the Acknowledgments section, as a way of assuring that nuances of the terminology were not lost. It is my fervent hope that this strategy was adequate to assure an appropriate level of quality overall.

Another goal in creating the dictionary was to make it as complete as possible. Completeness was a challenging goal. I found that there was no easy way to identify errors of omission. To address this, we enlisted the help of two doctoral students to find terms that were not included in an early draft of the dictionary. They were successful in identifying a number of additional terms; in the meantime, I continued adding terms until the moment the publisher pried the final draft from my hands.

One of the biggest challenges in creating this dictionary was to define its boundaries. For example, much of our terminology about hearing aids is generated by hearing instrument manufacturers about their own devices. I tried to include only those terms that I felt were generic enough to stand the test of time or that I thought might be useful from a historic perspective. Speech audiometric tests were handled similarly. Medical terminology was included as it related to hearing disorders or if it was used in a definition to describe a disease or disorder affecting the auditory system. However, no serious student would be without a *Stedman's Medical Dictionary* to supplement the terminology included in this audiology dictionary. I treated speech and language terminology similarly.

Margaret Prey was my 7th and 8th grade English teacher. She was famous for giving Dictation, a painful exercise in which we students were required to write the sentences that she dictated. She expected perfection. She was wonderfully tough and was quite quick to point out our errors. But we learned to expect perfection in our own writing. In that context, the task of writing a dictionary was exquisitely humbling—it provided me with over 6000 opportunities to be less than perfect. Although she has since passed away, Mrs. Prey would undoubtedly have gotten out her red pen as she read every word. If you as a reader find yourself doing the same, I hope that you will share your suggestions with me. I also hope that you will point out any omissions that you notice or any new terms that you create so that we can include them in future editions of the dictionary.

B.A.S.

ACKNOWLEDGMENTS

I am profoundly grateful to Charlotte Destino for her assistance in the initial phase of this project. Charlotte, a very talented audiologist and a favorite cousin, spent many hours consolidating the initial lists of terms from indices, glossaries, tables of contents, and appendices. She was responsible for compiling and distilling the list into an electronic database from which the definitions were ultimately generated. Although her task was an arduous one, she set as her goal the completion of the project prior to the birth of her first child. She delivered the database first, and then she and her husband, Tom, delivered a perfect child, Alexander Julian Destino. I would probably still be working on this project if it were not for the gracious assistance of Charlotte and the timeliness of Alex.

The first step in compiling this dictionary was to generate a database of terms to be defined. Numerous sources were used to accomplish this task. An electronic version of *Stedman's Medical Dictionary* served as a basis for the list. Relevant terms from *Terminology of Communication Disorders* by Nicolosi, Harryman, and Kresheck were added, as were relevant terms from the Delk dictionary. Indices, appendices, and glossaries were then compiled from a number of textbooks and journals, and missing terms were added to the database from these many sources. Textbooks from which terms were extracted included: Alpiner and McCarthy's *Rehabilitative Audiology;* Bess and Hall's *Screening Children for Auditory Function;* Bess and Humes's *Audiology: The Fundamentals;* Borden and Harris's *Speech Science Primer;* Carpenter's *Core Text of Neuroanatomy;* Davis and Hardick's *Rehabilitative Audiology for Children and Adults;* Davis and Silverman's *Hearing and Deafness;* Durrant and Lovrinic's *Bases of Hearing Science;* Gulick, Gescheider, and Frisina's *Hearing: Physiological Acoustics, Neural Coding, and Psychoacoustics;* Hall's *Handbook of Auditory Evoked Responses;* Hodgson's *Hearing Aid Assessment and Use in Audiologic Habilitation;* Jacobson and Northern's *Diagnostic Audiology;* Jerger and Jerger's *Auditory Disorders;* Jacobson's *Principles and Applications in Auditory Evoked Potentials;* Katz's *Handbook of Clinical Audiology;* Kryter's *Effects of Noise on Man;* Lipscomb's *Noise and Audiology;* Lipscomb's *Hearing Conservation,* Martin's *Introduction to Audiology;* Minifie's *Communication Sciences and Disorders;* Mueller, Hawkins, and Northern's *Probe Microphone Measurements;* Northern's *Hearing Disorders;* Northern and Downs's *Hearing in Children;* Olishifski and Harford's *Industrial Noise and Hearing Conservation;* Palmer's *Anatomy for Speech and Hearing;* Palmer and Yantis's *Survey of Communication Disorders;* Pollack's *Amplification for the Hearing Impaired;* Richard's *Basic Experimentation in Psychoacoustics;* Ross and Giolas's *Auditory Management of Hearing-Impaired Children;* Sandlin's *Handbook of Hearing Aid Amplification;* Sandlin's *Understanding Digitally Programmable Hearing Aids;* Schow and Nerbonne's *Introduction to Aural Rehabilitation;* Schuknecht's *Pathology of the Ear,* Speaks's *Introduction to Sound;* Silman and Silverman's *Auditory Diagnosis;* Tyler's *Cochlear Implants;* Valente's *Hearing Aids: Standards, Options, and Limitations;* Valente's *Strategies for Selecting and Verifying Hearing Aid Fittings,* and Zemlin's *Speech and Hearing Science Anatomy and Physiology.* Journals from which terms were extracted included: *American Journal of Audiology; American Journal of Otology; Archives of Otolaryngology—Head and Neck Surgery; Audiology; Audiology Today; Ear and Hearing; Journal of the American Academy of Audiology; Scandinavian Audiology; Seminars in Hearing;* and *The Hearing Journal.*

As definitions were being developed, the need arose to consult authoritative sources for clarification of terminology and the nuances of meaning. I found myself relying on a small group of sources for this purpose. For medical terms, I consulted *Stedman's* and, if necessary, *Dorland's Medical Dictionary.* I consulted the Durrant and Lovrinic book regularly for terminology related to anatomy and hearing science, the Schuknecht book regularly for auditory disorders, and the Northern and Downs book often for syndromes. For neuroanatomy questions, I referred to the Carpenter book, and for general questions, the Katz handbook. In addition, I cross-checked my understanding of the meaning of words with the Nicolosi et al. and Delk dictionaries. If I had questions about the meaning of more general terms, I consulted *Webster's New World Dictionary*. To compile the list of syndromes and associations, I referred often to a special issue of *Journal of the American Academy of Audiology,* edited by John Jacobson. Finally, whenever possible, I hunted for the original source of a term in journal articles too numerous to mention.

Once a draft of the dictionary was completed, it was reviewed by two doctoral students, George Lindley from the University of Pittsburgh, and Kiara Ebinger from Vanderbilt University. Their combined effort identified over 100 omissions that were included in the final version. I am indebted to these individuals for their efforts.

Appendix F, the report-writing glossary, consists of a number of descriptors of audiometric outcomes that can be used for computer generated reports. These descriptors were first developed around 1980 by Dr. James Jerger and his colleagues at the Baylor College of Medicine/Methodist Hospital. The audiology staff at The Methodist hospital and I fine-tuned them over the years. In addition, the audiology staffs at Georgetown University Medical Center and the California Ear Institute at Stanford contributed by adding descriptors of their own.

David Kirkwood, editor of *The Hearing Journal,* was responsible for the conceptualization of this project and its overall orchestration. He also edited the content and copy, an unquestionably tedious task, but one that enhanced the quality considerably. Cara Kaufman, from Williams & Wilkins, provided oversight of the project. Also from Williams & Wilkins, Raymund Didyk assisted in the initial coordination of the dictionary and Kathleen Gaffney and Wendi Neenan saw it to its completion. Their assistance was invaluable.

Casey Stach provided her audiologic expertise in two ways. First, she was often consulted about the nuances of a term and particularly about the wording of a definition. Second, she understood the value of the project despite its impact on early mornings, late evenings, and weekends. I am grateful.

CONTENTS

USER'S GUIDE TO THE DICTIONARY

Organization of the Vocabulary

Stach's *Comprehensive Dictionary of Audiology* is organized in a manner used commonly in general English dictionaries. All words, acronyms, and abbreviations are organized alphabetically and set in **bold face**. Alphabetization is letter by letter as spelled, ignoring punctuation and spaces.

Stach's *Comprehensive Dictionary* uses a format for multiple-word terms that is traditional in general dictionaries. For example, the definition of **immittance audiometry** is located in the **I**'s, **Békésy audiometry** is located in the **B**'s, and the chief noun **audiometry** is located in the **A**'s. Stach's *Comprehensive* also uses the traditional format of a specialty dictionary in which multiple-word terms are grouped under the chief noun as the main entry. Thus **immittance audiometry, pure-tone audiometry,** and **Békésy audiometry** also all appear under the chief noun **audiometry.** Both formats are used on the assumption that readers will be able to locate terms more efficiently.

Cross-References

Cross-referencing is used sparingly as a service to the reader. Most dictionaries use cross-referencing to avoid defining a term twice. We chose to limit the use of cross-referencing so that the reader can access most definitions at a first glance. For example, for concepts that have two or three terms, a definition is included under each. However, in the case of concepts that have an excessive number of terms, the terms are cross-referenced to a single entry. For example, we chose the term **auditory brainstem response** as the main referent for **brainstem evoked response, brainstem auditory evoked response,** etc.

Cross-referencing is also used to direct the reader to synonyms, antonyms, complementary terms, and colloquial terms.

Synonyms are words or terms that are equivalent. The label **SYN:** is used in the text to identify synonyms. For example:

> **audibility index** AI; measure of the proportion of speech cues that are audible; **SYN:** articulation index, speech intelligibility index

Antonyms are words or terms that are opposites. The label **ANT:** is used in the text to identify antonyms. For example:

> **abduction** away from the midline of the body or away from each other; **ANT:** adduction

Complementary words or terms are those that help to complete the meaning by designating an alternative. The label **COM:** is used in the text to identify complementary terms. For example:

> **continuous tracing** C tracing; graph that results from threshold tracking in Békésy audiometry to a continuous pure tone at a fixed or swept frequency; **COM:** interrupted tracing

Colloquial words or terms are those that are used only in informal speech or writing. The label **COL:** is used in the text to identify colloquial terms. For example:

> **cerebral vascular accident** CVA; interruption of blood supply to the brain due to aneurysm, embolism, or clot, resulting in sudden loss of function related to the affected portion of the brain; **COL:** stroke

Acronyms and Abbreviations

Acronyms and abbreviations are an integral part of the vocabulary of audiology. They appear in three locations in the dictionary: as entries, in the text of the definitions of the terms to which they apply, and in a separate appendix. The appendix includes all acronyms and abbreviations that appear in the body of the dictionary. An acronym or abbreviation appears as an entry, followed by the term to which it applies, followed by a definition of that term. For example:

> **BILL**   bass increase at low levels; type of automatic signal processing in a hearing aid that uses level-dependent control of frequency response, reducing low frequencies in response to high-intensity input

Acronyms and abbreviations also appear in the definition of the term to which they apply. For example:

> **benign paroxysmal positioning vertigo** BPPV; a recurrent, acute form of vertigo occurring in clusters in response to positional changes

Appendices

The appendices are designed to serve as a source for those words, terms, and concepts that are useful to have easily accessible. Acronyms, abbreviations, and symbols are included as described previously. The ear anatomy charts are labeled with terms that are also included in the body of the dictionary. Audiometric symbols show standards and suggested formats for audiometric data presentations. Ototoxic drugs are listed in a format that should be helpful in identifying the types and variations of drugs that are known to have a deleterious effect on the auditory system. Auditory disorders, including syndromes associated with hearing impairment, are included as a quick reference guide. The report writing glossary is a compilation of outcomes of the various audiometric test measures. These have been used successfully in report writing and are easily integrated into automated report generation systems.

LIST OF ILLUSTRATIONS AND TABLES

(In order of appearance)

Many of the figures in this dictionary have been reprinted from other sources, with the permission of the publisher. The sources of these reprinted figures are included in the following list. They are listed in the order of appearance.

Audiometric Symbols (Appendix)

Normal hearing sensitivity
Mild conductive hearing loss
Severe mixed hearing loss
High-frequency sensorineural hearing loss

A

A-weighted scale sound level meter filtering network weighted to approximate an equal loudness contour at 40 phons; decibel level measured with this scale is usually designated dBA or dB(A)

A1 left (1) earlobe (a) electrode location, typically used for inverting-electrode placement in auditory evoked potential testing, according to the 10–20 International Electrode System nomenclature

A2 right (2) earlobe (a) electrode location, typically used for inverting-electrode placement in auditory evoked potential testing, according to the 10–20 International Electrode System nomenclature

AAA American Academy of Audiology; professional association of audiologists founded in 1988

AAMD American Association on Mental Deficiency; professional organization of specialists from many fields who provide care for individuals with mental retardation

AAO-HNS American Academy of Otolaryngology—Head and Neck Surgery; professional organization of otolaryngologists

AAOHN American Association of Occupational Health Nurses

AAOO American Academy of Ophthalmology and Otolaryngology; former professional association that divided into two organizations, the American Academy of Ophthalmology and the AAO-HNS

AAP American Academy of Pediatrics; professional organization of pediatricians

AARP American Association of Retired Persons; consumer organization of people over the age of 55

AAS American Auditory Society; multidisciplinary association of professionals in audiology, otolaryngology, hearing science, and the hearing industry; formerly American Audiology Society

Abbreviated Profile of Hearing Aid Benefit APHAB; self-assessment questionnaire used for evaluating benefit received from amplification, consisting of four subscales—the aversiveness scale, background noise scale, ease of communication scale, and reverberation scale

abducens nerve Cranial Nerve VI; cranial nerve that provides efferent innervation to the lateral rectus muscles involved in eye movement

abducens nucleus nucleus of Cranial Nerve VI, responsible for controlling the lateral rectus muscles for horizontal eye movement

abduction away from the midline of the body or away from each other; ANT: adduction

aberrant differing from the normal

ABESPA American Board of Examiners in Speech-Language Pathology and Audiology; independent organization responsible for the national examination in audiology and speech-language pathology

ABI 1. auditory behavior index; 2. auditory brainstem implant

abiotrophy premature loss of vitality or degeneration of tissue

ablation surgical removal of a body part or destruction of its function

ABLB alternate binaural loudness balance test; auditory test designed to measure loudness growth or recruitment in the impaired ear of a patient with unilateral hearing loss

ABO American Board of Otolaryngology

ABR auditory brainstem response; auditory evoked potential, originating from Cranial Nerve VIII and auditory brainstem structures, consisting of five to seven identifiable peaks that represent neural function of auditory pathways and nuclei

Abruzzo-Erickson syndrome orofacial clefting syndrome, characterized by cleft palate, eye anomalies, short stature, and mixed or sensorineural hearing loss

abscess circumscribed collection of pus resulting from localized infection in a tissue or organ

abscess, subdural collection of purulent fluid between the dura mater and brain that can occur secondary to chronic otitis media

abscissa horizontal or X axis on a graph, such as frequency axis on an audiogram

absolute bone conduction early term used to describe bone-conduction thresholds established with the ears occluded; COM: relative bone conduction

absolute latency in auditory brainstem response analysis, the time in msec from signal onset to a waveform peak; COM: interpeak latency, interaural latency

1

absolute pitch   rare capability of identifying the pitch of a note; SYN: perfect pitch

absolute sensitivity   the capacity of the auditory system to detect faint sound; SYN: absolute threshold; COM: differential sensitivity

absolute threshold   1. psychophysical term used to denote the value of stimulus magnitude that elicits a desired response and is often related to detection threshold of a signal; 2. in audiometry, the lowest intensity level at which an acoustic signal can be detected

absorption   in acoustics, reduction of sound intensity by materials that prevent reflection

absorption coefficient   ratio of sound energy absorbed by a surface to sound energy reflected by the surface

absorption loss   transmission loss due to the dissipation of sound energy into other forms of energy

AC   1. air conduction; 2. alternating current

Academy of Dispensing Audiologists   ADA; organization of audiologists with a particular interest in dispensing hearing aids

Academy of Rehabilitative Audiology   ARA; association of audiologists with a particular interest in rehabilitation issues

accelerated speech   recorded speech signals that has been temporally altered to increase the speed of playback; COM: time-compressed speech

acceleration   rate of change in velocity of an object in motion

acceptable risk   in determining damage risk criteria for noise exposure, the proportion of the population that will be allowed to become materially impaired

accessory auricle   craniofacial anomaly characterized by an additional auricle or additional auricular tissue

accessory nerve   Cranial Nerve XI; cranial and spinal nerve that provides efferent innervation to muscles of the larynx and neck

acclimatization, auditory   systematic change in auditory performance over time due to a change in the acoustic information available to the listener; e.g., an ear becoming accustomed to processing sounds of increased loudness following introduction of a hearing aid

accutane   retinoic acid drug prescribed for cystic acne that can have a teratogenic effect on the auditory system of the developing embryo when taken by the mother during pregnancy, resulting in congenital hearing loss

ACE   Award for Continuing Education; certificate given by the American Speech-Language-Hearing Association for completion of a prescribed number of continuing education units

acetylcholine   ACh; excitatory neurotransmitter, released in synaptic regions, that controls the action of muscles and nervous system receptors

acetylsalicylic acid   analgesic and anti-inflammatory agent that can cause temporary ototoxicity in high doses; SYN: aspirin

ACh   acetylcholine

achondroplasia   1. abnormality in the conversion of cartilage to bone; 2. autosomal dominant disorder characterized by short stature, short limbs, large head, and middle and inner ear anomalies with associated hearing loss; SYN: chondrodystrophia fetalis

ACOEM   American College of Occupational and Environmental Medicine

acouesthesia   unusually acute sense of hearing

acoumeter   predecessor of the audiometer

acoupedics   method of auditory training that emphasizes acoustic stimulation of residual hearing without visual training

acouphone   early generic name for an electronic hearing aid

acousmatagnosia   loss of recognition of sounds

acousmatamnesia   loss of memory for sounds

acoustic   pertaining to sound and its perception

acoustic admittance   total energy flow through the middle ear system expressed in mhos; reciprocal of impedance

acoustic analysis   detailed study of sound in a specified environment

acoustic compliance   ease of energy flow through the middle ear system that is principal component of reactance at low frequencies; reciprocal of stiffness

acoustic conductance   energy flow through the middle ear system associated with resistance; reciprocal of resistance

acoustic coupling   an arrangement that joins parts together for the transference of sound waves

acoustic cue   segment of speech providing the necessary identifying information

acoustic damper a valve that provides smoothing of the frequency characteristics of an acoustic signal

acoustic damping reduction in sound energy by absorption

acoustic dispersion spreading of sound or change of speed of sound

acoustic feedback sound produced when an amplification system goes into oscillation, produced by amplified sound from the receiver reaching the microphone and being reamplified; e.g., hearing aid squeal

acoustic gain 1. increase in sound output; 2. in a hearing aid, the difference in dB between the input to the microphone and the output of the receiver

acoustic immittance global term representing acoustic admittance (total energy flow) and acoustic impedance (total opposition to energy flow) of the middle ear system

acoustic impedance total opposition to energy flow of sound through the middle ear system

acoustic inertance inertia of a sound medium, or the tendency of that medium to remain at rest or continue in a fixed direction

acoustic insulation material designed to absorb sound waves

acoustic mho unit of measure of conductance of sound wave flow through a medium; reciprocal of acoustic ohm

acoustic muscle reflex reflexive contraction of the tensor tympani and stapedius muscles in response to sound; SYN: acoustic reflex

acoustic nerve Cranial Nerve VIII; auditory nerve, consisting of a vestibular and cochlear branch

acoustic neurilemoma; neurilemmoma cochleovestibular Schwannoma; benign encapsulated neoplasm composed of Schwann cells arising from the intracranial segment of Cranial Nerve VIII; SYN: acoustic neuroma; acoustic neurinoma; acoustic tumor

acoustic neurinoma cochleovestibular Schwannoma

acoustic neuritis inflammation of the auditory portion of Cranial Nerve VIII, often of a viral nature, resulting in acute retrocochlear disorder; SYN: cochlear neuritis

acoustic neuroma AN; generic term referring to a neoplasm of Cranial Nerve VIII, most often a cochleovestibular Schwannoma; SYN: acoustic tumor

acoustic ohm unit of measurement of acoustic impedance equal to 1 dyne per square centimeter producing a volume velocity of 1 cc per second

acoustic output sound emanating from an amplification system

acoustic phonetics branch of phonetics devoted to the study of sound and auditory perception of speech sounds

acoustic reactance opposition to energy flow through the middle ear system due to storage

acoustic reflex AR; reflexive contraction of the intra-aural muscles in response to loud sound, dominated by the stapedius muscle in humans; SYN: acoustic stapedial reflex

acoustic reflex, contralateral crossed acoustic reflex

acoustic reflex, crossed acoustic reflex occurring in one ear as a result of stimulation of the other ear

acoustic reflex, ipsilateral uncrossed acoustic reflex

acoustic reflex, uncrossed acoustic reflex occurring in one ear as a result of stimulation of the same ear; SYN: ipsilateral acoustic reflex

acoustic reflex decay perstimulatory reduction in the magnitude of the acoustic reflex, considered abnormal if it is reduced by over 50% of initial amplitude within 10 seconds of stimulus onset

acoustic reflex latency time interval between the presentation of an acoustic stimulus and detection of an acoustic reflex

acoustic reflex pattern patterns of relations among crossed and uncrossed acoustic reflex thresholds for the right and left ears that describe abnormalities of the efferent, afferent, and central portions of the reflex arc

acoustic reflex threshold ART; lowest intensity level of a stimulus at which an acoustic reflex is detected

acoustic resistance opposition to energy flow through the middle ear system due to dissipation

acoustic spectrum magnitude and frequency composition of a sound

acoustic stapedial reflex reflexive contraction of the stapedius muscle in response to loud sound; SYN: acoustic reflex

acoustic stria, dorsal DAS; nerve fiber bundle that emanates from the dorsal cochlear nucleus and synapses in the contralateral lateral lemniscus and inferior colliculus, bypassing the superior olivary complex

acoustic stria, intermediate IAS; nerve bundle, the fibers of which emanate from the posterior ventral cochlear nucleus and synapse on the ipsilateral and contralateral periolivary nuclei and the contralateral lateral lemniscus

acoustic stria, ventral second-order fiber bundle leaving the AVCN and projecting ventrally and medially to distribute fibers to the ipsilateral LSO and MSO and continuing across midline to distribute fibers to the contralateral MSO and MNTB; SYN: trapezoid body

acoustic striae second-order fiber bundles that leave the cochlear nucleus toward higher brainstem levels, the ventral acoustic stria from the AVCN, intermediate a.s. from the PVCN, and dorsal a.s. from the DCN

acoustic susceptance energy flow through the middle ear system associated with reactance; reciprocal of reactance

acoustic trauma 1. damage to hearing from a transient, high-intensity sound; 2. long-term insult to hearing from excessive noise exposure

acoustic treatment use of materials or structural changes to alter sound transmission within a specified environment

acoustic tumor generic term referring to a neoplasm of Cranial Nerve VIII, most often a cochleovestibular Schwannoma; SYN: acoustic neuroma

acoustical acoustic

acousticolateralis organs collective reference to the lateral line organs, organs of balance, and organs of hearing

acousticopalpebral reflex auropalpebral reflex

acousticovestibular pertaining to the combined cochlea and vestibular end organ

acousticovestibular ganglia embryologic precursor to the vestibular and auditory ganglia

acoustics the study and science of sound and its perception

acoustics, earmold the influence of an earmold's dimensions, such as bore length and diameter, on the spectral content of sound reaching the tympanic membrane

acquired obtained after birth; ANT: congenital

acquired hearing loss hearing loss that occurs after birth as a result of injury or disease; not congenital; SYN: adventitious hearing loss

acquired immunodeficiency syndrome AIDS; disease compromising the efficacy of the immune system, characterized by opportunistic infectious diseases that can affect the middle ear and mastoid as well as peripheral and central auditory nervous system structures

acquired syphilis venereal disease, caused by the spirochete Treponema pallidum, which in its secondary and tertiary stages may result in auditory and vestibular disorders due to membranous labyrinthitis

acquired syphilis, secondary secondary stage of a syphilis infection, which can result in membranous labyrinthitis associated with acute meningitis

acquired syphilis, tertiary late stage of development of syphilis infection, occurring within 3 years to 10 years of initial infection, often resulting in otosyphilis

acrocephalosyndactyly, type I congenital syndrome characterized by a peaked head, fused digits, low-set ears, otitis media, stapes fixation, and associated conductive hearing loss; SYN: Apert syndrome

acrodysostosis skeletal dysplasia syndrome with recurrent otitis media and associated conductive hearing loss

acrofacial dysostosis syndrome of mandibulofacial dysostosis, or Treacher Collins syndrome, with absence of thumbs, often associated with ear and facial anomalies similar to those in Treacher Collins; SYN: Nager syndrome

actin protein complex that provides stiffness to the stereocilia of cochlear hair cells

action level level of noise exposure that requires a worker to be enrolled in an occupational hearing conservation program; defined by OSHA as 85 dBA for a time-weighted average of 8 hours

action potential AP; 1. synchronous change in electrical potential of nerve or muscle tissue; 2. in auditory evoked potential measures, whole-nerve or compound action potential of Cranial Nerve VIII, the main component of ECochG and Wave I of the ABR

action potential, cochlear nerve CNAP; compound action potential recorded from an electrode placed directly on Cranial Nerve VIII

action potential, electrically evoked EAP; compound action potential generated by electrical stimulation of the cochlea with either an extracochlear promontory electrode or a cochlear implant

action potential, whole-nerve 1. synchronous change in electrical potential of the fibers of a nerve; 2. in auditory-evoked potential measures, compound action potential of Cranial Nerve VIII, represented as the main component of the ECochG and Wave I of the ABR

active electrode 1. electrode that is attached to the positive-voltage, noninverting side of a differential amplifier; 2. vertex electrode in conventional auditory brainstem response recordings; COM: reference electrode, ground electrode

active filter filter circuit in which the response varies with gain of the amplifier

active tone control potentiometer on a hearing aid that permits frequency response alteration

acuity 1. sharpness or distinctness of a sense; 2. in audition, differential sensitivity to loudness and pitch; 3. often inaccurately used to describe absolute threshold of hearing sensitivity

acuity, temporal the ability to distinguish or resolve small time intervals or order of occurrence

acusis sense of hearing

acute of sudden onset and short duration; ANT: chronic

acute circumscribed external otitis reddened, pustular lesion surrounding a hair follicle, usually due to staphylococci infection during hot, humid weather; SYN: furunculosis

acute diffuse external otitis diffuse reddened, pustular lesions surrounding hair follicles, usually due to gram-negative bacterial infection during hot, humid weather and often initiated by swimming; COL: swimmer's ear

acute labyrinthitis inflammation of the labyrinth resulting in acute vertigo, vegetative symptoms, sensorineural hearing loss, and tinnitus

acute mastoiditis inflammation of the mastoid, secondary to acute suppurative otitis media, which can lead to acute suppurative labyrinthitis, facial nerve paralysis, meningitis, and brain abscess

acute myringitis short-duration inflammation of the tympanic membrane, usually associated with infection of the middle ear or external auditory meatus; SYN: acute tympanitis

acute otitis media AOM; inflammation of the middle ear having a duration of fewer than 21 days

acute serous otitis media acute inflammation of middle ear mucosa, with serous effusion

acute suppurative labyrinthitis acute inflammation of the labyrinth with infected effusion containing pus

acute suppurative otitis media acute inflammation of the middle ear with infected effusion containing pus

acute tympanitis short-duration inflammation of the tympanic membrane; SYN: acute myringitis

acute vermis syndrome central vestibular disorder caused by pressure on the vertebral artery resulting in paroxysmal vertigo and vegetative symptoms

AD [L. *auris dextra*] right ear

ADA 1. Academy of Dispensing Audiologists; 2. Americans with Disabilities Act

adaptation 1. property of sensory receptors in which they become less responsive to repeated or continuous stimuli; 2. adjustment of the auditory system to a change in the acoustic environment, such as the addition of a hearing aid

adaptation, auditory process by which a constant audible tone becomes inaudible after a time; SYN: tone decay

adaptive compression hearing aid circuit technique that incorporates output-limiting compression with automatically variable release time; SYN: variable compression

adaptive frequency response AFR; hearing aid circuitry technique in which frequency response changes as input level changes

adaptive high-frequency filter nonlinear automatic signal processing circuit in a hearing aid in which gain at high frequencies decreases as input level increases; SYN: BILL

adaptive low-frequency filter nonlinear automatic signal processing circuit in a hearing aid in which gain at low frequencies decreases as input level increases; SYN: TILL

adaptive noise canceler ANC; multiple microphone instrument that attempts to reduce background noise by changing the hearing aid microphone's directionality adaptively

adaptive procedure psychophysical method in which changes are automatically made to some signal parameter based on the subject's response

adaptive signal processing ASP; automatic signal processing

ADC analog-to-digital conversion; the process of turning a continuously varying (analog) waveform into a numerical (digital) representation of the waveform

ADD attention deficit disorder; cognitive disorder involving reduced ability to focus on an activity, task, or sensory stimulus, characterized by restlessness and distractibility; SYN: ADHD

adduction toward the midline of the body or toward each other; ANT: abduction

adenoid a hypertrophic mass of glandular tissue on the posterior wall of the nasopharynx

adenoidectomy surgical excision of adenoids

adenoma glandular tumor; ordinarily benign neoplasm of epithelial tissue in which the tumor cells form glandlike structures

adenosine triphosphate ATP; neurochemical substance produced by the stria vascularis

ADHD attention deficit hyperactivity disorder; cognitive disorder involving reduced ability to focus on an activity, task, or sensory stimulus, characterized by restlessness and distractibility; SYN: ADD

adhesions inflammatory fibrous bands of new tissue that abnormally connect opposing serous surfaces

adhesive otitis media inflammation of the middle ear caused by prolonged eustachian tube dysfunction resulting in severe retraction of the tympanic membrane and obliteration of the middle ear space

aditus opening in the middle ear cavity that connects the epitympanic recess to the mastoid antrum

aditus ad antrum orifice in the posterior wall of the epitympanic recess that serves as a passage from the tympanic cavity to the tympanic antrum

adjustment, method of psychophysical procedure for determining absolute or differential threshold in which the observer controls the changes in the stimulus necessary to measure a threshold

administrative noise control reduction of noise exposure by limiting employee exposure time; COM: engineering noise control

admittance Y; total energy flow through a system, expressed in mhos; reciprocal of impedance

adult-onset auditory deprivation the apparent decline in word-recognition ability in the unaided ear of an adult fitted with a monaural hearing aid following a period of asymmetric stimulation; SYN: late-onset auditory deprivation

advantage, binaural the cumulative benefits of using two ears over one, including enhanced threshold and better hearing in the presence of background noise

advantage, right-ear tendency in most individuals for right-ear performance on speech-perception measures to be better than left-ear performance

adventitious not inherited; acquired

adventitious hearing loss loss of hearing sensitivity occurring after birth; ANT: congenital hearing loss

AEF auditory evoked field; electromagnetic response of the auditory nervous system

AEP auditory evoked potential; electrophysiologic response to sound, usually distinguished according to latency, including ECoG, ABR, MLR, LVR, SSEP, P3

AER auditory evoked response

AERA averaged evoked response audiometry; audiometry using auditory evoked potentials to predict hearing sensitivity

aerate to expose to air

aerotitis media traumatic inflammation disorder of the middle ear caused by sudden changes in air pressure in the pneumatized spaces of the temporal bone on descent from high altitude or ascent from underwater diving; SYN: otitic barotrauma

afferent pertaining to the conduction of the ascending nervous system tracts from peripheral to central; ANT: efferent

AFR adaptive frequency response; hearing aid circuitry technique in which frequency response changes as input level changes

afterhearing aftersound

aftersound perception of sound after cessation of the stimulus; SYN: afterhearing

AGC automatic gain control; nonlinear hearing aid compression circuitry designed to automatically change gain as signal level changes or limit output when signal level reaches a specified criterion; SYN: automatic volume control

AGC-I automatic gain control—input; circuitry of a hearing aid in which the volume control follows the AGC

AGC-O automatic gain control—output; circuitry of a hearing aid in which the AGC follows the volume control

age, chronologic CA; age of an individual from date of birth

age, developmental age at which children acquire specific skills

age, educational EA; grade-level equivalent age of a student based on standardized achievement tests

age, gestational age since conception, measured in weeks and days from the first day of the last normal menstrual period

age, mental MA; intellectual age, as measured on standardized tests

ageism persecution or discrimination based on age

agenesis absence of a body structure due to failure of formation or incomplete development

ageotropic nystagmus positional nystagmus that beats in a direction that is away from the ground

aggregation embryologic process in which young neurons cluster into what later will become specific auditory nuclei

agnosia lack of sensory-perceptual ability to recognize stimuli

agnosia, auditory impairment in the ability to recognize speech or other sounds as a result of auditory cortex disorder

agnosia, auditory verbal inability to recognize spoken language due to central nervous system disorder

AI articulation index or audibility index; measure of the proportion of speech cues that are audible; SYN: speech intelligibility index

AICA anterior inferior cerebellar artery; large vessel arising from the basilar artery, a branch of which is the labyrinthine artery, which supplies blood to the cochlea

aided fitted with or assisted by the use of a hearing aid

aided gain, real-ear REAG; measurement of the difference, in decibels as a function of frequency, between the SPL in the ear canal and the SPL at a field reference point for a specified sound field with the hearing aid in place and turned on

aided response, real-ear REAR; probe-microphone measurement of the sound pressure level, as a function of frequency, at a specified point near the tympanic membrane with a hearing aid in place and turned on; expressed in absolute SPL or as gain relative to stimulus level

aided threshold lowest level at which a signal is audible to an individual wearing a hearing aid

AIDS acquired immunodeficiency syndrome; disease compromising the efficacy of the immune system, characterized by opportunistic infectious diseases

AIDS-related hearing impairment hearing disorder in a patient with AIDS, resulting from opportunistic infectious diseases of the middle ear, mastoid, and labyrinth, as well as of peripheral and central auditory nervous system structures

air-bone gap difference in dB between air-conducted and bone-conducted hearing thresholds for a given frequency in the same ear, used to describe the magnitude of conductive hearing loss

air cells air-filled spaces within bone

air cells, mastoid air-filled spaces throughout the mastoid, which are highly variable in number and shape

air conduction transmission of sound, delivered by an earphone, through the outer and middle ear to the cochlea; COM: bone conduction

air-conduction threshold absolute threshold of hearing sensitivity to pure-tone stimuli delivered via earphone

air-dielectric microphone type of condenser microphone that derives its electrical output from changes in distance between two polarized plates, with air serving as the dielectric between the two plates

Albers-Schönberg disease autosomal recessive craniofacial and skeletal disorder characterized by brittle bones; may include disarticulated ossicular chain and progressive sensorineural hearing loss; SYN: osteopetrosis

albinism syndrome autosomal recessive deficiency or absence of pigment in the skin, hair, and eyes often associated with sensorineural hearing loss of varying severity

Albrecht syndrome hereditary, sensorineural hearing loss occurring during childhood, with progression that is suggestive of early presbyacusis

alcoholic nystagmus positional nystagmus that occurs regularly after moderate ingestion of alcohol

ALD assistive listening device; hearing instrument or class of hearing instruments, usually with a remote microphone for improving signal-to-noise ratio, including FM systems, personal amplifiers, telephone amplifiers, television listeners

alerting devices assistive devices, such as doorbells, alarm clocks, smoke detectors, telephones, etc., that use light flashes or vibration instead of sound to alert individuals with deafness to a particular sound

alexia, auditory disorder characterized by difficulty perceiving similarities and differences in sounds

algorithm systematic protocol or set of instructions used to accomplish a goal or perform a certain task

aliasing distortion that occurs in the process of converting a signal from analog to digital form when the frequency of a signal being sampled exceeds that of one-half of the sampling rate

allogeneic pertaining to tissue from another individual of the same species

allogeneic middle ear implant tissue, such as tympanic membrane and ossicles, from another individual used in reconstructive middle ear surgery

alloplastic pertaining to inert material used for implantation into tissue

alloplastic middle ear implant ossicular prosthesis made of inert material, such as ceramic or plastic, used in reconstructive middle ear surgery

alpha rhythm or waves fundamental EEG waves of 8 Hz to 13 Hz

alphabet, manual finger positions and hand movements used in fingerspelling to represent letters of the alphabet

alphabet, phonetic alphabet containing symbols that represent speech sounds

Alport syndrome genetic syndrome characterized by progressive kidney disease and sensorineural hearing loss, probably resulting from X-linked inheritance through a gene that codes for collagen, identified as COL4A5

ALR auditory late response; evoked potential, originating from the cortex and having two main waveform peaks, a vertex negative peak at approximately 90 msec and a vertex positive peak at approximately 180 msec following signal presentation; SYN: LLAEP

Alstrom syndrome autosomal recessive metabolic disorder with delayed-onset progressive sensorineural hearing loss

alternate binaural loudness balance test ABLB; auditory test designed to measure loudness growth or recruitment in the impaired ear of a patient with unilateral hearing loss

alternate monaural loudness balance test AMLB; auditory test designed to measure loudness growth or recruitment in an ear with normal hearing sensitivity at some frequencies and sensorineural hearing loss at others

alternating current ac; electric current that periodically changes its value or direction of flow

alternating polarity characteristic of auditory evoked potential stimuli in which the rarefaction and condensation polarity of a click or tone burst are alternated successively

Alzheimer's disease presenile dementia with progressive neuronal degeneration, cerebral atrophy, and associated mental deterioration

AM amplitude modulation; the process of varying the magnitude of a radio wave or sound wave in relation to the strength of the carrier wave; COM: frequency modulation

AMA American Medical Association

ambient surrounding

ambient noise surrounding sounds in an acoustic environment

amblyacousia blunt or dull sense of hearing; hearing sensitivity loss

ameliorate to make or become better; to improve

amelioration process of improving or making something better

American Academy of Audiology AAA; professional association of audiologists founded in 1988

American Academy of Ophthalmology and Otolaryngology AAOO; former professional association that divided into two organization—the American Academy of Ophthalmology and the AAO—HNS

American Academy of Otolaryngology— Head and Neck Surgery AAO—HNS; professional organization of otolaryngologists

American Academy of Pediatrics AAP; professional organization of pediatricians

American Association of Retired Persons AARP; consumer organization of people over the age of 50

American Association On Mental Deficiency AAMD; professional organization of specialists from many fields who provide care for individuals with mental retardation

American Auditory Society AAS; multidisciplinary association of professionals in audiology, otolaryngology, hearing science, and the hearing industry; formerly American Audiology Society

American Board of Examiners in Speech Pathology and Audiology ABESPA; independent organization responsible for the national examination in audiology and speech-language pathology

American Medical Association AMA; national association of physicians

American National Standards Institute ANSI; association of specialists, manufacturers, and consumers that determines standards for measuring instruments, including audiometers; formerly ASA

American Neurotology Society ANS; professional organization of otolaryngologists who have a special interest in neurotology

American Sign Language ASL, Ameslan; common form of manual communication used in the United States

American Speech and Hearing Association ASHA; former name of the American Speech-Language-Hearing Association

American Speech-Language-Hearing Association ASHA; professional organization of audiologists, speech-language pathologists, and speech and hearing scientists; formerly American Speech and Hearing Association

American Standards Association ASA; former name of American National Standards Institute

American Tinnitus Association ATA; consumer organization of people with tinnitus

Americans with Disabilities Act ADA; United States law enacted to provide equal access for individuals with disabilities

Ameslan American Sign Language; common form of manual communication used in the United States

amg aminoglycoside

amikacin ototoxic, semisynthetic aminoglycocide antibiotic with a broad antibacterial spectrum, particularly effective against gentamicin-resistant bacteria

amimia loss of ability to communicate by gestures or signs

aminoglycoside antibiotics group of bacteriocidal antibiotics, which are often cochleotoxic and/or vestibulotoxic, derived from streptomyces or micromonosporum used primarily against gram-negative bacteria, including streptomycin, neomycin, kanamycin, and gentamicin

AMLB alternate monaural loudness balance test; auditory test designed to measure loudness growth or recruitment in an ear with normal hearing sensitivity at some frequencies and sensorineural hearing loss at others

AMLR auditory middle latency response; auditory evoked potential, originating from the region of the auditory radiations and cortex, having as a primary component a vertex positive peak at 25 msec to 40 msec following signal presentation; SYN: MLR

amperage the power of electrical current expressed in amperes

ampere unit of electric current equal to 1 volt applied across a 1-ohm resistance

ampicillin antibiotic used in the treatment of gram-negative infections, including meningitis and urinary tract infections, which may be ototoxic in certain cases

amplification 1. increasing of the intensity of sound; 2. generic description of a hearing aid or assistive listening device

amplification, binaural use of a hearing aid in both ears

amplification, compression hearing aid with compression-limiting and/or wide-dynamic-range-compression circuitry

amplification, dichotic seldom used fitting technique in which high-frequency emphasis amplification is fitted to the right ear and flat-frequency response to the left ear, in an effort to exploit the right ear advantage for processing speech; SYN: split-band amplification

amplification, linear hearing aid amplification in which the gain is the same for all input levels until the maximum output is reached

amplification, nonlinear amplification whose gain is not the same for all input levels

amplification, selective hearing aid response with gain limited over a restricted frequency range, selected to match the audiometric configuration

amplification, sound field amplification of a classroom or other open area with a public address system or other small-room system to enhance the signal-to-noise ratio for all listeners

amplification, split-band seldom-used hearing aid fitting strategy in which a high-frequency response is fitted to the right ear and flat-frequency response to the left ear, in an effort to exploit the right-ear advantage for processing speech; SYN: dichotic amplification

amplification system, loop assistive listening device in which a microphone/amplifier delivers signals to a loop of wire encircling a room; the signals are received by the telecoil of a hearing aid via magnetic induction

amplified speech spectrum electroacoustic output of a hearing aid in response to speech-weighted noise or other signals representative of the speech spectrum

amplifier device that increases the intensity of a sound

amplifier, Class A type of single-ended hearing aid amplifier used in low-power applications that has a constant current drain across input levels; Class A refers to the operational characteristic of the output or power stage of the amplifier

amplifier, Class B push-pull type of hearing aid amplifier used in high-power applications that draws current in proportion to signal level; Class B refers to the operational characteristic of the output or power stage of the amplifier

amplifier, Class D pulse-width modulated type of hearing aid amplifier built inside a receiver, the use of which results in reduced battery current, smaller size, and higher saturation levels; Class D refers to operational characteristic of the output or power stage

amplifier, differential amplifier used in evoked potential measurement to eliminate extraneous noise; the voltage from one electrode's input is inverted and subtracted from another input, so that any electrical activity that is common to both electrodes is rejected

amplifier, telephone any of several types of assistive devices designed to increase the intensity level output of a telephone receiver

amplify to increase the intensity of sound

amplitude magnitude of a sound wave, acoustic reflex, evoked potential, etc.

amplitude, peak maximum instantaneous displacement of a waveform in a specified time interval

amplitude, peak-to-peak difference in amplitude between the positive and negative extremes of a waveform

amplitude distortion inaccurate reproduction of sound waves when the limits of an amplifier are exceeded and the output is no longer proportional to the input; SYN: harmonic distortion, nonlinear distortion

amplitude distribution representation of noise that varies over time as the percentage of time that a level is present at specified amplitude intervals

amplitude modulation AM; the process of varying the magnitude of a radio wave or sound wave in relation to the strength of the carrier wave; COM: frequency modulation

amplitude-sensitive hearing protection device nonlinear hearing protection device that provides little or no attenuation of low-intensity sound and significant attenuation of high-intensity sound

amplitude spectrum expression of an acoustic waveform as amplitude as a function of component frequencies

ampulla 1. flasklike structure or dilation of a tube; 2. bulbous portion at the end of each of the three semicircular canals leading into the utricle

ampulla, horizontal bulging portion of the horizontal semicircular canal that contains the crista ampullaris

ampulla, lateral vestibular end organ of the lateral (horizontal) semicircular canal

ampulla, posterior bulging portion of the posterior semicircular canal that contains the crista ampullaris

ampulla, superior bulging portion of the superior semicircular canal that contains the crista ampullaris

ampullary nerve, horizontal nerve fiber bundle from the hair cells of the crista ampullaris of the horizontal semicircular canal that joins with similar bundles from the other semicircular canals, the utricle, and the saccule to form the vestibular branch of Cranial Nerve VIII

ampullary nerve, lateral horizontal ampullary nerve

ampullary nerve, posterior nerve fiber bundle from the hair cells of the crista ampullaris of the posterior semicircular canal that joins with similar bundles from the other semicircular canals, the utricle, and the saccule to form the vestibular branch of Cranial Nerve VIII

ampullary nerve, superior   nerve fiber bundle from the hair cells of the crista ampullaris of the superior semicircular canal that joins with similar bundles from the other semicircular canals, the utricle, and the saccule to form the vestibular branch of Cranial Nerve VIII

ampullofugal   flow of endolymph and deflection of kinocilia away from the ampulla and utricle; SYN: utriculofugal

ampullopetal   flow of endolymph and deflection of kinocilia toward the ampulla and utricle; SYN: utriculopetal

amusia   loss of ability to produce or recognize musical sounds

amygdaloid nuclear complex   part of the basal ganglia portion of the cerebrum that receives olfactory input and is involved in visceral function

AN   1. acoustic neuroma; 2. auditory nerve

anacusis   total lack of hearing; deafness

analgesia   reduction or abolition of sensitivity to pain

analgesic   drug that relieves pain

analog   continuously varying over time; ANT: digital

analog hearing aid   amplification device that uses conventional, continuously varying signal processing

analog-to-digital conversion   ADC; the process of turning continuously varying (analog) signals into a numerical (digital) representation of the waveform

analytic speechreading method   a speechreading technique that emphasizes the visual recognition of individual speech sounds

anastomosis   connection or opening between two spaces or vessels

anatomic frequency scale   modification of the frequency scale, designed to correlate pathology with hearing loss, in which audiometric frequencies are represented on the abscissa in accordance with the spatial distribution of maximum excitation along the basilar membrane

ANC   adaptive noise canceler; multiple microphone instrument that attempts to reduce backgn round noise by changing the hearing aid microphone's directionality adaptively

anechoic   without echo or reverberation

anechoic chamber   room designed for acoustic research with sound-absorbing material on all surfaces designed to enhance sound absorption and reduce reverberation

anencephaly   congenital malformation of the brain, characterized by the absence of cerebral and cerebellar hemispheres, often associated with malformed temporal bones and severe anomalies of the outer, middle, and inner ear

anesthesia   a state characterized by loss of sensation, usually in reference to pharmacologic applications of anesthetics

anesthetic   an agent that produces anesthesia

aneurysm   circumscribed dilation of a blood vessel

angioma   tumor made up of blood or lymph cells

angiotitis   inflammation of blood vessels

angular acceleration   in vestibular assessment, term referring to head rotation

angular velocity   time rate of change of rotational motion

ankylosis   stiffening or fixation of a joint with a fibrous or bony union, such as fixation of the stapes in otosclerosis

ankylosis, malleus   stiffness or fixation of the malleus at its abutment to the tegmen tympani

anlage   embryologic cell group indicating the first trace of a structure or organ

annoyance level   intensity level at which noise is judged subjectively to be disturbing or a nuisance

annular ligament   ring-shaped ligament that holds the footplate of the stapes in the oval window

annular ring   annular ligament

annulus   fibrocartilaginous ring on the periphery of the pars tensa portion of the tympanic membrane that fits into the tympanic sulcus of the temporal bone

annulus tympanicus   annulus

anode   1. positive electrode in an electrolytic cell; 2. negative terminal in a battery; COM: cathode

anomaly   structure or function that is unusual, irregular, or deviates from the norm

anomaly, craniofacial   congenital malformation of the face and/or cranium

anotia   congenital absence of the pinna; SYN: auricular aplasia

anoxia   absence or deficiency of oxygen in body tissues

ANS 1. American Neurotology Society; 2. autonomic nervous system

ANSI American National Standards Institute; association of specialists, manufacturers, and consumers that determines standards for measuring instruments, including audiometers; formerly ASA

antenatal occurring before birth; SYN: prenatal

anterior anatomical direction, referring to structures that are located toward the front or forward; SYN: ventral; ANT: posterior

anterior epitympanic recess pneumatized space that lies anterior to the main epitympanic cavity

anterior inferior cerebellar artery AICA; large vessel arising from the basilar artery, a branch of which is the labyrinthine artery, which supplies the cochlea

anterior malleolar fold one of two ligamentous bands on the tympanic membrane, coursing superiorly and anteriorly from the lateral process of the malleus to the tympanic sulcus

anterior malleolar ligament one of several ligaments responsible for maintaining the position of the ossicles, extending from the anterior process of the malleus to the anterior wall of the middle ear cavity

anterior tympanic artery branch of the maxillary artery giving rise to three main branches, which supply the bone and mucosa of the epitympanum, medial aspect of the tympanic membrane, and the malleus and incus

anterior ventral cochlear nucleus AVCN; portion of the cochlear nucleus that receives primary afferent projections from Cranial Nerve VIII and sends second-order fibers via the ventral acoustic stria to the superior olivary complex

anterior vertical canal superior semicircular canal

anterior vestibular artery branch of the labyrinthine artery that supplies the macula of the utricle, a portion of the macula of the saccule, the cristae and membranous canals of the superior and lateral semicircular canals, and the superior surfaces of the utricle and saccule

anterior vestibular vein vessel that drains the utricle and the ampullae of the superior and lateral semicircular canals

anterograde moving forward along an afferent neural pathway

anterograde degeneration neural degeneration forward along afferent pathways, secondary to deafferentation

anthropocentrism the bias that everything is centered around human beings

anti-aliasing filter low-pass filter designed to reduce aliasing distortion that can occur in the conversion of a signal from analog to digital form

antibiotic a chemical compound that is antagonistic to pathogenic or noxious organisms

antibiotic prophylaxis the use of antibiotics as a preventive measure, as in their application to children who are prone to otitis media

antigen substance that induces a state of sensitivity or resistance to an infection or toxic substance as a result of coming into contact with appropriate body tissue

antihelix; anthelix auricular ridge of cartilage anterior and parallel to the helix

antilobium tragus portion of the auricle

antiphasic of opposite phase

antitoxin, tetanus antibody formed in response to a specific neurotropic toxin, which when used prophylactically or therapeutically has been associated with bilateral profound sensorineural hearing loss

antitragus projection on the auricle opposite, or posterior to, the tragus

Antley-Bixler syndrome craniosynostosis syndrome that can include dysplastic ears, low-set protruding ears, external canal atresia, and associated conductive hearing loss

antrotympanic pertaining to the mastoid antrum and tympanic cavity

antrum any nearly closed cavity or hollow space, especially in bone

antrum, mastoid enlarged space in the mastoid portion of the temporal lobe extending posteriorly from the epitympanic recess and connected via the aditus

antrum auris external auditory canal

antrum tympanicum mastoid antrum

anvil colloquial term for incus

AOM acute otitis media; inflammation of the middle ear having a duration of fewer than 21 days

AOR audito-oculogyric reflex; rapid turning of the eyes toward the source of a sudden sound

AP action potential; 1. synchronous change in electrical potential of nerve or muscle tissue; 2. in auditory evoked potential measures, whole-nerve or compound action potential of Cranial Nerve VIII, the main component of ECochG and Wave I of the ABR

APD auditory processing disorder; reduction in the ability to manipulate acoustic signals, despite normal hearing sensitivity and regardless of language, attention, and cognition ability; SYN: central auditory processing disorder

aperiodic occurring at irregular intervals; not periodic

aperiodic wave wave form that does not regularly repeat itself in a given period of time and that is not restricted to components at multiples of the fundamental frequency

Apert syndrome congenital syndrome characterized by a peaked head, fused digits, low-set ears, otitis media, stapes fixation, and associated conductive hearing loss; SYN: acrocephalosyndactyly, Type 1

apex tip or uppermost point of a conical structure

Apgar score numeric value, ranging from 0 to 10, designed to describe a newborn's physical status, based on the assignment of values to five criteria: color, heart rate, respiration, muscle tone, and response to stimuli

APHAB Abbreviated Profile of Hearing Aid Benefit; self-assessment questionnaire consisting of four subscales used for evaluating benefit received from amplification

aphasia complete or partial loss of language ability due to brain dysfunction

aphasia, auditory impairment in the comprehension of spoken language; SYN: fluent aphasia, receptive aphasia, Wernicke's aphasia

apical near or at an apex

aplasia congenital absence of an organ

aplasia, auricular congenital absence of an auricle; SYN: anotia

aplasia, cochleosaccular congenital malformation of the membranous portion of the cochlea and saccule, including atrophy of the striae vascularis and abnormalities of the tectorial membrane

apoplectiform vertigo single or recurring, sudden, severe attack of vertigo accompanied by nausea and vomiting, often caused by vestibular neuritis

apoplexia cerebelli central vestibular disorder caused by a lesion of the cerebellar artery resulting in acute, severe vertigo accompanied by symptoms of cerebellar paralysis

apoplexy effusion of blood into a tissue or organ, as in a cerebral vascular accident

APR auropalpebral reflex; eyeblink or twitch at the canthus caused by a sudden loud sound

apraxia movement disorder, characterized by an incapacity to execute purposeful movement in the presence of normal muscle function

apraxia of speech impaired capacity to purposefully program and sequence speech musculature movement

aprosexia inability to pay attention; inattention

AR acoustic reflex; reflexive contraction of the intra-aural muscles in response to loud sound, dominated by the stapedius muscle in humans; SYN: acoustic stapedial reflex

ARA Academy of Rehabilitative Audiology; association of audiologists with a particular interest in rehabilitation issues

arachnoid cobweb-like membrane covering the brain and spinal cord

arachnoid cyst sac formed from abnormal splitting and duplication of the arachnoid membrane, often located in the middle cranial fossa with compression of the temporal lobe

arachnoiditis inflammation of the arachnoid membrane and subarachnoid space

arachnoiditis pontocerebellaris central vestibular disorder caused by inflammation of the arachnoid membrane of the posterior fossa, resulting in attacks of rotary vertigo, headache, and vegetative symptoms; SYN: Barany syndrome

areflexia absence of reflexes

armamentarium entire collection of methods and equipment available to a practitioner

Arnold-Chiari malformation cerebellomedullary malformation syndrome, characterized by congenital deformity of the cerebellum and medulla oblongata

Arnold's nerve nerve formed by a portion of Cranial Nerve X, the inferior branch of which is joined by fibers from the facial nerve to provide cutaneous sensation to a region of the posterior surface of the external auditory canal

ARO Association for Research in Otolaryngology; professional organization devoted to research related to ear, nose, and throat diseases and functions

arousal response   a stirring or increase in activity in response to auditory stimulation

arsacetin   ototoxic drug used in the treatment of syphilis and parasitic infections, which can cause degenerative changes in cochlear hair cells, supporting cells, and the stria vascularis

ART   acoustic reflex threshold; lowest intensity level of a stimulus at which an acoustic reflex is detected

arteria cerebelli superior syndrome   central vestibular disorder caused by an obstruction of the superior cerebellar artery resulting in acute vertigo, vegetative symptoms, cerebellar hemiataxia, hypotonia, and intentional tremor

arterioles   minute vessels, such as those that supply capillary beds in the cochlea

arterioles, external radiating   branch of the main cochlear artery that divides to form capillary networks supplying the scala vestibuli, Reissner's membrane, stria vascularis, spiral prominence, and spiral ligament

arterioles, internal radiating   a group of arterioles constituting a branch of the main cochlear artery that divides to form capillary networks supplying the basilar membrane and hair cells

arterioles, radiating   two sets of blood vessels, branching from the main cochlear artery, that supply the internal and external walls of the cochlea

artery, anterior inferior cerebellar   AICA; large vessel arising from the basilar artery, a branch of which is the labyrinthine artery, which supplies the cochlea

artery, anterior tympanic   branch of the maxillary artery giving rise to three main branches, which supply the bone and mucosa of the epitympanum, medial aspect of the tympanic membrane, and the malleus and incus

artery, anterior vestibular   branch of the labyrinthine artery that supplies the macula of the utricle, a portion of the macula of the saccule, the cristae and membranous canals of the superior and lateral semicircular canals, and the superior surfaces of the utricle and saccule

artery, auricular   1. posterior branch originating from the external carotid that distributes blood to the middle ear, mastoid cells, and auricle; 2. deep branch originating from the maxillary that distributes to the tympanic membrane and external auditory meatus

artery, basilar   vessel giving rise to the anterior inferior cerebellar artery, which supplies blood to the cochlea

artery, caroticotympanic   one of two separate branches arising from the internal carotid artery that connect with branches of the tympanic and tubal arteries to supply blood to the anterior portion of the middle ear

artery, common cochlear   branch of the labyrinthine artery that divides into the main cochlear artery and vestibulocochlear artery

artery, deep auricular   branch of the internal maxillary artery that divides into posterior and anterior branches to supply a large portion of the tympanic membrane

artery, inferior cerebellar   large vessel arising from the basilar artery, a branch of which is the labyrinthine artery, which supplies the cochlea; SYN: anterior inferior cerebellar artery

artery, inferior tympanic   branch of the ascending pharyngeal artery that supplies the mucosa and bone of the hypotympanum and promontory

artery, internal auditory   labyrinthine artery

artery, internal carotid   vessel providing the main blood supply to the cerebral hemisphere, located in the petrous apex region of the temporal bone; often encountered in temporal bone resection for tumor removal

artery, labyrinthine   blood vessel arising from the anterior inferior cerebellar artery and distributing to the dura and nerves of the internal auditory canal before dividing into the common cochlear artery and the anterior vestibular artery; SYN: internal auditory artery

artery, main cochlear   branch of the common cochlear artery that supplies the apical three-fourths of the cochlea, including the modiolus

artery, mastoid   artery in the mastoid portion of the temporal bone, branching from the occipital artery and supplying the posterior part of the mastoid bone

artery, posterior vestibular   branch of the vestibulocochlear artery that supplies the macula of the saccule, the crista and membranous canal of the posterior semicircular canal, and the inferior surface of the utricle and saccule

artery, stylomastoid branch of the posterior auricular artery that supplies the facial nerve, bone and mucosa of adjacent mastoid region and otic capsule, and the stapedius muscle

artery, superior tympanic vessel arising from the middle meningeal artery and entering the middle ear to supply the tensor tympani muscle, the medial half of the roof, and the medial wall of the epitympanic space

artery, vestibulocochlear branch of the common cochlear artery that divides into the posterior vestibular artery and the cochlear ramus, supplying the saccule, posterior semicircular canal, and the basal end of the cochlea

articulated connected together loosely to allow motion between parts

articulation 1. a joint or juncture of bones connected together loosely to allow motion between parts; 2. movement and placement of tongue, lip, hard and soft palate, and teeth during speech production

articulation curve obsolete term for performance-versus-intensity function in word-recognition testing

articulation index AI; early term for the numerical prediction of the quantity of speech signal available or audible to the listener, based on speech importance weightings of various frequency bands; SYN: audibility index; speech intelligibility index

artifact unwanted signal that can interfere with the measurement of desired signals

artifact, blooming inaccurate frequency response observed in an output-AGC hearing aid when tonal rather than broad-band signals are used; results from failure of tonal stimuli to activate frequency-dependent compression

artifact, muscle in the recording of auditory evoked potentials, the unwanted myogenic electrical activity generated from neck or other muscles

artificial ear standardized device used to couple the earphone of an audiometer to a sound level meter microphone for the purpose of calibrating an audiometer

artificial mastoid standardized device that simulates the mechanical impedance of the mastoid process, used to couple the bone vibrator of an audiometer to a sound

level meter microphone for the purpose of calibrating an audiometer

AS [L. *auris sinistra*] left ear

ASA 1. Acoustical Society of America; 2. American Standards Association

ascending auditory pathways central auditory nervous system pathway composed of primary afferent fibers, conveying nerve impulses from the periphery to higher centers

ascending-descending method audiometric technique used in establishing hearing sensitivity thresholds by varying signal intensity from inaudible to audible and then from audible to inaudible

ascending method audiometric technique used in establishing hearing sensitivity thresholds by varying signal intensity from inaudible to audible; ANT: descending method

ASHA American Speech-Language-Hearing Association; professional organization of audiologists and speech-language pathologists; formerly American Speech and Hearing Association

ASL American Sign Language; common form of manual communication used in the United States

ASNHL asymmetric sensorineural hearing loss

ASP 1. automatic signal processing; 2. adaptive signal processing

aspartate amino acid that is thought to play a role as a neurotransmitter from Cranial Nerve VIII fibers to neurons of the cochlear nucleus

aspergillosis infectious lung disease caused by aspergillus, often involving the middle ear by direct extension of the infection from the upper respiratory tracts

aspergillus a genus of fungi

aspergillus auricularis fungus that grows in the external ear canal and on the tympanic membrane

asphyxia 1. impaired or absent exchange of oxygen and carbon dioxide in breathing; 2. apparent or actual cessation of life due to oxygen deprivation to the lungs

aspirate substance removed by aspiration

aspiration removal, by suction, of fluid or a foreign body

aspiration, needle removal by suction of fluid from the middle ear via a needle placed through the tympanic membrane; SYN: myringotomy

aspirin analgesic and anti-inflammatory agent, which can cause temporary ototoxicity in high doses; SYN: acetylsalicylic acid

aspirin ototoxicity temporary threshold shift and tinnitus caused by excessive doses of aspirin

assay 1. to test or examine; 2. an analysis

assistive listening device ALD; hearing instrument or class of hearing instruments, usually with a remote microphone for improving signal-to-noise ratio, including FM systems, personal amplifiers, telephone amplifiers, television listeners

assistive listening device, FM an assistive listening device, designed to enhance signal-to-noise ratio, in which a remote microphone/transmitter worn by a speaker sends signals via FM to a receiver worn by a listener

assistive listening device, infrared assistive listening device consisting of a microphone/transmitter placed near the sound source of interest that broadcasts over infrared light waves to a receiver/amplifier, thereby enhancing the signal-to-noise ratio

association in genetics, the occurrence of two or more traits in a population, at least one of which is of genetic origin

Association for Research in Otolaryngology ARO; professional organization devoted to research related to ear, nose, and throat diseases and functions

astasia inability to stand, due to lack of motor coordination

asthenia weakness

astrocytoma central nervous system tumor characterized as a well-differentiated glioma consisting of astrocytes, which are star-shaped neuroglia cells

asymmetric denoting a dissimilarity between two or more like parts that are normally similar

asymmetry dissimilarity between two or more like parts that are normally similar; e.g., lack of symmetry between ears on some auditory measure

asymptote level of maximum function or performance

at-risk having an increased likelihood of having or developing a disease or impairment

ATA American Tinnitus Association; consumer organization of people with tinnitus

ataxia condition characterized by lack of muscle coordination, often affecting gait and balance

ataxia-hypogonadism syndrome autosomal recessive nervous system disorder, characterized by ataxia, muscle wasting, and severe mental retardation, with early-onset, progressive sensorineural hearing loss; SYN: Richards-Rundle syndrome

atelectasis 1. absence or lack of air in a cavity, as in the middle ear space and mastoid cavity after eustachian tube dysfunction; 2. incomplete expansion or collapse of a structure

atelectasis, vestibular vestibular disorder, characterized by collapse of the walls of the utricle and ampullae and compression of the sensory epithelia, resulting in acute severe vertiginous episodes with nausea and vomiting

atelolalia imperfect development of speech

athreotic cretinism type of congenital hypothyroidism resulting from failure of thyroid embryogenesis, often accompanied by sensorineural hearing loss

athymia morbid impassivity

atmospheric pressure static pressure of the atmosphere

atonia absence or lack of normal muscle tone

atopic dermatitis inflammation of the skin due to allergic reaction, which has strong hereditary influence

atoxyl ototoxic drug used in the treatment of syphilis and parasitic infections, which can cause outer hair cell loss and degenerative changes in Reissner's membrane, stria vascularis, and auditory nerve endings

ATP adenosine triphosphate; neurochemical substance produced by the stria vascularis

atresia congenital absence or pathologic closure of a normal anatomical opening

atresia, aural absence of the opening to the external auditory meatus

atresia, bilateral congenital absence of the external auditory meatus on both ears

atresia, bony congenital absence of the external auditory meatus due to a wall of bone separating the external auditory meatus from the middle ear space

atresia, congenital absence or pathologic closure at birth of a normal anatomical opening, such as the external auditory meatus

atresia, membranous congenital absence of the external auditory meatus due to a dense soft tissue plug between the external auditory canal and middle ear space

atretic   abnormally closed

atrium   1. a chamber or cavity; 2. portion of the middle ear cavity below the malleus

atrophic   pertaining to atrophy

atrophy   wasting away or shrinking of a normally developed organ or tissue

attack time   latency of a compression circuit from detection of a signal to engagement to its steady-state value

attention   mental focus or readiness

attention, auditory   perceptual process by which an individual focuses on specific sounds

attention deficit disorder   ADD; attention deficit hyperactivity disorder

attention deficit hyperactivity disorder   ADHD; cognitive disorder involving reduced ability to focus on an activity, task, or sensory stimulus, characterized by restlessness and distractibility

attenuate   to reduce in magnitude; to decrease

attenuation   reduction in magnitude

attenuation, interaural   IA; reduction in the sound energy of a signal as it is transmitted by bone conduction from one side of the head to the opposite ear

attenuation, linearity of   condition in which a change in an attenuator setting results in a comparable change in output

attenuation, real-ear   probe-microphone measurement of the attenuation characteristic of hearing protection devices, expressed as the difference between the real-ear unaided response and the real-ear occluded response

attenuator   1. device used to reduce voltage, current, or power; 2. intensity level control of an audiometer

attic   upper portion of the middle ear cavity above the tympanic membrane, which contains the head of the malleus and the body of the incus

attic perforation   perforation of the pars flaccida portion of the tympanic membrane

atticitis   inflammation of the attic

atticoantral   pertaining to the attic and mastoid antrum of the middle ear

atticoantrotomy   surgical exposure of the attic and mastoid antrum by partial removal of a portion of the bony tympanic annulus and lateral wall of the epitympanum while preserving the pars tensa and ossicles

atticotomy   surgical opening into the attic

atypical   not normal

AU   [L. *auris uterque*] each ear; [L. *aures unitas*] both ears together

AuD   Doctor of Audiology; designator for professional doctorate degree in audiology

audi(o)-   combining form: hearing

audibility   state of being audible

audibility, homogeneity of   uniformity in terms of audibility throughout, as in lists of spondaic words used in speech-threshold testing

audibility index   AI; measure of the proportion of speech cues that are audible; SYN: articulation index, speech-intelligibility index

audibility threshold   threshold of hearing sensitivity

audible   of sufficient magnitude to be heard

audible frequency range   range of frequencies that can be heard, which, in young humans, is from approximately 15 Hz to 20,000 Hz

audible range   audible frequency range

audile   pertaining to hearing

auding   reception, perception, and comprehension of acoustic information

audio boot   device used with a behind-the-ear hearing aid for coupling with direct audio input cord

audio dosimeter   a body-worn instrument used to measure accumulated level and duration of noise to which a person is exposed over a specified time period

audioanalgesia   a state of reduction in the sensitivity to pain by the use of sound, particularly in dentistry

audiofrequency   a sound wave frequency within the audible frequency range

audiogenic   produced by sound, especially a loud sound

audiogenic seizure   seizure that is caused by sound

audiogram   graphic representation of threshold of hearing sensitivity as a function of stimulus frequency

audiogram, baseline   initial audiogram obtained for comparison with later audiograms to quantify any change in hearing sensitivity

audiogram, behavioral   audiogram obtained by means of behavioral audiometry

audiogram, cookie bite   colloquial term referring to the audiometric configuration characterized by a hearing loss in the middle frequencies and normal or nearly normal hearing in the low and high frequencies

audiogram, corner audiometric configuration characterized by a profound hearing loss with measurable thresholds only in the low-frequency region

audiogram, flat audiogram configuration in which hearing sensitivity is similar across the audiometric frequency range

audiogram, pure-tone graph of the threshold of hearing sensitivity, expressed in dB HL, as determined by pure-tone air-conduction and bone-conduction audiometry at octave and half-octave frequencies ranging from 250 Hz to 8000 Hz

audiogram, serial one of a series of audiograms obtained at regular intervals, usually on an annual basis as part of a hearing conservation program

audiogram, shadow an audiogram reflecting cross hearing from an unmasked nontest ear with normal or nearly normal hearing, obtained while testing an ear with a severe or profound hearing loss; indicative of the organicity of the loss in the test ear

audiogram, U-shaped audiometric configuration with poorest thresholds in the middle frequencies, often associated with congenital hearing loss

audiogram configuration audiometric configuration

audiograph early term for audiogram

audiography early term for audiometry

audiologic, audiological pertaining to audiology

audiologic evaluation assessment of hearing ability

audiologic habilitation aural habilitation or rehabilitation

audiologist healthcare professional who is credentialed in the practice of audiology to provide a comprehensive array of services related to prevention, evaluation, and rehabilitation of hearing impairment and its associated communication disorder

audiologist, dispensing an audiologist who dispenses hearing aids

audiologist, educational audiologist with a subspecialty interest in the hearing needs of school-age children in an academic setting

audiologist, pediatric audiologist with a subspecialty interest in the evaluation and treatment of hearing disorders in children

audiology branch of healthcare devoted to the study, diagnosis, treatment, and prevention of hearing disorders

audiology, educational audiology subspecialty devoted to the hearing needs of school-age children in an academic setting

audiology, forensic audiology subspecialty devoted to legal proceedings related to hearing loss and noise matters

audiology, pediatric audiology subspecialty devoted to the study, evaluation, and treatment of hearing disorders in children

audiology, recreational audiology subspecialty devoted to the conservation of hearing during recreational activities, such as shooting, listening to music, boating, etc.

audiometer electronic instrument designed for measurement of hearing sensitivity and for calibrated delivery of suprathreshold stimuli

audiometer, automatic audiometer that does not require an operator, such as a Békésy audiometer in which the patient controls intensity with a continuously variable attenuator or a computer-based audiometer in which signal presentation level is under software control

audiometer, Békésy automatic audiometer in which the patient controls attenuation of signal intensity with a push-button switch at a fixed frequency or as frequency is swept

audiometer, clinical diagnostic audiometer; wide-range audiometer

audiometer, continuous-frequency early term used to describe a Békésy audiometer in which signal frequency changes automatically in small steps (1 cycle per second) throughout the frequency range

audiometer, discrete-frequency audiometer in which pure-tone frequencies are separate and distinct

audiometer, extended high-frequency high-frequency audiometer

audiometer, high-frequency audiometer with a frequency range extended beyond 8000 Hz

audiometer, limited-range audiometer limited in frequency range and in function, used mostly in identification audiometry

audiometer, microprocessor automatic audiometer characterized by its ability to carry out pure-tone audiometry under microprocessor control

audiometer, peep show early visual-reinforcement device used in pure-tone audiometry with small children, in which the appearance of a puppet served to reinforce a correct response

audiometer, pure-tone   instrument for presenting pure-tone stimuli of selected frequencies at calibrated output levels for the determination of an audiogram

audiometer, Rudmose   early automatic audiometer in which the patient controlled the intensity level of the signal

audiometer, speech   early term for an audiometer that had the capacity to deliver speech, via microphone, tape recorder, or turntable, with a controlled output level

audiometer, wide-range   early term describing an audiometer with a full range of audiometric frequencies and air- and bone-conduction capabilities

audiometric   pertaining to audiometry

audiometric configuration   shape of the audiogram, e.g., flat, rising, steeply sloping

audiometric simulator   computer-based instrument designed to simulate responses of patients with various audiometric configurations for training in audiometric skills

audiometric technician   audiometrist

audiometric tests   procedures used to determine the nature and degree of hearing disorder

audiometric Weber   Weber test in which the bone-conduction vibrator of an audiometer (rather than a tuning fork) is placed on the forehead at midline, and the patient indicates the location of sound in the head

audiometric zero   lowest sound pressure level at which a pure tone at each of the audiometric frequencies is audible to the average normal hearing ear, designated as 0 dB Hearing Level, or audiometric zero, according to national standards

audiometrist   a technician trained in the use of an audiometer to establish hearing thresholds, usually under the supervision of an audiologist or otologist; SYN: audiometric technician

audiometry   measurement of hearing by means of an audiometer

audiometry, auditory brainstem response   ABR measure used to predict hearing sensitivity and to assess the integrity of Cranial Nerve VIII and auditory brainstem structures

audiometry, automatic   automated measurement of hearing by means of either a Békésy audiometer or a computer-based audiometer

audiometry, averaged evoked response   AERA; audiometry using auditory evoked potentials to predict hearing sensitivity

audiometry, behavioral   pure-tone and speech audiometry involving any type of behavioral response, in contrast to electrophysiologic or electroacoustic audiometry

audiometry, behavioral observation   BOA; pediatric assessment of hearing by observation of a child's unconditioned responses to sounds

audiometry, Békésy   automatic audiometry in which a Békésy audiometer is used to determine threshold of hearing to both interrupted tones and continuous tones; patterns of tracings are generally classified into five types, consistent with various hearing disorders

audiometry, brainstem evoked response   BERA; brainstem response audiometry

audiometry, brainstem response   BRA; auditory brainstem response measure used to predict hearing sensitivity and to assess the integrity of Cranial Nerve VIII and auditory brainstem structures

audiometry, brief-tone   BTA; test developed to identify cochlear site of lesion, in which thresholds are obtained for 100-msec tone bursts and 10-msec tone bursts; normal threshold reduction is 10 dB for a tenfold decrease in duration

audiometry, cardiac evoked response   CERA; electrophysiologic technique for predicting hearing sensitivity by measuring changes in heart rate in response to auditory stimulation

audiometry, computerized   automated audiometry controlled by a computer program

audiometry, conditioned orientation reflex   COR audiometry; behavioral audiometry, designed to assess hearing sensitivity in a young child, in which an orienting head-turn response to a sound source is conditioned by visual reinforcement

audiometry, COR   conditioned orientation reflex audiometry

audiometry, cortical evoked response   CERA; electrophysiologic technique for predicting hearing sensitivity by measuring late-latency auditory evoked responses to auditory stimulation

audiometry, delayed feedback   DFA; the use of delayed auditory feedback in assessing the organicity of a suspected functional hearing loss; the delayed delivery of speech, if audible, interferes with fluency or rate of speech

audiometry, diagnostic measurement of hearing to determine the nature and degree of hearing impairment

audiometry, electric response ERA; evoked response audiometry

audiometry, electrocardiographic response early electrophysiologic measure designed to predict hearing sensitivity by monitoring heart-rate changes, via an electrocardiogram, in response to sound stimulation; SYN: cardiac evoked response audiometry

audiometry, electrodermal EDA; method of determining hearing sensitivity in cases of suspected functional hearing loss by measuring psychogalvanic skin response to sound, following conditioning to the sound paired with a mild shock

audiometry, electroencephalic EEA; earliest use of electrophysiologic responses to predict hearing sensitivity, involving observation of changes in EEG patterns in response to auditory stimulation

audiometry, electrophysiologic response ERA; prediction of hearing sensitivity based on the recording of physiologic electrical potentials in response to auditory stimulation

audiometry, evoked response ERA; electrophysiologic prediction of hearing sensitivity

audiometry, fixed-frequency the use of Békésy or automatic audiometry to track sensitivity threshold at a single, fixed frequency; COM: sweep-frequency audiometry

audiometry, galvanic skin response method of determining hearing sensitivity in cases of suspected functional hearing loss by measuring psychogalvanic skin response to sound, following conditioning to the sound paired with a mild shock; SYN: electrodermal audiometry

audiometry, group simultaneous hearing testing of several patients, usually by means of a network of automated audiometers

audiometry, heart-rate HRA; electrophysiologic technique for predicting hearing sensitivity by measuring heart-rate changes in response to auditory stimulation; SYN: cardiac evoked response audiometry

audiometry, identification testing designed to screen the hearing of large numbers of individuals, such as neonates and school-age children, with the goal of identifying those who need more comprehensive audiologic assessment; SYN: screening audiometry

audiometry, immittance battery of immittance measurements, including static immittance, tympanometry, and acoustic reflex threshold determination, designed to assess middle ear function

audiometry, impedance immittance audiometry

audiometry, in situ assessment of hearing in which pure-tone thresholds and loudness discomfort levels are measured and expressed in ear canal SPL

audiometry, industrial assessment of hearing, including determination of baseline sensitivity and periodic monitoring, to determine the effects of industrial noise exposure on hearing sensitivity

audiometry, manual any type of standard hearing measurement in which the examiner controls the stimulus presentation; ANT: automatic audiometry

audiometry, objective measurement of hearing sensitivity based on predictions made from physiological responses to sound

audiometry, PGSR method of determining hearing sensitivity in suspected functional hearing loss by measuring psychogalvanic skin response to sound, following conditioning of the patient to the sound paired with a mild shock; SYN: electrodermal audiometry

audiometry, play behavioral method of hearing assessment of young children in which the correct identification of a signal presentation is rewarded with the opportunity to engage in any of several play-oriented activities

audiometry, pure-tone measurement of hearing sensitivity thresholds to pure-tone stimuli by air and bone conduction

audiometry, screening rapid assessment of the ability of individuals to hear acoustic signals across a frequency range at a fixed criterion intensity level; designed to identify those who require additional audiometric procedures; SYN: identification audiometry

audiometry, sound field measurement of hearing sensitivity to signals presented in a sound field through loudspeakers; used especially in pediatric assessment

audiometry, speech measurement of the hearing of speech signals; includes measurement of speech awareness, speech reception, word and sentence recognition, sensitized speech processing, and dichotic listening

audiometry, sweep-frequency the use of Békésy or automatic audiometry to track sensitivity thresholds as the frequency of the signal slowly increases across the audiometric frequency range; COM: fixed-frequency audiometry

audiometry, tangible reinforcement operant conditioning TROCA; audiometric technique that uses a mechanical box from which the child or mentally disabled patient receives reinforcement, usually in the form of candy or cereal, for the correct identification of a signal presentation

audiometry, tracking automatic or Békésy audiometry in which the patient controls signal attenuation with a switch and adjusts the intensity alternately from a level of audibility to inaudibility to audibility and so on

audiometry, visual reinforcement VRA; audiometric technique used in pediatric assessment in which a correct response to signal presentation, such as a head turn toward the speaker, is rewarded by the activation of a light or lighted toy

audiometry, yes-no technique for establishing auditory thresholds in children or others who are exaggerating hearing loss by asking them to respond by saying "yes" when they hear the tone that is presented and "no" when they do not hear the tone that is presented

audiophile enthusiast of high-fidelity sound reproduction equipment

audioprosthetist audioprosthologist

audioprosthologist person credentialed in the fitting and dispensing of hearing aids

audioprosthology study of hearing aid fitting

audioreflexometry prediction of hearing levels by observation of involuntary responses to auditory stimulation, especially in infants

audiotherapy auditory training

audiovestibular pertaining to the combined function of the auditory and vestibular structures

audiovisual pertaining to instruction that uses both auditory and visual presentation of information

audition hearing

auditive auditory

audito-oculogyric reflex AOR; rapid turning of the eyes toward the source of a sudden sound

auditorally; auditorially in an auditory manner

auditory pertaining to the sense of hearing

auditory acclimatization systematic change in auditory preformance over time due to a change in the acoustic information available to the listener; e.g., an ear becoming accustomed to processing sounds of increased loudness following introduction of a hearing aid

auditory adaptation process by which a constant audible tone becomes inaudible after a time; SYN: tone decay

auditory agnosia impairment in the ability to recognize speech or other sounds as a result of cortical disorder

auditory alexia disorder characterized by difficulty perceiving similarities and differences in sounds

auditory analysis perceptual process by which an auditory sequence is identified as a whole and separated into its component parts

auditory aphasia impairment in the comprehension of spoken language; SYN: fluent aphasia, receptive aphasia, Wernicke's aphasia

auditory area primary auditory cortex (Brodmann's area 41) located at the transverse gyrus (Heschl's gyrus) of the temporal lobe

auditory attention perceptual process by which an individual focuses on specific sounds

auditory behavior index ABI; classification of expected behavioral responses from infants and young children

auditory blending perceptual process by which phonemes of a word are combined into the whole word

auditory boundaries, natural sound discrimination ability present at birth, attributable to the natural operation of the auditory perceptual mechanism

auditory brainstem implant ABI; electrode implanted at the juncture of Cranial Nerve VIII and the cochlear nucleus that receives signals from an external processor and sends electrical impulses directly to the brainstem

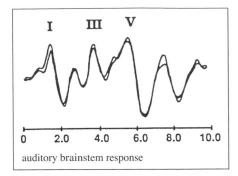

auditory brainstem response

auditory brainstem response ABR; auditory evoked potential, originating from Cranial Nerve VIII and auditory brainstem structures, consisting of five to seven identifiable peaks that represent neural function of auditory pathways and nuclei

auditory brainstem response, electrically evoked EABR; auditory brainstem response generated by electrical stimulation of the cochlea with either an extracochlear promontory electrode or a cochlear implant

auditory brainstem response audiometry ABR measure used to predict hearing sensitivity and to assess the integrity of Cranial Nerve VIII and auditory brainstem structures

auditory canal external auditory meatus

auditory capsule vesicle or otocyst in the human embryo that develops from the otic placode and becomes the cochlea; SYN: otic capsule

auditory closure perceptual process by which partial auditory information is integrated into a whole, so that a word can be recognized when some of its phonemes are missing or not perceived

auditory comprehension understanding of spoken language

auditory cortex auditory area of the cerebral cortex located on the transverse temporal gyrus (Heschl's gyrus) of the temporal lobe

auditory cue verbal information provided to prompt a response as an aid to communication

auditory deprivation diminution or absence of sensory opportunity for neural structures central to the end organ, due to a reduction in auditory stimulation resulting from hearing loss

auditory deprivation, adult-onset late-onset auditory deprivation

auditory deprivation, delayed-onset late-onset auditory deprivation

auditory deprivation, late-onset decline in word-recognition ability in the unaided ear of a person fitted with one hearing aid, resulting from asymmetric stimulation

auditory deprivation effect systematic decrease over time in auditory performance associated with the reduced availability of acoustic information

auditory differentiation auditory figure-ground discrimination

auditory discrimination perceptual process by which an individual distinguishes and differentiates among sounds or words

auditory disorder disturbance in auditory structure, function, or both

auditory disorder, central CAD; functional disorder resulting from diseases of or trauma to the central auditory nervous system

auditory disorder, peripheral functional disorder resulting from diseases of or trauma to the external ear, middle ear, cochlea, and Cranial Nerve VIII

auditory evoked field AEF; electromagnetic response of the auditory nervous system

auditory evoked potential AEP; electrophysiologic response to sound, usually distinguished according to latency, including ECoG, ABR, MLR, LVR, SSEP, P3

auditory evoked response AER; auditory evoked potential

auditory evoked response, brainstem BAER; auditory brainstem response

auditory evoked response, late late-latency auditory evoked response

auditory evoked response, long-latency LLAEP; auditory evoked potential, having two main waveform peaks—a vertex negative peak at approximately 90 msec and a vertex positive peak at approximately 180 msec following signal presentation; SYN: ALR

auditory evoked response, middle-latency MLAER; auditory evoked potential, originating from the region of the auditory radiations and cortex, having as a primary component a vertex positive peak at 25 msec to 40 msec following signal presentation; SYN: auditory middle latency response

auditory evoked response, slow negative SN10; averaged auditory electrical potential evoked by tone bursts, characterized as a broad vertex negative peak occurring around 10 msec following signal onset

auditory fatigue temporary elevation of hearing thresholds following exposure to sound; SYN: temporary threshold shift

auditory feedback perception of one's own vocalizations

auditory feedback, delayed DAF; condition in which a listener's speech is delayed by a controlled amount of time and delivered back to the listener's ears, interfering with the rate and fluency of the speech

auditory field area or distance that defines the limits of audibility of a definite sound

auditory figure-ground relation of relevant acoustic information to competing background noise

auditory figure-ground discrimination perceptual process by which relevant acoustic information is differentiated from background noise

auditory flutter fusion auditory fusion

auditory fusion process by which interrupted sound is perceived as continuous

auditory ganglia cell bodies of the auditory nerve fibers, clustered in the modiolus; SYN: spiral ganglia

auditory hallucination the apparent perception of sound that has no basis in external stimulation

auditory imperception impairment in the recognition or interpretation of sound

auditory late response ALR; auditory evoked potential, originating from the cortex and having two main waveform peaks, a vertex negative peak at approximately 90 msec and a vertex positive peak at approximately 180 msec following signal presentation; SYN: LLAEP

auditory lateralization perceptual process of determining the location of a sound within the head

auditory localization perceptual process of determining the location of a sound source in an acoustic environment

auditory meatus, external EAM; canal extending from the auricle to the tympanic membrane

auditory meatus, internal IAM; an opening on the posterior surface of the petrous portion of the temporal bone through which the auditory and facial nerves pass

auditory memory assimilation, storage, and retrieval of previously experienced sound

auditory memory span number of items that can be recalled following presentation of speech or other sounds

auditory method form of aural rehabilitation that stresses optimization of the use of residual hearing by focusing on listening skills training

auditory middle latency response AMLR; auditory evoked potential, originating from the region of the auditory radiations and cortex, having as a primary component a vertex positive peak at 25 msec to 40 msec following signal presentation; SYN: MLR

auditory nerve AN; Cranial Nerve VIII, consisting of a vestibular and cochlear branch; SYN: vestibulocochlear nerve

auditory nervous system, central CANS; portion of the central nervous system that involves hearing, including the cochlear nucleus, superior olivary complex, lateral lemniscus, inferior colliculus, medial geniculate, and auditory cortex

auditory nervous system, peripheral hearing mechanism of the peripheral nervous system, including the cochlea and Cranial Nerve VIII

auditory neurons, primary first-order neurons of the cochlear branch of Cranial Nerve VIII, with dendrites from the inner hair cells to cell bodies of the spiral ganglion to axons synapsing on the cochlear nucleus

auditory oculogyric reflex AOR; audito-oculogyric reflex

auditory pathway peripheral and central auditory nerve fibers and nuclei from Cranial Nerve VIII to the auditory cortex

auditory pathway, primary neural pathway in the central nervous system that carries the primary afferent input from the cochlea to the cortex

auditory pattern sequence of speech sounds in words that is specific to a particular language

auditory perception awareness, recognition, and interpretation of auditory stimuli received in the brain

auditory pit depression for the formation of an ear on the side of the head of an embryo; SYN: otic pit

auditory placode thickened plate of cells on the lateral aspect of the neural fold in the human embryo that develops into the otic capsule and inner ear; SYN: otic placode

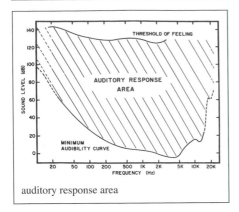

auditory response area

auditory plate bony roof of the external auditory meatus

auditory process edge of the auditory plate to which the cartilaginous portion of the external auditory meatus attaches

auditory processes specific auditory skills such as analysis, blending, closure, discrimination, localization

auditory processing peripheral and central auditory system manipulation of acoustic signals

auditory processing disorder APD; reduction in the ability to manipulate acoustic signals, despite normal hearing sensitivity and regardless of language, attention, and cognition ability; SYN: central auditory processing disorder

auditory processing disorder, central CAPD; disorder in function of central auditory structures, characterized by impaired ability of the central auditory nervous system to manipulate and use acoustic signals, including difficulty understanding speech in noise and localizing sounds

auditory processing dysfunction auditory processing disorder

auditory radiations bundle of nerve fibers emanating from the medial geniculate body to the primary auditory cortex

auditory receptor cochlear hair cell

auditory response area dynamic range of hearing from the threshold of audibility to the threshold of pain across the audiometric frequency range; SYN: auditory sensation area

auditory sensation area auditory response area

auditory sequencing perceptual process

by which sounds and words are properly ordered

auditory synthesis perceptual process by which discrete phonemes are integrated into syllables or whole words

auditory threshold lowest intensity level at which a specified sound is perceptible

auditory trainer electronic amplification device used in the classroom to supplement conventional hearing aid use

auditory trainer, FM classroom amplification system in which a remote microphone/transmitter worn by the teacher sends signals via FM to a receiver worn by the student

auditory trainer, hard-wired early type of amplification device in which the listener's receiver was attached to a desk and the speaker's microphone was connected to an amplifier

auditory trainer, loop-induction loop amplification system in which an auditory training unit receives signals via magnetic induction through its telecoil from a loop of wire encircling a room that is sending signals generated by a microphone and amplifier

auditory training aural rehabilitation methods designed to maximize use of residual hearing by structured practice in listening, environmental alteration, hearing aid use, etc.

auditory tube passageway leading from the nasopharynx to the anterior wall of the middle ear, which opens to equalize middle ear air pressure; SYN: eustachian tube

auditory verbal agnosia inability to recognize spoken language due to central nervous system disorder

auditory vertex response auditory late response; late vertex response

auditory vesicle saclike cavity formed by closure of the auditory pit in the human embryo from which the cochlea develops; SYN: otic vesicle

auditory-vocal association development of the relation between perception of auditory stimuli and vocal expression of same

aura sensation that occurs preceding the occurrence of more definitive symptoms or preceding an epileptic seizure

aural pertaining to the ear or hearing

aural adenoma, benign glandular tumor of the external auditory canal and middle ear, which appears as a painless mass and may be accompanied by conductive hearing loss

aural adenoma, malignant   rare malignant glandular tumor of the external auditory canal and middle ear, which is accompanied by hearing loss, otorrhea, pain, and cranial nerve palsies

aural atresia   absence of the opening to the external auditory meatus

aural habilitation   treatment of persons with congenital hearing impairment to improve the efficacy of overall oral/aural communication ability, including the use of hearing aids, auditory training, speech and language therapy, speechreading, manual communication

aural harmonics   perception of harmonics of tones that are not present in the tonal stimuli, related to distortion generated within the cochlea due to its nonlinearity

aural murmurs   noises originating within the ear; SYN: tinnitus

aural myiasis   infection due to invasion of the external, middle, or inner ear by larvae of certain insects

aural-oral method   aural habilitation approach of teaching children with hearing impairment using hearing, speech, and speechreading, but not manual communication; SYN: oral-aural method

aural overload   cochlear distortion of a signal due to excessive intensity

aural polyp   benign lesion in the external auditory meatus, protruding from a perforation of the tympanic membrane

aural rehabilitation   treatment of persons with adventitious hearing impairment to improve the efficacy of overall communication ability, including the use of hearing aids, auditory training, speech reading, counseling, and guidance

aural speculum   funnel-shaped instrument for enlarging the opening of the external auditory meatus to facilitate inspection of the ear canal and tympanic membrane

aural vertigo   nonspecific term for sensation of motion caused by labyrinthine disorders

auralism   oralism

aurally   by ear

aures unitas   AU; both ears together

auricle   external or outer ear, which serves as a protective mechanism, as a resonator, and as a baffle for directional hearing of front-versus-back and in the vertical plane; SYN: pinna

auricle, accessory   craniofacial anomaly characterized by an additional auricle or additional auricular tissue

auricula   auricle

auricular   pertaining to the auricle

auricular aplasia   congenital absence of an auricle; SYN: anotia

auricular artery   1. posterior branch originating from the external carotid and distributing blood to the middle ear, mastoid cells, and auricle; 2. deep branch originating from the maxillary and distributing to the tympanic membrane and external auditory meatus

auricular ligament   any of several ligaments that attach the auricle to the temporal bone

auricular perichondritis   inflammation of the connective tissue membrane around the cartilage of the auricle

auricular point   auriculare

auriculare   center of the concha or opening to the external auditory meatus

auricularis anterior muscle   muscle innervated by the facial nerve that inserts into the cartilage of the ear and may draw the auricle forward

auricularis posterior muscle   muscle innervated by the facial nerve that originates at the mastoid process and inserts into the cartilage of the ear and may draw the auricle backward

auricularis superior muscle   muscle innervated by the facial nerve that inserts into the cartilage of the ear and may raise the auricle

auricularis transverse muscle   muscle innervated by the facial nerve that inserts into the cartilage of the ear

auriculate   resembling an ear

auriform   shaped like an ear

auris   ear

auris dextra   AD; right ear

auris sinistra   AS; left ear

auris uterque   AU; each ear

auriscope   otoscope

auristics   treatment of ear diseases

auropalpebral reflex   APR; eyeblink or twitch at the canthus caused by a sudden loud sound

auscultate   to examine by listening to sounds of the body

auscultation   listening to sounds made by various body structures

auscultatory   relating to auscultation

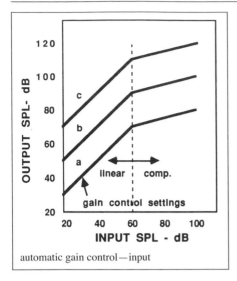

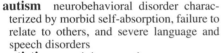

automatic gain control—input

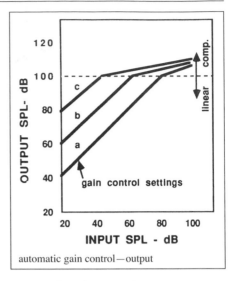

automatic gain control—output

autism neurobehavioral disorder characterized by morbid self-absorption, failure to relate to others, and severe language and speech disorders

autistic pertaining to autism

autogenic originating within oneself; e.g., functional hearing loss

autoimmune arising from and directed against the body's own tissue

autoimmune hearing loss auditory disorder characterized by bilateral, asymmetric, progressive, sensorineural hearing loss in patients who test positively for autoimmune disease

automatic audiometer audiometer that does not require an operator, such as a Békésy audiometer in which the patient controls intensity with a continuously variable attenuator or a computer-based audiometer in which signal presentation level is under software control

automatic audiometry automated measurement of hearing by means of either a Békésy audiometer or a computer-based audiometer

automatic gain control AGC; nonlinear hearing aid compression circuitry designed to automatically change gain as signal level changes or limit output when signal level reaches a specified criterion; SYN: automatic volume control

automatic gain control—input AGC-I; circuitry of a hearing aid in which the volume control follows the AGC

automatic gain control—output AGC-O; circuitry of a hearing aid in which the AGC follows the volume control

automatic signal processing ASP; process in which hearing aid circuitry adjusts some parameter of the amplified output automatically or adaptively as the input signal reaches a certain criterion

automatic volume control AVC; automatic gain control

autonomic not under voluntary control; functionally independent

autonomic nervous system ANS; that portion of the nervous system that regulates glandular and visceral responses

autophonia autophony

autophony sensation of abnormally increased loudness or resonance of one's own voice as a result of middle ear disorder

autosomal pertaining to autosomes

autosomal dominant inheritance transmission of a genetic characteristic or mutation in which only one gene of a pair must carry the characteristic in order for it to be expressed, and both sexes have an equal chance of being affected

autosomal inheritance genetic inheritance related to non-sex-linked chromosomes; COM: X-linked inheritance

autosomal recessive inheritance transmission of a genetic characteristic or mutation in which both genes of a pair must share the characteristic in order for it to be expressed

autosome any of the 22 pairs of chromosomes not related to the determination of sex

AVC automatic volume control

AVCN anterior ventral cochlear nucleus; portion of the cochlear nucleus that receives primary afferent projections from Cranial Nerve VIII and sends second-order fibers via the ventral acoustic stria to the superior olivary complex

average, high-frequency HFA; an ANSI hearing aid specification, expressed as the average of decibel response values at 1000 Hz, 1600 Hz, and 2500 Hz

average, pure-tone PTA; average of hearing sensitivity thresholds to pure-tone signals at 500 Hz, 1000 Hz, and 2000 Hz

average, time-weighted TWA; measure of daily noise exposure, expressed as the product of durations of exposure at particular sound levels to the allowable durations of exposure for those levels

averaged evoked response audiometry AERA; audiometry using auditory evoked potentials to predict hearing sensitivity

aviator's ear traumatic inflammation disorder of the middle ear caused by sudden changes in air pressure in the pneumatized spaces of the temporal bone on descent from high altitude; SYN: aerotitis media

Award for Continuing Education ACE; certificate given by the American Speech-Language-Hearing Association for completion of a prescribed number of continuing education units

axoaxonic pertaining to the synapse between the axon of one nerve cell and that of another

axodendritic pertaining to the synapse between an axon and a dendrite

axon efferent process of a neuron that conducts impulses away from the cell body and other cell processes

axonotmesis damage to axons of a nerve followed by complete degeneration of the peripheral segment without damage to the supporting structures of the nerve

azimuth direction of a sound source measured in angular degrees in a horizontal plane in relationship to the listener; e.g., 0° azimuth is directly in front of the listener, 180° azimuth is directly behind

azimuth, loudspeaker direction of a loudspeaker, measured in angular degrees in the horizontal plane, in relationship to the listener

Aztec ear an auricle with no lobule; SYN: Cagot ear

B

B susceptance; energy flow associated with reactance; reciprocal of reactance

B-weighted scale sound level meter filtering network weighted to approximate an equal loudness contour at 70 phons; frequencies below 300 Hz are reduced by approximately 4 dB per octave

babble competing message that contains multiple talkers

babbling prelinguistic verbal behavior of infants within the first 6 months of life

Babinski reflex normal extension and fanning of the toes on stimulation of the sole of the foot, a lack of a which is consistent with neurologic disorder

back-end noise source of noise located in the power amplifier or receiver segments of a hearing aid

background noise extraneous surrounding sounds of the environment; SYN: ambient noise

backward masking the masking of a sound by another sound that occurs milliseconds later

bacterial labyrinthitis inflammation of the membranous labyrinth due to bacterial invasion

BADGE test Békésy ascending descending gap evaluation test; variation of Békésy audiometry, used to detect functional hearing loss, in which the tracking levels obtained with an ascending and descending approach are compared for discrepancies

BAEP brainstem auditory evoked potential; SYN: auditory brainstem response

BAER brainstem auditory evoked response; SYN: auditory brainstem response

baffle a shielding partition designed to reduce sound wave transmission between two points in an acoustic system

baffle effect, head relative enhancement of high-frequency sound due to the acoustic diffraction of low-frequency sound by the auricle and head combining to form a wall or baffle

balance harmonious adjustment of muscles against gravity to maintain equilibrium

balance mechanism biological system that, in conjunction with the ocular and proprioceptive systems, functions to maintain equilibrium; SYN: vestibular system

Baller-Gerold syndrome craniosynostosis syndrome that may include auricular malformation, characterized by low-set dysplastic auricles

band range of frequencies

band, octave division of the frequency range into octave intervals

band, side a group of frequencies on either side of a carrier frequency

band frequency range of frequencies between specified limits

band-pass filter an electronic filter that allows a specified band of frequencies to pass, while reducing or eliminating frequencies above and below the band; SYN: passband filter

band spectrum graphic representation of sound, displayed as sound pressure levels of specified frequency bands

bandwidth range of frequencies within a specified band

BAPP bleomycin, adriamycin, cisplatin, prednisone; potentially ototoxic chemotherapy regimen used in the treatment of malignant thymoma

bar unit of force equal to 1 megadyne

Barany caloric test irrigation of the external auditory meatus with warm and cool water to stimulate the vestibular labyrinth, resulting in nystagmus as an indicator of vestibular function

Barany chair early rotating chair designed to test vestibular function

Barany noise box early mechanical device operated by a key-wound spring to produce broad-band noise for masking

Barany sign reduction or absence of nystagmus in response to caloric stimulation of the vestibular system

Barany syndrome central vestibular disorder caused by inflammation of the arachnoid membrane of the posterior fossa, resulting in attacks of rotary vertigo, headache, and vegetative symptoms; SYN: arachnoiditis pontocerebellaris

barbula hirci hairs growing at the opening of the external auditory meatus

barotitis media traumatic inflammation disorder of the middle ear caused by sudden changes in air pressure in the pneumatized spaces of the temporal bone on descent from high altitude or ascent from underwater diving; SYN: aerotitis media

barotrauma traumatic injury caused by a rapid marked change in atmospheric pressure resulting in a significant mismatch in air pressure in the pneumatized spaces of the body, including the temporal bone

barotrauma, otitic barotitis media

barrier penetration the transmission of sound through barriers; penetration is greater for sounds with longer wave lengths

Barry five-slate system early aural rehabilitative approach to teaching syntax and grammar to hearing-impaired persons by using five slates that represent the principal parts of a sentence

basal denoting the lowest level possible; near the base

basal cell carcinoma slow-growing malignant skin cancer which can occur on the pinna and external auditory meatus as a flat, painless, slightly raised lesion followed by the development of a penetrating bleeding ulcer

basal ganglia large subcortical nuclei of the cerebrum, including the caudate and lentiform nuclei of the corpus striatum and the amygdaloid nuclear complex

basal turn of the cochlea lowest or first turn of the cochlea wherein high frequencies are represented

baseline starting point or level of functioning

baseline audiogram initial audiogram obtained for comparison with later audiograms to quantify any change in hearing sensitivity

basement membrane thin membranous portion of Reissner's membrane that separates the mesothelial cell layer in the scala vestibuli from the epithelial cell layer in the scala media

basic frequency fundamental frequency

basilar pertaining to the base

basilar artery vessel giving rise to the anterior inferior cerebellar artery, which supplies blood to the cochlea

basilar crest shelflike prominence of the spiral ligament near the basilar membrane; SYN: spiral prominence

basilar macula cluster of cells in the embryonic otic vesicle that develops into the basilar membrane

basilar membrane base of the membranous labyrinth of the cochlea, dividing it into the scala vestibuli and scala tympani, that supports the scala media and organ of Corti

basilar papilla organ of Corti

bass increases at low levels BILL; type of automatic signal processing in a hearing aid that uses level-dependent control of the frequency response, reducing low frequencies in response to high-intensity input

battery 1. a cell that stores an electrical charge and furnishes a current; 2. group of diagnostic tests

battery drain amount of electrical current being drawn from a battery

BBN broad-band noise; sound with a wide bandwidth, containing a continuous spectrum of frequencies, with equal energy per cycle throughout the band

BC bone conduction; transmission of sound to the cochlea by vibration of the skull

BC-HIS board-certified in hearing instrument sciences; credential awarded to qualifying hearing instrument specialists by the National Board for Certification in Hearing Instrument Sciences

BCL test Békésy comfortable loudness test; variant of Békésy audiometry, used to detect functional hearing loss, in which pulsed and continuous tracings are obtained at comfortable loudness rather than threshold

beamformer noise canceler consisting of two or more microphones that are oriented spacially relative to the locations of the desired signal and the undesired noise

Beasley report study from the 1935–1936 U.S. Public Health Survey that established audiometric zero levels that later became the ASA 1951 standards

beat perception of periodic loudness changes when two tones of very similar frequencies are presented simultaneously

beat-frequency oscillator electronic instrument that generates pairs of pure tones that combine to produce difference tones or beats

Beckwith-Weidemann syndrome overgrowth syndrome, which may include auricular malformations, characterized by earlobe grooves and indented lesions on the helix or concha and associated conductive hearing loss

behavioral pertaining to externally observable activity of a person

behavioral audiogram audiogram obtained by means of behavioral audiometry

behavioral audiometry pure-tone and speech audiometry involving any type of behavioral response, in contrast to electrophysiologic or electroacoustic audiometry; COM: objective audiometry

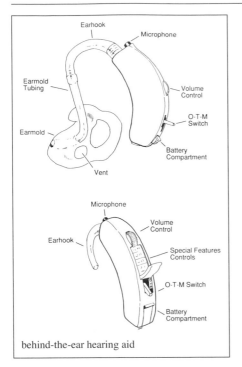

behind-the-ear hearing aid

behavioral criterion   standard by which to judge behavioral responses

behavioral observation audiometry BOA; pediatric assessment of hearing by observation of a child's unconditioned responses to sounds

behind-the-ear hearing aid   BTE hearing aid; a hearing aid that fits over the ear and is coupled to the ear canal via an earmold; SYN: postauricular hearing aid

Békésy ascending descending gap evaluation test BADGE test; variation of Békésy audiometry, used to detect functional hearing loss, in which the tracking levels obtained with an ascending and descending approach are compared for discrepancies

Békésy audiometer   automatic audiometer in which the patient controls attenuation of signal intensity with a push-button switch at a fixed frequency or as frequency is swept

Békésy audiometry   automatic audiometry in which a Békésy audiometer is used to determine threshold of hearing to both interrupted tones and continuous tones; patterns of tracings are generally classified into five types, consistent with various hearing disorders; after George von Békésy, a Hungarian

physicist who received a Nobel prize for his description of the traveling wave

Békésy comfortable loudness test   BCL test; variant of Békésy audiometry, used to detect functional hearing loss, in which pulsed and continuous tracings are obtained at comfortable loudness rather than threshold

Békésy forward-reverse test   a test in which two continuous-tone Békésy threshold tracings, one from low to high frequencies and the other from high to low frequencies, are compared; differences in thresholds are found in patients with functional hearing loss

Békésy tracing types   patterns of interrupted and continuous tracings, classified into five types: Types I and II are associated with normal neural function, Types III and IV with retrocochlear pathology, and Type V with functional hearing loss

Békésy traveling wave   sound-induced displacement pattern along the basilar membrane that describes fundamental cochlear processing

bel   unit expressing the intensity of a sound relative to a reference intensity; intensity in bels is the logarithm (to the base 10) of the ratio of the power of a sound to that of a reference sound; after Alexander Graham Bell

bell-shaped curve   description of the graphic representation of a normal distribution

Bell's palsy   acute unilateral facial paralysis due to facial nerve disorder of idiopathic origin

belled bore   enlarged bowl-shaped canal opening of an earmold or custom hearing aid

belt region   portion of the inferior colliculus, medial geniculate, and auditory cortex that surrounds the core areas of each center, through which parallel auditory information travels

benign   1. denoting mild character of an illness; 2. denoting nonmalignant character of a neoplasm

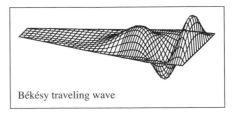

Békésy traveling wave

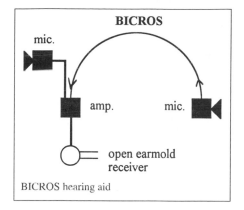

BICROS hearing aid

benign aural adenoma   glandular tumor of the external auditory canal and middle ear, which appears as a painless mass and may be accompanied by conductive hearing loss

benign paroxysmal nystagmus   sudden, transient burst of nystagmus during the Dix-Hallpike maneuver, which disappears within 10 seconds once the head position is achieved

benign paroxysmal positioning vertigo   BPPV; a recurrent, acute form of vertigo occurring in clusters in response to positional changes

BEP   bleomycin, etoposide, platinol (cisplatin); potentially ototoxic chemotherapy regimen used in the treatment of testicular cancer

BERA   brainstem evoked response audiometry; brainstem electric response audiometry

Berger prescriptive procedure   first comprehensive hearing aid selection algorithm designed to prescribe gain and frequency response based on the pure-tone audiogram, with different weighting factors at each of six frequencies from 500 Hz to 6000 Hz

beta rhythm or waves   EEG waves of 14 Hz to 25 Hz

Bezold triad   triad of clinical findings in otosclerosis including low-frequency air-conduction hearing loss, better bone conduction, and negative Rinne test

BHI   Better Hearing Institute

biauricular   pertaining to both auricles

BICROS   bilateral contralateral routing of signals; a hearing aid system with one microphone contained in a hearing aid at each ear; the microphones lead to a single amplifier

and receiver in the better hearing ear of a person with bilateral asymmetric hearing loss

BIFROS   bilateral frontal routing of signals; hearing aid system with microphones placed in the front of eyeglass hearing aids

bifurcate   divide into two branches

bifurcation   1. division into two branches; 2. point at which the division into two branches occurs

bilateral   pertaining to both sides, hence to both ears

bilateral atresia   congenital absence of the external auditory meatus in both ears

bilateral contralateral routing of signals   BICROS; a hearing aid system with one microphone contained in a hearing aid at each ear; the microphones are connected to a single amplifier and receiver in the better ear of a person with bilateral asymmetric hearing loss

bilateral horizontal gaze nystagmus   nystagmus that beats to the right on right gaze and beats to the left on left gaze

bilateral unequal gaze nystagmus   nystagmus that is present in both gaze directions, but of different magnitude in one direction, consistent with central nervous system pathology

bilateral weakness   BW; hypoactivity of vestibular system to caloric stimulation in both ears, consistent with bilateral peripheral vestibular disorder

bilirubin   a pigment in the blood serum produced by degeneration of hemoglobin

bilirubinemia   presence of bilirubin in the blood

BILL   bass increase at low levels; type of automatic signal processing in a hearing aid that uses level-dependent control of the frequency response, reducing low frequencies in response to high-intensity input

bimastoid   pertaining to both mastoid processes

bimodal   pertaining to the combined use of two modalities

bimodal distribution   data distribution having two distinct peaks

bimodal method   aural rehabilitation method combining auditory and visual communication

binaural   pertaining to both ears

binaural advantage   the cumulative benefits of using two ears over one, including enhanced threshold and better hearing in the presence of background noise

binaural amplification   use of a hearing aid in both ears

binaural beats   perception of beats due to central nervous system interaction resulting from the presentation of a tone to one ear and a tone of a slightly different frequency (<5 Hz) to the other ear

binaural CROS   hearing aid system that separates the microphone from the receiver to reduce feedback; microphones are mounted in hearing aids on both sides of the head, and amplified signals are routed across the head to the opposite ear; SYN: criss-CROS

binaural diplacusis   condition in which tones of identical frequency are perceived to be of dissimilar pitch in the right and left ears

binaural fusion   1. phenomenon wherein different sounds presented to the two ears fuse into a single sound image somewhere in the head; 2. integration of simultaneous but different speech signals presented to the two ears

binaural integration   fusion of simultaneous but different speech signals presented to the two ears; SYN: binaural fusion

binaural lateralization   perception of movement of a sound image within the head resulting from binaural auditory stimulation

binaural localization   use of two ears for locating sounds in space

binaural masking level difference   BMLD; measure of binaural release from masking in which binaural thresholds are determined in noise for tones that are in phase and 180° out of phase; SYN: masking level difference

binaural release from masking   enhancement in threshold in noise for binaurally presented tones as noise or tones are changed from being in phase to being out of phase; basis for the masking level difference (MLD) test

binaural resynthesis   binaural fusion

binaural separation   ability to perceive stimuli presented to one ear while ignoring stimuli presented to the opposite ear

binaural squelch   improvement in speech intelligibility in noise of two ears over one because of interaural phase and intensity differences

binaural summation   cumulative effect of sound reaching both ears, resulting in enhancement in hearing with both ears over one ear, characterized by binaural improve-ment in hearing sensitivity of approximately 3 dB over monaural sensitivity

binauricular   pertaining to both ears

Bing test   tuning fork test that measures the occlusion effect by applying a fork or other bone vibrator to the head while the ear canal is open and closed, with absence of change in perceived loudness indicating conductive hearing loss

binotic   binaural

bioacoustics   the science pertaining to the effects of sound on living organisms

bioelectric   pertaining to electric phenomena in living cells

biologic calibration   the determination of audiometric zero for a particular signal based on average thresholds from a sample of normal-hearing subjects

biologic check   assessment of the functioning of various parameters of an audiometer by performing a listening check

biphasic pulse   square wave having equal positive and negative amplitude

bipolar electrode   an electrode array with two poles that are active for recording or delivering electrical signals; COM: monopolar electrode

bipolar stimulation   1. delivery of an electrical signal across two poles of an electrode array; 2. cochlear implant stimulation in which both the active and indifferent electrodes are intracochlear; COM: monopolar stimulation;

bisensory method   aural rehabilitation approach that combines visual (speechreading) and auditory training

bisyllabic   having two syllables

bithermal caloric stimulation test   assessment of vestibular function by irrigation of the external auditory meatus with warm and cool water or air

Björnstad syndrome   autosomal dominant disorder with low penetrance, characterized by congenital sensorineural hearing loss and pili torti

Blainville ears   asymmetry in size or shape of the auricles

bleb   blister

blending, auditory   perceptual process by which phonemes of a word are combined into the whole word

block   1. arrest in the passage of a nervous impulse; 2. a plug

block, oto   a small piece of plastic foam or other material that is inserted in the external auditory meatus before an earmold impression is made to prevent impression material from reaching the tympanic membrane

blooming artifact   inaccurate frequency response observed in an output-AGC hearing aid when tonal rather than broad-band signals are used; results from failure of tonal stimuli to activate frequency-dependent compression

blue eardrum   bluish appearance of the tympanic membrane due to a variant of otitis media with effusion, idiopathic hemotympanum, in which the fluid is bluish in color caused by bleeding of granulomas

BMC   bleomycin, methotrexate, cisplatin; potentially ototoxic chemotherapy regimen used in the treatment of head and neck cancer

BMLD   binaural masking level difference; measure of binaural release from masking in which binaural thresholds are determined in noise for tones that are in phase and 180° out of phase

BMT   bilateral myringotomy tube

BOA   behavioral observation audiometry; pediatric assessment of hearing by observation of a child's unconditioned responses to sounds

board-certified in hearing instrument sciences   BC-HIS; credential awarded to qualifying hearing instrument specialists by the National Board for Certification in Hearing Instrument Sciences

body baffle effect   change in the response of a hearing aid when worn on the body; the body produces acoustic changes in a sound field that impact the frequency response of the hearing aid, especially a body-worn device

body hearing aid   body-worn hearing aid

body-worn hearing aid   hearing aid with its components encased in a small box worn on the chest with a cord connected to a receiver worn on the ear, for use in cases of severe and profound hearing loss

BOE   bilateral otitis externa

boilermaker's ear   early term for noise-induced hearing loss, after workers who were exposed to excessive noise levels for many years making or repairing boilers

BOM   bilateral otitis media

BOMA   bilateral otitis media, acute

BOMP   bleomycin, vincristine, mitomycin, platinol (cisplatin); potentially ototoxic chemotherapy regimen used in the treatment of cervical cancer

bone-air gap   difference in dB between bone-conducted and air-conducted hearing thresholds for a given frequency in the same ear, used to describe the condition in which bone conduction is paradoxically poorer than air conduction

bone-anchored hearing aid   surgically implanted bone-conduction receiver that interfaces with an external amplifier, designed to provide amplification for those with intractable middle ear disorder

bone conduction   transmission of sound to the cochlea by vibration of the skull

bone conduction, absolute   early term used to describe bone-conduction thresholds established with the ears occluded; COM: relative bone conduction

bone conduction, compressional   distortional bone conduction

bone conduction, distortional   component of bone conducted hearing created by alternating compressions and expansions of the bony labyrinth, resulting in fluid displacement in the membranous labyrinth

bone conduction, inertial   stimulation of the cochlear labyrinth by the lag of the ossicular chain when the bones of the skull are set into motion by a bone vibrator, resulting in relative movement between the stapes and the oval window, contributing to bone-conducted hearing

bone conduction, osseotympanic   minor contribution to bone-conducted hearing from the cochlear reception of sound energy radiated into the osseous external auditory meatus

bone conduction, relative   early term used to describe bone-conduction thresholds established with the ears unoccluded; COM: absolute bone conduction

bone-conduction hearing aid   hearing aid, used most often in patients with bilateral atresia, in which amplified signal is delivered to a bone vibrator placed on the mastoid, thereby bypassing the middle ear and stimulating the cochlea directly

bone-conduction oscillator   electromechanical vibrator designed to stimulate the cochlea via transmission of vibrations through the bones of the skull

bone-conduction receiver   vibrator or oscillator used to transmit sound through vibration of the bones of the skull

bone-conduction threshold   absolute threshold of hearing sensitivity to pure-tone stimuli delivered via bone-conduction oscillator

bone-conduction vibrator bone-conduction oscillator

bone vibrator bone-conduction oscillator

bonelet an ossicle or small bone

bony atresia congenital absence of the external auditory meatus due to a wall of bone separating the external auditory meatus from the middle ear space; COM: membranous atresia

bony labyrinth cavity in the temporal bone that contains the fluids and membranous labyrinth of the cochlea and vestibular system; SYN: osseous labyrinth

boom microphone microphone that is suspended above a speaker's head

boot, audio device used with a behind-the-ear hearing aid for coupling with direct audio input cord

boot, FM small bootlike device containing an FM receiver that attaches to the bottom of a behind-the-ear hearing aid

border cells cells of the organ of Corti providing support for the inner hair cells

bore, belled enlarged bowl-shaped canal opening of an earmold or custom hearing aid

bore, earmold hole in an earmold through which amplified sound is directed into the ear canal; SYN: sound bore

bore, horn tapered bore in an earmold that is widest in diameter at its medial aspect, designed to enhance high-frequency amplification

bore, reverse horn tapered bore in an earmold that is widest in diameter at its lateral aspect, designed to reduce high-frequency amplification

bore, sound earmold bore

boundary noise limit maximum level of noise allowed at a boundary line, most often pertaining to the interface between industrial and residential areas

BP bipolar

BPPN benign paroxysmal positioning nystagmus; sudden, transient burst of nystagmus during the Dix-Hallpike maneuver, which disappears within 10 seconds once the head position is achieved

BPPV benign paroxysmal positional vertigo; a recurrent, acute form of vertigo occurring in clusters in response to positional changes

BRA brainstem response audiometry

bradyacusia dullness of hearing

brain mapping electrophysiologic technique designed to measure distribution of electrical activity across the scalp, in which voltages from ongoing EEG or AEPs are measured at multiple electrodes and represented as different colors in a map of the brain's activity

brainstem portion of the brain between the spinal cord and cerebrum, including the diencephalon, midbrain, pons, and medulla oblongata

brainstem auditory evoked potentials BAEP; SEE: auditory brainstem response

brainstem auditory evoked response BAER; SEE: auditory brainstem response

brainstem evoked response audiometry BERA, BSERA; brainstem response audiometry

brainstem evoked response BSER; SEE: auditory brainstem response

brainstem response audiometry BRA; auditory brainstem response measure used to predict hearing sensitivity and to assess the integrity of Cranial Nerve VIII and auditory brainstem structures

branchial pertaining to gills, particularly the embryonic gill arches

branchial arch embryonic gill-like structure from which the outer and middle ear structures develop

branchio-oto-renal syndrome autosomal dominant disorder consisting of branchial clefts, fistulas, and cysts, renal malformation, and conductive, sensorineural, or mixed hearing loss

bridge original term for an immittance meter, when the instrumentation was based on a bridge circuit

brief-tone audiometry BTA; test developed to identify cochlear site of lesion, in which thresholds are obtained for 100-msec tone bursts and 10-msec tone bursts; normal threshold reduction is 10 dB for a tenfold decrease in duration

broad-band noise BBN; sound with a wide bandwidth, containing a continuous spectrum of frequencies, with equal energy per cycle throughout the band

Broca's area motor speech area of the brain, located in the inferior convolution of the frontal lobe

Brodmann's area 41 transverse temporal gyrus of the cerebral cortex, associated with auditory perception

Bruhn method early analytic speechreading method based upon careful observation of the movements of the lips from one sound position to another

bruit an auscultatory sound, as of blood moving in an ear

BSAER brainstem auditory evoked response

BSER brainstem evoked response

BSERA brainstem evoked response audiometry

BSOM bilateral serous otitis media

BTA brief-tone audiometry; test developed to identify cochlear site of lesion, in which thresholds are obtained for 100-msec tone bursts and 10-msec tone bursts; normal threshold reduction is 10 dB for a tenfold decrease in duration

BTE behind-the-ear hearing aid; a hearing aid that fits over the ear and is coupled to the ear canal via an earmold; SYN: postauricular hearing aid

bullae blisters

bullous myringitis acute painful viral inflammation of the tympanic membrane accompanied by bullae formation between layers of the tympanic membrane, commonly occurring in association with influenza

bumetanide potentially ototoxic diuretic used in the treatment of edema associated with cardiac, liver, and renal disease

bundle of Rasmussen group of efferent nerve fibers, of the medial olivocochlear bundle, coursing from the periolivary nuclei near the medial superior olive across the brainstem to the outer hair cells of the contralateral cochlea; SYN: crossed olivocochlear bundle

bursa a sac filled with fluid

BW bilateral weakness; hypoactivity of vestibular system to caloric stimulation in both ears, consistent with bilateral peripheral vestibular disorder

C

C compliance; measure of the ease of energy transfer through the outer and middle ear; reciprocal of stiffness

C tracing continuous tracing; graph that results from threshold tracking in Békésy audiometry to a continuous pure tone at a fixed or swept frequency; ANT: interrupted tracing

C-weighted scale sound level meter filtering network designed to provide a uniform frequency response over the frequency range from 20 Hz to 10,000 Hz

C8 Cranial Nerve VIII

CA 1. chronological age; 2. compressed analog

CA processing compressed analog processing; cochlear implant processing strategy in which speech signals are divided into frequency bands and delivered to corresponding implant electrodes

Ca++ chemical symbol for calcium

CAD central auditory disorder; functional disorder resulting from diseases of or trauma to the central auditory nervous system

Cagot ear an auricle having no lobulus; SYN: Aztec ear

cal tone calibration tone

calcium Ca++; chemical found in high concentration in perilymph

calibrate 1. to adjust the output of an instrument to a known standard; 2. in audiometry, to adjust the intensity levels of an audiometer to correspond with ANSI standard levels for audiometric zero

calibration the act of calibrating the output of an instrument, such as an audiometer

calibration, biologic the determination of audiometric zero for a particular signal based on average thresholds from a sample of normal-hearing subjects

calibration tone cal-tone; a 1000-Hz tone preceding recorded speech materials that is used to adjust an audiometer's VU meter to insure identical output calibration of speech signals from one test session to the next

California Consonant Test CCT; adult speech audiometric test of monosyllabic word recognition that is particularly useful in assessing the influence of high-frequency hearing loss on speech recognition

caloric pertaining to heat

caloric inversion condition in which nystagmus beats in a direction opposite of that expected following caloric stimulation, consistent with brainstem disorder

caloric irrigation introduction of warm and cool water into the ear canal for caloric testing of vestibular function

caloric irrigation, closed-loop method of warm or cool stimulation of the vestibular system in which water is delivered into a balloonlike catheter in the ear canal

caloric irrigation, open-loop method of warm or cool stimulation of the vestibular system in which water is delivered directly into the ear canal

caloric nystagmus characteristic nystagmus eye movement pattern induced by vestibular labyrinthine stimulation with warm or cold water in the external auditory meatus

caloric reversal, premature caloric nystagmus that reverses its direction prior to 140 seconds following onset of irrigation, consistent with central vestibular pathology; SYN: secondary phase nystagmus

caloric stimulation introduction of warm or cool water or air into the external auditory meatus to stimulate the vestibular system

caloric stimulation, bithermal assessment of vestibular function by irrigation of the external auditory meatus with warm and cool water or air

caloric stimulation, monothermal assessment of vestibular function by irrigation of the external auditory meatus with warm, cool, or ice water only

caloric test irrigation of the external auditory meatus with warm and cool water to stimulate the vestibular labyrinth, resulting in nystagmus as an indicator of vestibular function

caloric test, Barany caloric test

caloric test, Kobrak minimal early test of vestibular function in which the external auditory meatus was irrigated with cool water or ice water injected with a syringe and nystagmus was observed using Frenzel glasses

caloric test position CTP; conventional head position for caloric testing in which the patient lies in a supine position with the head angled at 30°

canal passage or duct in the body

canal earmold type of earmold that uses only the canal portion of the ear impression with the helix and concha areas removed

canal hearing aid hearing aid that fits mostly in the external auditory meatus with a small portion extending into the concha; SYN: ITC hearing aid; in-the-canal hearing aid

canal-lock earmold canal earmold with a fingerlike projection along the bottom of the concha to retain the earmold in place

canal mold colloquial term for canal earmold

canales semicirculares ossei bony superior, posterior, and lateral semicircular canals

canalicular pertaining to a canaliculus

canaliculi perforantes system of small channels in the tympanic shelf of the osseous spiral lamina connecting the scala tympani with the fluid spaces surrounding cochlear nerve dendrites and the organ of Corti

canaliculus a small canal or channel

canaliculus cochleae minute canal in the temporal bone that contains the endolymphatic duct

canaliculus mastoideus canal that travels through the mastoid process containing the auricular branch of the vagus nerve

canaliculus tympanicus minute canal that passes through the temporal bone to the floor of the tympanic cavity containing the tympanic branch of the glossopharyngeal nerve

canalis a canal or channel

canalis spiralis cochleae cochlear canal; bony labyrinth of the cochlea

canalis spiralis modioli spiral canal of the modiolus in which the spiral ganglia of the cochlear nerve are located

cancellation in acoustics, the reduction of a sound-wave amplitude to zero, resulting from two tones of identical frequency and amplitude occurring 180 degrees out of phase

CANS central auditory nervous system; portion from Cranial Nerve VIII to the auditory cortex that involves hearing, including the cochlear nucleus, superior olivary complex, lateral lemniscus, inferior colliculus, medial geniculate, and auditory cortex

CAOHC Council for Accreditation in Occupational Hearing Conservation; multidisciplinary coordinating body involved in the training and certification of occupational hearing conservationists

CAP 1. central auditory processing; 2. compound action potential

CAP cyclophosphamide, adriamycin, platinol (cisplatin); potentially ototoxic chemotherapy regimen used in the treatment of various cancers

capacitance quantity of electric charge stored by two conducting surfaces separated by a dielectric

capacitor electric component consisting of two conducting surfaces separated by a dielectric, used to store and control electric charges; SYN: condenser

capacitor microphone microphone in which the variation of capacitance in response to sound level controls the electrical signal, including air-dielectric and electret microphones; SYN: condenser microphone

CAPD central auditory processing disorder; disorder in function of central auditory structures, characterized by impaired ability of the central auditory nervous system to manipulate and use acoustic signals

capitation managed care reimbursement system wherein the provider receives a fixed payment per member per month for carrying out specified services

capitulum protrusion on the head of a bone

capitulum malleus head of the malleus

capitulum stapes head of the stapes

CAPS communication assessment procedure for seniors; a self-assessment inventory used for evaluating the communication needs of aging patients

capsule, otic osseous portion of the cochlea containing the membranous labyrinth

captioning, closed CC; printed text of the dialogue or narrative on television or video that is available only with an adapter or special circuitry

captioning, open printed text of the dialogue or narrative on television or video that is available without the use of an adapter or special circuitry

captioning, real-time computerized captioning of a person's speech with little or no time delay

carbon hearing aid obsolete hearing aid that used a carbon microphone

carbon microphone obsolete microphone that used carbon granules to convert sound pressure into electrical energy

carboplatin often ototoxic drug used as chemotherapy treatment for cancer

carcinoma any of various types of cancerous tumors derived from epithelial tissue

carcinoma, basal-cell slow-growing malignant skin cancer, which can occur on the pinna and external auditory meatus as a flat, painless, slightly raised lesion followed by the development of a penetrating bleeding ulcer

carcinoma, epidermoid cancerous neoplasms of the auricle, external auditory canal, middle ear, and/or mastoid

carcinoma, squamous cell most common malignant tumor of the auricle, characterized by a progression of skin thickening with scaling, painless out-growth, and formation of an ulcer with a raised edge

cardiac evoked response audiometry CERA; electrophysiologic technique for predicting hearing sensitivity by measuring changes in heart rate in response to auditory stimulation

cardioid response heart-shaped pattern of response of a directional microphone

cardiotachometry measure of changes in heart rate

Carhart procedure early hearing aid selection procedure, involving the comparison of aided word-recognition ability with various amplification configurations, in an effort to determine differences in aided performance

Carhart's notch pattern of bone-conduction audiometric thresholds associated with otosclerosis, characterized by reduced bone-conduction sensitivity predominantly at 2000 Hz

caroticotympanic arteries two separate branches arising from the internal carotid artery that connect with branches of the tympanic and tubal arteries to supply blood to the anterior portion of the middle ear

carotid wall anterior surface of the tympanic cavity, containing the opening through which the chorda tympani exits the middle ear

Carpenter syndrome autosomal recessive craniosynostosis disorder, which may include low-set ears, preauricular pits, and associated conductive hearing loss

carrier phrase in speech audiometry, phrase preceding the target syllable, word, or sentence to prepare the patient for the test signal

cartilage connective tissue characterized by firm consistency and absence of blood vessels

cartilago auriculae auricular cartilage

case history patient report regarding relevant communication and medical background

CAT scan computerized axial tomography (scan); sectional radiographs of specified areas of the brain presented as a computer-generated image representing a synthesis of x-rays obtained from different directions on a given plane

catarrh inflammation of a mucous membrane

catarrhal deafness conductive hearing loss resulting from catarrh of the nasopharynx with congestion of the eustachian tube

catarrhal otitis media middle ear inflammation resulting from catarrh of the nasopharynx with congestion of the eustachian tube

cathode 1. negative electrode in an electrolytic cell; 2. positive terminal in a battery; COM: anode

caudal anatomical direction, referring to structures that are located away from the head or, more accurately, toward the tail; ANT: rostral

caudate nucleus elongated, arched mass of gray matter that is part of the basal ganglia or inner portion of the cerebrum

cauliflower ear thickening and malformation of the auricle following repeated trauma, commonly related to injury caused by the sport of wrestling

cavernous hemangioma benign tumor consisting of newly formed blood vessels that may involve the external auditory canal, tympanic membrane, and middle ear, with associated hearing loss and pulsatile tinnitus

cavity a hollow or space within or between structures

cavum inferior aspect of the concha bowl

CBM cisplatin, bleomycin, mitomycin; potentially ototoxic chemotherapy regimen used in the treatment of head and neck cancer

cc cubic centimeter; measure of volume; 1 cc equals 1 ml

CC closed captioning; printed text of the dialogue or narrative on television or video that is available only with an adapter or special circuitry

CCC-A Certificate of Clinical Competence in Audiology; certification awarded by the American Speech-Language-Hearing Association to individuals who have met the academic and clinical requirements necessary to become audiologists

CCM contralateral competing message; in speech audiometry, noise or other competing signal that is delivered to the ear opposite the ear receiving the target signal; ANT: ICM or ipsilateral competing message

CCS Crippled Children's Services; state-funded organization that provides financial assistance for healthcare and other services to children with disabilities

CCT California Consonant Test; adult speech audiometric test of monosyllabic word recognition that is particularly useful in assessing the influence of high-frequency hearing loss on speech recognition

CD communication disorder; impairment in communication ability, resulting from speech, language, and/or hearing disorders

CDP computerized dynamic posturography; quantitative assessment of integrated function of the balance system for postural stability during quiet and perturbed stance, using a computer-based moving platform and motion transducers

CEC Council on Exceptional Children

ceiling effect in data analysis, reduction of information that results when maximum performance obscures differences in ability among those scoring at the highest, or ceiling, level

cell mass of protoplasm, enclosed in a membrane and containing a nucleus, that is the active basis of all living organisms

cells of Henson supporting cells in the organ of Corti, adjacent to the outer side of the Deiter cells

cellulitis inflammatory lesion of the pinna, characterized by redness, warmth to touch, tenderness, and tenseness on palpation

center frequency frequency at the center of a bandwidth

center of gravity COG; point in a body around which weight is evenly balanced

central associated with the central nervous system

central auditory disorder CAD; functional disorder resulting from diseases of or trauma to the central auditory nervous system

central auditory nervous system CANS; portion from Cranial Nerve VIII to the auditory cortex that involves hearing, including the cochlear nucleus, superior olivary complex, lateral lemniscus, inferior colliculus, medial geniculate, and auditory cortex

central auditory nuclei central nervous system nuclei that receive primary afferent auditory input; include the cochlear nucleus, superior olivary complex, lateral lemniscus, inferior colliculus, and medial geniculate body

central auditory processing CAP; function of the central auditory nervous system, including sound localization, lateralization, binaural processes, speech perception, etc.

central auditory processing disorder CAPD; disorder in function of central auditory structures, characterized by impaired ability of the central auditory nervous system to manipulate and use acoustic signals, including difficulty understanding speech in noise and localizing sounds

central deafness central auditory disorder related to bilateral brainstem or temporal lobe lesions, often characterized by difficulty in recognizing auditory signals or understanding speech despite normal or near-normal cochlear function; SYN: cortical deafness

Central Institute for the Deaf CID; residential school for the deaf in St. Louis, founded in 1914

central masking elevation in hearing sensitivity of the test ear, on the order of 5 dB, as a result of introducing masking noise in the non-test ear, presumably due to the influence of masking noise on central auditory function

central nervous system CNS; that portion of the nervous system to which sensory impulses and from which motor impulses are transmitted, including the cortex, brainstem, and spinal cord

central nucleus central core of the inferior colliculus

centrifugal denoting motion away from a center or axis of rotation

centripetal denoting motion toward a center or axis of rotation

cephalad anatomical direction, referring to structures that are located toward the head; ANT: caudal; SYN: cranial, rostral

cephalic pertaining to the head

CERA 1. cardiac evoked response audiometry; 2. cortical evoked response audiometry

ceramic microphone type of piezoelectric microphone in which electric current is generated by applied mechanical stress

cerebellar pertaining to the cerebellum

cerebellopontine angle CPA; anatomical angle formed by the proximity of the cerebellum and the pons from which Cranial Nerve VIII exits into the brainstem

cerebellopontine angle tumor CPA tumor; most often a cochleovestibular Schwannoma located or growing outside the internal auditory canal at the juncture of the cerebellum and pons

cerebellum large posterior brain structure behind the pons and medulla, consisting of two hemispheres united by a median portion (the vermis), serving to coordinate motor function and maintain equilibrium

cerebral pertaining to the cerebrum

cerebral cortex outer layer of the cerebrum

cerebral dominance functional prominence of one hemisphere of the brain over the other

cerebral palsy motor-control disorder caused by damage to the motor cortex of the brain

cerebral vascular accident cerebrovascular accident

cerebrospinal fluid CSF; clear liquid filling the ventricles and the subarachnoid space surrounding the brain and spinal cord that supports and cushions the central nervous system against trauma and may serve to remove waste products of neuronal metabolism

cerebrovascular accident CVA; interruption of blood supply to the brain due to aneurysm, embolism, or clot, resulting in sudden loss of function related to the affected portion of the brain; COL: stroke

cerebrum cerebral cortex and basal ganglia

Certificate of Clinical Competence in Audiology CCC-A; certification awarded by the American Speech-Language-Hearing Association to individuals who have met the academic and clinical requirements necessary to become audiologists

cerumen waxy secretion of the ceruminous glands in the external auditory meatus; COL: ear wax

cerumen, impacted cerumen that causes blockage of the external auditory meatus

ceruminal pertaining to cerumen

cerum:nectomy extraction of impacted cerumen from the external auditory meatus

ceruminolytic pertaining to substances placed into the external auditory meatus to soften impacted cerumen

ceruminoma benign tumor of ceruminous glands

ceruminosis excessive cerumen in the external auditory meatus

ceruminous characterized by or full of cerumen

ceruminous glands glands in the external auditory meatus that secrete cerumen

cervico-oculo-acoustic syndrome congenital branchial arch syndrome, occurring primarily in females, characterized by fusion of two or more cervical vertebrae; similar to Klippel-Feil syndrome, with retraction of eyeballs, lateral gaze weakness, and hearing loss; SYN: Wildervanck syndrome

CES Competing Environmental Sounds; test of dichotic processing of familiar non-speech sounds

CF characteristic frequency; the frequency to which an auditory neuron is most sensitive

CFA continuous flow adapter; earmold with a constant interior tubing diameter designed to permit high-frequency amplification with a smooth frequency response

CHAMPUS Civilian Health and Medical Programs of the Uniformed Services

channel in a hearing aid, a frequency region that is processed independently of other regions

CHAP cyclophosphamide, hexamethylmelamine, adriamycin, platinol (cisplatin); potentially ototoxic chemotherapy regimen used in the treatment of ovarian cancer

characteristic frequency CF; the frequency to which an auditory nerve fiber is most sensitive

characteristic impedance impedance that occurs naturally based on a system's characteristics

CHARGE association genetic association featuring *c*oloboma, *h*eart disease, *at*resia choanae (nasal cavity), *r*etarded growth and development, *g*enital hypoplasia, and *e*ar anomalies and/or hearing loss that can be conductive, sensorineural, or mixed

chemoreceptor cell or organ that is activated by chemical stimulation, originating the flow of nerve impulses

chemotherapy   treatment of disease with chemical substances or drugs

CHI   closed head injury; brain injury in which the primary cause is blunt trauma, rather than penetrating wound, CVA, neoplasms, etc.

chloral hydrate   hypnotic drug commonly used for sedation of young children during ABR audiometry; typical dosage is 50 mg/kg to 75 mg/kg of body weight

chloropromazine   drug used as a tranquilizer and to enhance the effects of analgesics

chloroquine   synthetic drug with a molecular structure similar to quinine, used chiefly as an antimalarial agent, which may be ototoxic with prolonged treatment

cholesteatoma   tumorlike mass of squamous epithelium and cholesterol in the middle ear that may invade the mastoid and erode the ossicles, usually secondary to chronic otitis media or marginal tympanic membrane perforation

cholesteatosis   condition resulting from lipid metabolism disturbance, characterized by deposits of cholesterol in tissue

cholesterol granuloma   circumscribed mass, formed in reaction to cholesterol deposits occurring in fluid-filled cells that are usually pneumatized, occurring in either the tympanomastoid compartment or the petrous apex, resulting in conductive or retrocochlear disorder

cholinergic   relating to peripheral and central nervous system receptors that involve acetylcholine as their neurotransmitter

chondroblastoma   neoplasm occurring occasionally in the temporal bone, consisting of highly cellular material resembling fetal cartilage

chondrodermatitis nodularis chronica helicis   tender, benign, pea-shaped, nodular lesion on the free edge of the pinna

chondrodysplasia   disorder in the development of early embryonic aggregation of cartilage cells, leading to deformities associated with arrested growth of the long bones; SYN: chondrodystrophy, dyschondroplasia

chondrodystrophia fetalis   autosomal dominant disorder characterized by short stature, short limbs, large head, and middle and inner ear anomalies with associated hearing loss; SYN: achondroplasia

chondrodystrophy   chondrodysplasia

chondrogenesis   formation of cartilage

chondroma   benign cartilaginous tumor

chorda tympani   branch of the facial nerve that passes through the middle ear and conveys taste sensation from the anterior two-thirds of the tongue and carries fibers to the submandibular and sublingual salivary glands

chromosomal   pertaining to chromosomes

chromosome   structure composed of long strands of DNA and protein in the cell nucleus that is the carrier of genes

chromosome 21-trisomy syndrome   congenital genetic abnormality, characterized by mental retardation and characteristic facial features, with high incidence of chronic otitis media and associated conductive, mixed, and sensorineural hearing loss; SYN: Down syndrome

chronic   of long duration

chronic adhesive otitis media   longstanding inflammation of the middle ear caused by prolonged eustachian tube dysfunction resulting in severe retraction of the tympanic membrane and obliteration of the middle ear space

chronic atticoantral suppurative otitis media   persistent purulent inflammation of the attic and mastoid antrum of the middle ear

chronic diffuse external otitis   inflammation of the external auditory meatus, characterized by itching and a persistent or recurring scaling or weeping dermatitis, caused by bacterial infection

chronic interstitial salpingitis   persistent inflammation of the eustachian tube

chronic otitis media   COM; persistent inflammation of the middle ear having a duration of greater than 8 weeks

chronic otitis media with effusion   COME; persistent inflammation of the middle ear, accompanied by fluid in the middle ear space

chronic suppurative otitis media   CSOM; persistent inflammation of the middle ear with infected effusion containing pus

chronic tubotympanic catarrh   persistent inflammation of the mucosal membrane of the eustachian tube and middle ear

chronologic age   CA; age of an individual from date of birth

CIC   1. completely-in-the-canal hearing aid; 2. commissure of the inferior colliculus

CID   Central Institute for the Deaf; residential school for the deaf in St. Louis, founded in 1914

CID Auditory Test W-1   list of 36

spondaic words, developed at the Central Institute for the Deaf, commonly used in the determination of speech-reception threshold

CID Auditory Test W-2   version of the CID Auditory Test W-1 in which the 36 spondees were recorded with 3 dB of attenuation for every three words

CID Auditory Test W-22   word-recognition test developed at CID consisting of four lists of 50 monosyllabic words

cilia   plural of cilium

ciliated   having cilia

ciliotoxic   having a poisonous action on cilia

cilium   motile, threadlike extension of a cell surface, such as the processes of the sensory hair cells in the cochlear and vestibular endorgans

cinchonism   1. poisoning from cinchona bark; 2. in hearing, the temporary hearing loss related to ingestion of quinine, an alkaloid derivative of cinchona

circuit   1. path or line of an electric current; 2. combination of electronic components that carry an electric current

circuit, integrated   IC; electronic circuit with its many interconnected elements formed on a single body of semiconductor material

circuit noise   unwanted signal in the output of a circuit created by the functioning of the circuit

circuitry   the system or components of an electric circuit

circumambient   ambient; surrounding

circumaural   around the ear

circumaural earphones   headphone with cushions that encircle the pinna; COM: insert earphone

circumscribed labyrinthitis   inflammation of the labyrinth restricted to a defined, limited area

CIS processing   continuous interleaved sampling processing; cochlear implant processing strategy designed to deliver nonsimultaneous pulses at a high rate of stimulation to multiple implant electrodes

CISCA   cisplatin, cyclophosphamide, adriamycin; potentially ototoxic chemotherapy regimen used in the treatment of genito-urinary cancer

cisplatin; cis-diamminedichloroplatinum   ototoxic antimitotic and antineoplastic drug often used as part of a chemotherapy regimen for cancer treatment

Class A amplifier   a type of single-ended hearing aid amplifier used in low-power applications that has a constant current drain across input levels; Class A refers to the operational characteristic of the output or power stage of the amplifier

Class B amplifier   a push-pull type of hearing aid amplifier used in high-power applications that draws current in proportion to signal level; Class B refers to the operational characteristic of the output or power stage of the amplifier

Class D amplifier   a pulse-width modulated type of hearing aid amplifier built inside a receiver, the use of which results in reduced battery current, smaller size, and higher saturation levels; Class D refers to operational characteristic of the output or power stage

Claudius cells   cells in the organ of Corti that support the outer hair cells on their lateral side

cleft   fissure or opening

cleft lip   congenital fissure of the upper lip

cleft palate   congenital fissure of the palate

cleft pinna   congenital fissure of the pinna

cleidocranial dysostosis   autosomal dominant disorder of the skeleton due to retarded bone formation, characterized by absence of clavicles and irregular formation of bones, with associated conductive and sensorineural hearing loss

click   rapid-onset, short-duration, broadband sound, produced by delivering an electric pulse to an earphone; used to elicit an auditory brainstem response and transient-evoked otoacoustic emissions

click, compression   condensation click

click, condensation   rapid-onset, short-duration, broad-band sound produced by delivering a positive-polarity electric pulse to an earphone

click, rarefaction   rapid-onset, short-duration, broad-band sound produced by delivering a negative-polarity electric pulse to an earphone

click-evoked otoacoustic emission   transient otoacoustic emission elicited by click stimuli

clicking tinnitus   tinnitus, either subjective or objective, characterized by a clicking sound; present in cases of chronic middle ear disorder. presumably caused by an opening and closing of the eustachian tube; SYN: Leudet tinnitus

clinical pertaining to diagnosis and treatment of a patient on the basis of observation or measurement of symptoms; COM: laboratory

clinical audiometer diagnostic audiometer; wide-range audiometer

clinician healthcare professional engaging in clinical practice

clipping, peak 1. process of limiting maximum output intensity of a hearing aid or amplifier by removing alternating current amplitude peaks at a fixed level; 2. distortion of an acoustic waveform resulting from hearing aid amplifier saturation

clonus abnormal movement marked by rapid contractions and relaxations of a muscle in response to forcible flexion or extension

closed captioning CC; printed text of the dialogue or narrative on television or video that is available only with an adapter or special circuitry

closed head injury CHI; brain injury in which the primary cause is blunt trauma, rather than penetrating wound, CVA, neoplasms, etc.

closed-loop caloric irrigation method of warm or cool stimulation of the vestibular system in which water is delivered into a balloonlike catheter in the ear canal; ANT: open-loop caloric irrigation

closed-set test speech audiometric test with multiple-choice format in which the targeted syllable, word, or sentence is chosen from among a limited set of foils; ANT: open-set test

closure, auditory perceptual process by which partial auditory information is integrated into a whole, so that a word can be recognized when some of its phonemes are missing or not perceived

CM cochlear microphonic; minute alternating-current electrical potential of the hair cells of the cochlea that resembles the input signal

CMB cisplatin, methotrexate, bleomycin; potentially ototoxic chemotherapy regimen used in the treatment of cervical cancer

CMOS complementary metal oxide semiconductor; integrated circuitry used in hearing aid design

CMR common mode rejection; noise-rejection strategy used in electrophysiologic measurement in which noise that is identical (common) at two electrodes is subtracted by a differential amplifier

CMRR common mode rejection ratio; amount of reduction in dB of signals determined to be common at two electrodes

CMV cytomegalovirus; intrauterine-prenatal or postnatal herpetoviral infection, usually transmitted in utero, that can cause central nervous system disorder, including brain damage, hearing loss, vision loss, and seizures

CN 1. cochlear nucleus; 2. cranial nerve

CN-VIII Cranial Nerve VIII

CNAP cochlear nerve action potential; compound action potential recorded from an electrode placed directly on Cranial Nerve VIII

CNC consonant-nucleus-consonant; a word or syllable used in speech-recognition testing, consisting of a vowel or diphthong (nucleus) between two consonants; SYN: CVC

CNE could not evaluate; could not establish

CNR composite noise rating; a scale used to rate and predict the total noise environment in a specified geographic area, such as around an airport, for evaluating compatible land use

CNS central nervous system; that portion of the nervous system to which sensory impulses and from which motor impulses are transmitted, including the cortex, brainstem, and spinal cord

CNT could not test

CNV contingent negative variation; evoked potential, characterized by a low-frequency negative-voltage electrophysiologic response occurring in the 300 msec to 500 msec latency region; associated with anticipation of a stimulus condition

coarticulation the influence that a phoneme has on the phonemes that precede and follow in a word or phrase

COB cisplatin, oncovin, bleomycin; potentially ototoxic chemotherapy regimen used in the treatment of head and neck cancer

COCB crossed olivocochlear bundle; group of efferent nerve fibers of the medial olivocochlear bundle, coursing from the periolivary nuclei near the medial superior olive, across the brainstem, to the outer hair cells of the contralateral cochlea

cochlea auditory portion of the inner ear, consisting of fluid-filled membranous channels within a spiral canal around a central core

cochlear pertaining to the cochlea

cochlear ablation removal of the cochlea in animal research

cochlear aqueduct small channel in the temporal bone near the round window that connects the scala tympani of the cochlea to the subarachnoid space of the cranium, possibly allowing communication of perilymph and cerebrospinal fluid

cochlear artery, common branch of the labyrinthine artery that divides into the main cochlear artery and vestibulocochlear artery

cochlear artery, main branch of the common cochlear artery that supplies the apical three-fourths of the cochlea, including the modiolus

cochlear duct spiral membranous canal that is the cochlear portion of the membranous labyrinth, located between the osseous spiral lamina and external bony wall of the cochlea

cochlear epithelium membranous labyrinth of the cochlea

cochlear fenestra round opening on the medial wall of the middle ear leading into the cochlea and covered by the round window membrane; SYN: round window, cochlear window, fenestra rotunda

cochlear hydrops excessive accumulation of endolymph within the cochlear labyrinth, resulting in fluctuating sensorineural hearing loss, tinnitus, and a sensation of fullness

implant, cochlear device that enables persons with profound hearing loss to perceive sound, consisting of an electrode array surgically implanted in the cochlea, which delivers electrical signals to CN VIII, and an external amplifier, which activates the electrode

cochlear implant mapping representation of the threshold and suprathreshold parameters for each electrode or electrode combination in an individual cochlear implant user's speech-coding program

cochlear Ménière's disease atypical form of Ménière's disease in which only the characteristic auditory symptoms are present without vertiginous episodes; SYN: cochlear hydrops

cochlear microphonic CM; minute alternating-current electrical potential of the hair cells of the cochlea that resembles the input signal

cochlear nerve auditory branch of Cranial Nerve VIII, arising from the spiral ganglion of the cochlea and terminating in the cochlear nuclei of the brainstem

cochlear nerve action potential CNAP; compound action potential recorded from an electrode placed directly on Cranial Nerve VIII

cochlear neuritis inflammation of the auditory portion of Cranial Nerve VIII, often of a viral nature, resulting in acute retrocochlear disorder; SYN: acoustic neuritis

cochlear nucleus CN; cluster of cell bodies of second-order neurons on the lateral edge of the hindbrain in the central auditory nervous system at which fibers from Cranial Nerve VIII have an obligatory synapse

cochlear nucleus, anterior ventral AVCN; portion of the cochlear nucleus that receives primary afferent projections from Cranial Nerve VIII and sends second-order fibers via the ventral acoustic stria to the superior olivary complex

cochlear nucleus, dorsal DCN; dorsal portion of the cochlear nucleus that receives nerve fibers from the posterior branch of Cranial Nerve VIII after it bifurcates

cochlear nucleus, posterior ventral PVCN; portion of the cochlear nucleus that receives nerve fibers from the posterior branch of Cranial Nerve VIII and sends fibers, via the intermediate acoustic stria, to the periolivary nuclei and contralateral nuclei of the lateral lemniscus

cochlear otosclerosis disease process involving new formation of spongy bone near the oval window resulting in sensorineural or mixed hearing loss

cochlear partition scala media or cochlear duct, when it is represented schematically as a partition between the scala vestibuli and scala tympani

cochlear ramus branch of the vestibulocochlear artery that supplies the basal one-fourth of the cochlea and adjacent modiolus

cochlear recess round-window recess

cochlear reflex acoustic reflex

cochlear reserve ability of the inner ear to function; functionality of the cochlea at suprathreshold levels

cochlear window round opening on the medial wall of the middle ear leading into the cochlea and covered by the round window membrane; SYN: round window, cochlear fenestra, fenestra rotunda

cochleo-orbicular reflex auropalpebral reflex

cochleogram audiogram derived from electrophysiologic prediction of hearing sensitivity based on detection thresholds of cochlear microphonic responses to signals presented across a frequency range

cochleopalpebral reflex CPR; eyeblink or twitch at the canthus caused by a sudden loud sound; SYN: auropalpebral reflex

cochleosaccular aplasia congenital malformation of the membranous portion of the cochlea and saccule, including atrophy of the striae vascularis and abnormalities of the tectorial membrane

cochleosaccular degeneration, infantile idiopathic or viral selective degeneration of the cochlea and saccule with preservation of the utricle and cristae, occurring in infancy and resulting in unilateral or bilateral profound sensorineural hearing loss

cochleosacculotomy surgical procedure used to fistulize the membranous labyrinth by introducing a needle through the stapes footplate in an effort to puncture the dilated saccule in Ménière's disease; SYN: sacculotomy

cochleostapedial reflex acoustic reflex

cochleotoxic having a poisonous action on the hair cells of the organ of Corti; COM: ototoxic, vestibulotoxic

cochleotoxicity the property of being cochleotoxic; COM: ototoxicity, vestibulotoxicity

cochleovestibular pertaining to the cochlea and vestibule of the ear

cochleovestibular Schwannoma benign encapsulated neoplasm composed of Schwann cells arising from the intracranial segment of Cranial Nerve VIII, commonly the vestibular portion; SYN: acoustic neuroma; acoustic neurilemoma; Schwannoma

Cockayne syndrome rare autosomal recessive disorder characterized by delayed-onset dwarfism, mental and motor retardation, and retinal atrophy, with progressive sensorineural hearing loss

COG center of gravity; point in a body around which weight is evenly balanced

Cogan syndrome any autoimmune disorder characterized by nonsyphilitic interstitial keratitis, associated with Ménière-like symptoms

cognition the processes involved in knowing, including perceiving, recognizing, conceiving, judging, sensing, and reasoning

cognitive pertaining to cognition

cogwheeling abnormal presence of saccades during smooth pursuit in which the eyes cannot keep up with the oscillating target

coherence 1. the extent to which two conditions are connected or similar; 2. in hearing aid analysis, the extent to which the output of a circuit resembles the input; 3. in evoked potentials, the extent to which successive averages are similar

cold-opposite warm-same COWS; mnemonic term that describes the direction of nystagmus beating in response to caloric stimulation; stimulation of an ear with cold water results in nystagmus that beats in the direction of the opposite ear

cold-running speech connected or continuous discourse

collagen main protein of connective tissue, cartilage, and bone, the age-related loss of which can reduce auricular cartilage strength and result in collapsed ear canals

collapsed canal condition in which the cartilaginous portion of the external auditory meatus narrows, usually in response to pressure from a circumaural earphone against the pinna, resulting in apparent high-frequency conductive hearing loss

colliculus 1. small elevation; 2. midbrain nuclei of the visual (superior) and auditory (inferior) central nervous systems

colliculus, inferior IC; central auditory nucleus of the midbrain; its central nucleus receives ascending input from the cochlear nucleus and superior olivary complex, and its pericentral nucleus receives descending input from the cortex

coloboma lobuli congenital fissure of the earlobe

color hearing unusual subjective perception of color in response to certain sounds

columella small column of bone in the middle ear of birds that is equivalent to the ossicular chain in humans

COM chronic otitis media; persistent inflammation of the middle ear having a duration of greater than 8 weeks

coma state of profound unconsciousness from which one cannot be aroused

coma score, Glasgow GCS; method for grading depth of coma and severity of brain injury, based on eye opening, verbal response, and motor response

comatose in a coma

combination tone harmonic perceived when two pure tones are presented simultaneously

COME chronic otitis media with effusion; persistent inflammation of the middle ear, accompanied by fluid in the middle ear space

comfort level comfortable loudness level

comfortable loudness, range of difference, in decibels, between threshold of audibility and loudness discomfort level for a specified acoustic signal

comfortable loudness, upper limits of ULCL; measure of loudness comfort level describing the highest intensity level at which the loudness of sound remains comfortable

comfortable loudness level intensity level of a signal that is perceived as comfortably loud

commissure bundle of nerve fibers joining together one side of the brain to the other, as in commissure of the inferior colliculus

commissure of Probst bundle of nerve fibers passing from the dorsal nucleus of the lateral lemniscus on one side of the brain to that on the other side of the brain

commissure of the inferior colliculus bundle of nerve fibers passing from the dorsomedial portion of the inferior colliculus on one side of the brain to that on the other side of the brain

common cochlear artery branch of the labyrinthine artery that divides into the main cochlear artery and vestibulocochlear artery

common crus portion of the semicircular canal where the superior and posterior canals meet

common electrode in electrophysiologic measurement, the electrode that attaches the patient to ground; SYN: ground electrode

common mode rejection CMR; noise-rejection strategy used in electrophysiologic measurement in which noise that is identical (common) at two electrodes is subtracted by a differential amplifier

common mode rejection ratio CMRR; amount of reduction in dB of signals determined to be common at two electrodes

common modiolar vein vessel providing venous drainage of the cochlea

common phrases test a sentence-comprehension task for children in which short sentences are presented in three test modes: visual only, auditory only, and combined

communication the act of exchanging information by speech, sign language, writing, etc.

communication, manual method of communicating that involves the use of fingerspelling, gestures, and sign language

communication, oral-aural method of communicating that involves hearing, speaking, and speechreading

communication, total habilitative approach used in individuals with severe and profound hearing impairment consisting of the integration of oral/aural and manual communication strategies

communication assessment procedure for seniors CAPS; a self-assessment inventory used for evaluating the communication needs of aging patients

communication disorder CD; impairment in communication ability, resulting from speech, language, and/or hearing disorders

communication profile for the hearing impaired CPHI; self-assessment questionnaire designed to quantify a patient's perception of the communication disorder and acceptance of the hearing loss

communication sciences study of human communication and its disorders

communicologist speech-language pathologist: archaic

communicology communication sciences

community noise environmental noise, such as aircraft and traffic noise, that affects residents of a community

comodulation masking paradigm to measure release from masking by comparing perception of a stimulus in modulated noise to that in unmodulated noise

comparative hearing aid evaluation hearing aid selection procedure in which aided speech-recognition ability is assessed with various amplification configurations or types in an effort to determine differences in aided performance

compensation adjustment of behavior or nervous system function in response to change or to a disordered condition

compensation, motoric compensatory movement of the muscles in response to changes in gravitational pull

Competing Environmental Sounds test CES; test of dichotic processing of familiar nonspeech sounds

competing message speech signal that is used in speech audiometry as competition to the target signal

competing message, contralateral CCM; in speech audiometry, noise or other competing signal that is delivered to the ear opposite the ear receiving the target signal

competing message, ipsilateral ICM; in speech audiometry, noise or other competing signal that is delivered to the same ear as the target signal

Competing Sentence Test (CST) CST; test of dichotic processing of simple sentences

complete recruitment condition in which the loudness of a tone in an ear with hearing loss is equal to the loudness of a tone of the same intensity in an ear with normal hearing at high intensity levels; COM: partial recruitment, decruitment

completely-in-the-canal hearing aid CIC hearing aid; small amplification device, extending from 1 mm to 2 mm inside the meatal opening to near the tympanic membrane, which allows greater gain with less power due to the proximity of the receiver to the membrane

complex tone sound containing more than one frequency component

complex wave waveform of a complex tone

compliance C; measure of the ease of energy transfer through the outer and middle ear; reciprocal of stiffness

compliance, static static acoustic immittance

composite noise rating CNR; a scale used to rate and predict the total noise environment in a specified geographic area, such as around an airport, for evaluating compatible land use

compound action potential CAP; 1. synchronous change in electrical potential of nerve or muscle tissue; 2. in auditory evoked potential measures, whole-nerve potential of Cranial Nerve VIII, the main component of ECochG and Wave I of the ABR

comprehension, auditory understanding of spoken language

compressed analog processing CA processing; cochlear implant processing strategy in which speech signals are divided into frequency bands and delivered to corresponding implant electrodes

compressed speech speech that is accelerated, without alteration of the frequency characteristics, by removing segments and compressing the remaining segments; SYN: time-compressed speech

compression 1. in acoustics, portion of the sound-wave cycle in which particles of the transmission medium are compacted; ANT: expansion; 2. in hearing aid circuitry, nonlinear amplifier gain used either to limit maximum output (compression limiting) or to match amplifier gain to an individual's loudness growth (dynamic-range compression)

compression, adaptive hearing aid circuit technique that incorporates output-limiting compression with automatically variable release time; SYN: variable compression

compression, curvilinear hearing aid compression in which the compression ratio increases as input level increases, providing dynamic-range compression for low-level and mid-level inputs and compression limiting for high-level input

compression, dual-time-constant output-limiting technique in some hearing aids in which the release time of a compression circuit varies as a function of the duration of the input signal

compression, dynamic-range hearing aid compression algorithm with a low threshold of activation, designed to package signals between a listener's thresholds of sensitivity and discomfort level in a manner that matches loudness growth

compression, frequency-dependent hearing aid compression whose activation threshold varies by frequency

compression, frequency-independent hearing aid compression whose activation threshold is the same at all frequencies

compression, full-dynamic-range wide-dynamic-range compression

compression, high-level compression-limiting process of a hearing aid, characterized by a high threshold, high ratio, and long release time

compression, input process in which a hearing aid compresses a signal before it reaches the volume control, resulting in a constant dynamic range with a change in maximum output as gain is increased or decreased by the volume control

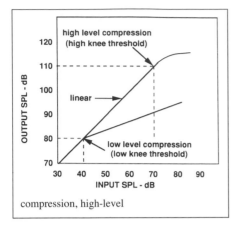

compression, high-level

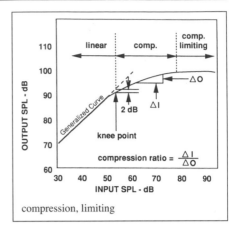

compression, limiting

compression, limiting method of limiting maximum output of a hearing aid with compression circuitry

compression, linear in hearing aids, amplifier gain that is linear at input levels that exceed the compression kneepoint

compression, low-level hearing aid compression circuitry that is activated in response to low-intensity input, such as wide-dynamic-range compression

compression, multichannel process in which a hearing aid separates the input signal into two or more frequency bands, each having independently controlled compression circuitry

compression, output process in which a hearing aid compresses a signal after the volume control, resulting in an expanded dynamic range for low gain settings and a lower kneepoint for high gain settings

compression, syllabic hearing aid compression algorithm that incorporates a low threshold of activation, short attack and release times, and a low compression ratio, resulting in a reduction of the dynamic range of the input

compression, two-channel process in which a hearing aid separates the input signal into two frequency bands, each having independently controlled compression circuitry

compression, wide-dynamic-range hearing aid compression that is activated throughout most of the dynamic range, typically resulting in greatest gain for soft sounds and least gain for loud sounds

compression amplification hearing aid

with compression limiting and/or wide-dynamic-range-compression circuitry

compression click condensation click

compression limiting limiting of maximum output in a hearing aid by use of compression circuitry

compression range the decibel range of sound input in which hearing aid compression is activated

compression ratio the decibel ratio of acoustic input to amplifier output in a hearing aid; e.g., a hearing aid with a compression ratio of 2:1 will increase output by 1 dB for every 2 dB increase in input

compression threshold the minimum input decibel level at which compression circuitry is activated in a hearing aid

compressional bone conduction component of bone-conducted hearing created by alternating compressions and expansions of the bony labyrinth, resulting in fluid displacement in the membranous labyrinth; SYN: distortional bone conduction

computed tomography CT; computerized axial tomography

computer averaging signal averaging with a computer; used in evoked potential measures

computerized audiometry automated audiometry controlled by a computer program

computerized axial tomography CAT; sectional radiographs of specified areas of the brain presented as a computer-generated image representing a synthesis of x-rays obtained from different directions on a given plane

computerized dynamic posturography CDP; quantitative assessment of integrated function of the balance system for postural stability during quiet and perturbed stance, using a computer-based moving platform and motion transducers

concha shell or bowl-like depression of the auricle, lying just above the lobule, that forms the mouth of or funnel to the external auditory meatus

concha bowl concha

concha rim portion of an earmold that fits inside the rim of the concha bowl

concurrent equalization in probe-microphone measurements, equalization performed concurrently with the measurement

concurrent validity extent to which test results agree with a specified criterion

condensation in the propagation of sound waves, the time during which the density of air molecules is increased above its static value; ANT: rarefaction

condensation click rapid-onset, short-duration, broad-band sound produced by delivering a positive-polarity electric pulse to an earphone; ANT: rarefaction click

condenser electric component consisting of two conducting surfaces separated by a dielectric, used to store and control electrical charges; SYN: capacitor

condenser microphone microphone in which the variation of capacitance in response to sound level controls the electrical signal; includes air-dielectric and electret microphones; SYN: electrostatic microphone, capacitor microphone

conditioned orientation reflex audiometry COR audiometry; behavioral audiometry, designed to assess hearing sensitivity in a young child, in which an orienting head-turn response to a sound source is conditioned by visual reinforcement

conditioned response behavior that is elicited or modified by conditioning

conditioned stimulus cue or stimulus that by conditioning becomes capable of eliciting a response

conditioning process of establishing new behaviors or changing existing behaviors in response to environmental influences

conductance G; ease of energy flow associated with resistance; reciprocal of resistance

conduction 1. transmission of energy through a medium; 2. the transmission of sound pressure waves from the ear canal to the cochlea via the middle ear mechanism

conductive pertaining to conduction

conductive hearing loss reduction in hearing sensitivity, despite normal cochlear function, due to impaired sound transmission through the external auditory meatus, tympanic membrane, and ossicular chain

conductivity capacity for conduction

cone of light bright triangular reflection on the surface of the tympanic membrane of the illumination used during otoscopic examination

configuration, audiometric shape of the audiogram, e.g., flat, rising, steeply sloping

congenital present at birth

congenital atresia absence or pathologic closure at birth of a normal anatomical opening, such as the external auditory meatus

congenital hearing loss reduced hearing sensitivity existing at or dating from birth, resulting from pre- or perinatal pathologic conditions

congenital rubella teratogenic disorder caused by maternal rubella, characterized by cataract or glaucoma, cardiovascular defects, mental retardation, psychomotor retardation, and severe to profound sensorineural hearing loss

conjugate eye movement paired movement of eyes in the same direction

connected discourse running or continuous speech, as in a talker reading a story, used in speech audiometry primarily as background competition; SYN: continuous discourse

consanguineous related by blood

consanguinity blood relationship; common ancestry

conscious sedation sedated state wherein the patient retains protective reflexes and breathes independently, commonly attained with chloral hydrate

consensual referring to a reflex or involuntary response to a stimulus

conservation protection from being damaged or depleted

conservation, hearing prevention or reduction of hearing impairment through a program of identification of risk, monitoring of hearing, protection from hazardous noise, and education

conservation, speech treatment designed to maintain speech-production ability following acquired hearing loss

consonant-nucleus-consonant CNC; a word or syllable used in speech-recognition testing, consisting of a vowel or diphthong (nucleus) between two consonants; SYN consonant-vowel-consonant

consonant-vowel CV; syllable used in speech audiometric measures that consists of a consonant followed by a vowel

consonant-vowel ratio relationship between the intensity of a consonant and its neighboring vowel

consonant-vowel-consonant CVC; a word or syllable used in speech-recognition testing, consisting of a vowel or diphthong between two consonants; SYN: consonant-nucleus-consonant

constant stimuli, method of psychophysical procedure for determining thresholds in which the same stimuli that fall into a discrete range about the threshold of interest are presented repeatedly until a 50% threshold is determined on a psychometric function

construct validity extent to which a test measures the nature of a trait

content validity extent to which a test represents an appropriate sampling of the trait it is intended to measure

contingent negative variation CNV; evoked potential, characterized by a low-frequency, negative-voltage electrophysiologic response occurring in the 300 msec to 500 msec latency region; associated with anticipation of a stimulus condition

continuous discourse running or connected speech, as in a talker reading a story, used in speech audiometry primarily as background competition; SYN: connected discourse

continuous flow adapter earmold CFA earmold; earmold with a constant interior tubing diameter designed to permit high-frequency amplification with a smooth frequency response

continuous frequency audiometer early term used to describe a Békésy audiometer in which signal frequency changes automatically in small steps (1 cycle per second) throughout the frequency range

continuous interleaved sampling processing CIS processing; cochlear implant processing strategy designed to deliver non-simultaneous pulses at a high rate of stimulation to multiple implant electrodes

continuous tracing C tracing; graph that results from threshold tracking in Békésy

audiometry to a continuous pure tone at a fixed or swept frequency; ANT: interrupted tracing

contraindication a condition that renders the use of a treatment or procedure inadvisable

contralateral pertaining to the opposite side of the body; SYN: heterolateral

contralateral acoustic reflex acoustic reflex occurring in one ear as a result of stimulation of the other ear; SYN: crossed acoustic reflex

contralateral competing message CCM; in speech audiometry, noise or other competing signal that is delivered to the ear opposite the ear receiving the target signal; ANT: ipsilateral competing message

contralateral delayed endolymphatic hydrops endolymphatic hydrops occurring in two phases—an initial profound hearing loss in one ear followed by development of fluctuating hearing loss and episodic vertigo in the previously normal-hearing ear

contralateral interference level, minimum on the Stenger test, the lowest intensity level of a signal presented to the allegedly poorer-hearing ear that causes the patient to stop responding, despite continued suprathreshold presentation to the better ear

contralateral masking the contralateralization of masking noise from the nontest ear to test ear once it exceeds interaural attenuation; SYN: overmasking

contralateral routing of signals CROS; hearing aid configuration designed for unilateral hearing loss, in which a microphone is placed on the poor ear, and the signal is routed to a hearing aid on the better ear

contralateral suppression reduction in the amplitude of transient otoacoustic emissions by the introduction of noise into the contralateral ear

contralateralization the result of sound presented to one ear through an earphone crossing the head via bone conduction and being perceived by the other ear; SYN: cross hearing, crossover

control, postural maintenance of body posture by the interaction of sensory perception, central nervous system integration, and motor function

control, remote hand-held unit that permits volume and/or program changes in a programmable hearing aid

control, volume VC; manual or automatic control designed to adjust the output level of a hearing instrument

control group in research, a group of individuals that serves as a standard against which observations of an experimental group can be compared

conversion, analog-to-digital ADC; the process of turning continuously varying (analog) signals into a numerical (digital) representation of the waveform

conversion, digital-to-analog DAC; the process of turning numerical (digital) representation of a waveform into a continuously varying (analog) signal

conversion deafness nonorganic hearing loss resulting from the transformation of severe anxiety into the physical manifestation of deafness; SYN: hysterical deafness; psychogenic deafness

cookie bite audiogram colloquial term referring to the audiometric configuration characterized by a hearing loss in the middle frequencies and normal or nearly normal hearing in the low and high frequencies

COR audiometry conditioned orientation reflex; behavioral audiometry, designed to assess hearing sensitivity in a young child, in which an orienting head-turn response to a sound source is conditioned by visual reinforcement

CORA conditioned orientation reflex audiometry

cord insulated electrical cable used to connect a body-worn hearing aid, FM-system, cochlear implant processor, etc. to a receiver or earmold

core area main portion of the inferior colliculus, medial geniculate, and auditory cortex through which primary afferent auditory information travels

CORFIG coupler response for flat insertion gain; frequency response that is added to a real-ear insertion response to obtain a prescribed 2-cc coupler response

Cornelia de Lange syndrome small-stature syndrome characterized by severe mental and growth retardation, abnormally shaped skull and face, and anomalies of the external ear and auditory meatus, with associated conductive, sensorineural, or mixed hearing loss

corneoretinal potential CRP; electrical potential generated by the voltage difference between the relatively positive cornea and the relatively negative retina

corner audiogram audiometric configuration characterized by a profound hearing loss with measurable thresholds only in the low-frequency region

coronal plane anatomic plane of reference that divides a structure into anterior (front) and posterior (back) portions; SYN: frontal plane

corpus the main portion of an organ or other anatomical structure

corpus callosum the prominent white-matter band of nerve fibers that connects the cerebral hemispheres

corpus geniculatum mediale medial geniculate; auditory nucleus of the thalamus, divided into central and surrounding pericentral nuclei, that receives primary ascending fibers from the inferior colliculus and sends fibers, via the auditory radiations, to the auditory cortex

corpus striatum part of the basal ganglia of the cerebrum responsible for somatic motor functions; includes the caudate nucleus and lenticular nucleus (globus pallidus, claustrum, and putamen)

correlation the tendency of two traits or physical quantities to vary together

correlation, negative inverse relationship of the values of two sets of measures

correlation, positive direct relationship of the values of two sets of measures

cortex outer layer; used most commonly to describe the cerebral cortex

cortex, auditory auditory area of the cerebral cortex located on the transverse temporal gyrus (Heschl's gyrus) of the temporal lobe

Corti's organ hearing organ, composed of sensory and supporting cells, located on the basilar membrane in the cochlear duct; SYN: organ of Corti

cortical pertaining to the cerebral cortex

cortical audiometry cortical evoked response audiometry

cortical deafness central auditory disorder related to bilateral temporal lobe lesions, often characterized by difficulty in recognizing auditory signals or understanding speech despite normal or near-normal cochlear function; SYN: central deafness

cortical evoked response audiometry CERA; electrophysiologic technique for predicting hearing sensitivity by measuring late-latency auditory evoked responses to auditory stimulation

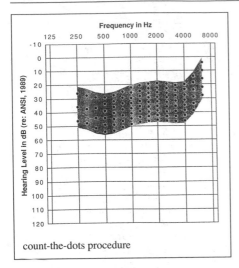

count-the-dots procedure

cortical lateralization cerebral dominance

cortical response, late long-latency auditory evoked response

cortilymph perilymph found within the spaces of the organ of Corti

Costen syndrome a symptom complex of otalgia, tinnitus, headache, and dizziness associated with temporomandibular joint disorder

COT critical off time; interval between pulsed tones at which threshold or loudness is equal to that of a continuous tone

Council for Accreditation in Occupational Hearing Conservation CAOHC; multidisciplinary coordinating body involved in the training and certification of occupational hearing conservationists

counseling, genetic advising of potential parents as to the probability of inherited disorders and conditions in their offspring

count-the-dots procedure a method for calculating audibility of speech in which dots corresponding to weighted speech information are plotted on an audiogram; aided responses superimposed on the audiogram reveal the proportion of the information that is audible

coupled joined or attached

coupled FM system personal FM amplification receiver coupled to a hearing aid telecoil by a neckloop

coupler any device that joins one part of an acoustic system to another

coupler, 0.5-cc device designed to replicate the volume of an ear canal fitted with a completely-in-the-canal hearing aid that joins the receiver of a hearing aid to the microphone of a sound level meter

coupler, HA-1 standard 2-cc coupler used to connect a hearing aid to an electroacoustic analyzer; the HA-1 device allows direct coupling of an earmold or an in-the-ear hearing aid, with putty used to seal the earmold or shell into the device

coupler, HA-2 standard 2-cc coupler used to connect a hearing aid to an electroacoustic analyzer; the HA-2 device has an earmold simulator and is used for testing earphones with nubs, such as an external receiver of a body aid

coupler, HA-3 standard 2-cc coupler used to connect a hearing aid to an electroacoustic analyzer; the HA-3 device is used for testing modular ITE hearing aids, earphones, and insert receivers that do not have nubs

coupler, HA-4 standard 2-cc coupler used to connect a hearing aid to an electroacoustic analyzer; the HA-4 device is a modification of the HA-2 with entrance tubing for use with postauricular or eyeglass hearing aids

coupler, 6-cc device designed to replicate the volume of an ear canal under a circumaural earphone that joins the earphone speaker to the microphone of a sound level meter

coupler, 2-cc device designed to replicate the volume of an ear canal fitted with a hearing aid or earmold that joins the receiver of a hearing aid to the microphone of a sound level meter

coupler, Zwislocki a hard-wall cylindrical cavity that connects a hearing aid receiver to the microphone of a sound level meter, with acoustic impedances designed to be more like those of a human ear across the frequency range than the conventional 2-cc coupler

COWS cold-opposite warm-same; mnemonic acronym that describes the direction of nystagmus beating in response to caloric stimulation; stimulation of an ear with cold water results in nystagmus that beats in the direction of the opposite ear

CP cerebral palsy; motor-control disorder caused by damage to the motor cortex of the brain

CPA cerebellopontine angle; anatomical

CN	Name	Function
I	olfactory	afferent innervation from the nose
II	optic	afferent innervation from the eyes
III	oculomotor	primarily efferent innervation to the extraocular muscles involved in eye movement
IV	trochlear	efferent innervation to the superior oblique muscle involved in eye movement
V	trigeminal	efferent innervation to the mastication muscles, including the tensor tympani, and afferent innervation from the face
VI	abducens	efferent innervation to the lateral rectus muscles involved in eye movement
VII	facial	efferent innervation to the facial muscles and afferent innervation from the soft palate and tongue
VIII	vestibulocochlear	afferent innervation from the cochlear and vestibular labyrinths
IX	glossopharyngeal	efferent innervation to pharyngeal muscles and the parotid gland and afferent innervation from the auricle, eustachian tube, and posterior one-third of the tongue
X	vagus	efferent and afferent innervation to the thoracic and abdominal viscera, pharynx, and larynx
XI	accessory	efferent innervation to muscles of the larynx and neck
XII	hypoglossal	efferent innervation to the muscles of the tongue

Cranial nerves

angle formed by the proximity of the cerebellum and the pons from which Cranial Nerve VIII exits into the brainstem

CPA tumor cerebellopontine angle tumor; most often a cochleovestibular Schwannoma located or growing outside the internal auditory canal at the juncture of the cerebellum and pons

CPHI communication profile for the hearing impaired; self-assessment questionnaire designed to quantify a patient's perception of the communication disorder and acceptance of the hearing loss

CPR cochleopalpebral reflex; eyeblink or twitch at the canthus caused by a sudden loud sound; SYN: auropalpebral reflex

cps cycles per second; measurement of sound frequency in terms of the number of complete cycles of a sinusoid that occur within a second; SYN: Hz

CPT codes current procedural terminology codes; numeric codes assigned to diagnostic and treatment procedures, used primarily for billing purposes

cranial 1. pertaining to the cranium; 2. anatomical direction, referring to structures that are located toward the head; ANT: caudal; SYN: cephalad, rostral

cranial nerve any of 12 pairs of neuron bundles exiting the brainstem above the first cervical vertebra

Cranial Nerve VIII CVIII; C8; CN-VIII; auditory nerve, consisting of a vestibular and a cochlear branch; SYN: vestibulocochlear nerve

craniocervical dysplasia primarily inherited disorder characterized by bony, vascular, and neural malformations of the craniocervical region, with associated unilateral fluctuating progressive sensorineural hearing loss

craniodiaphyseal dysplasia craniotubular disorder with mixed hearing loss as a predominant feature

craniofacial pertaining to both the face and cranium

craniofacial anomaly congenital malformation of the face and/or cranium

craniofacial dysostosis autosomal dominant disorder with manifestations related to premature fusion of the cranial sutures, including ear canal atresia, commonly with sensorineural, conductive, or mixed hearing loss; SYN: Crouzon syndrome

craniosynostosis premature closure of the sutures of the skull

cranium skull

crest factor difference in decibels between the peak sound pressure level of a signal and the root-mean-square sound pressure level of that signal

crib-o-gram pioneering method for automated neonatal hearing screening in which a motion-sensitive transducer in the mattress of a crib detected changes in movement in response to auditory stimuli presented through a loudspeaker

Crippled Children's Service CCS; state-funded organization that provides financial assistance for healthcare and other services to children with disabilities

criss-CROS version of a CROS hearing aid designed for bilateral severe hearing loss in which the microphone on each side transmits its signal to the hearing aid in the opposite ear, thereby permitting substantial gain without feedback

crista ampullaris; pl. cristae ampullares sense organ in the semicircular canal, containing stereocilia and kinocilia, which responds to angular acceleration

critical bandwidth for loudness range of frequencies over which complete loudness summation occurs and beyond which no further loudness growth occurs

critical bandwidth for masking in masking pure tones, the frequency range of the masking noise, centered around the pure tone, over which effective masking occurs and beyond which no further masking effect occurs

critical off time COT; interval between pulsed tones at which threshold or loudness is equal to that of a continuous tone

critical period early years of a child's development during which language is most readily acquired

critical ratio a measure of the limited effective bandwidth of a noise masker, taken as the difference in decibels between a masked threshold and the level per cycle of the masker

CROS contralateral routing of signals; hearing aid configuration designed for unilateral hearing loss, in which a microphone is placed on the poor ear, and the signal is routed to a hearing aid on the better ear

CROS-plus modification of a transcranial CROS arrangement in which traditional CROS aid is fitted to the better ear and a power in-the-ear hearing aid is fitted to the unaidable ear

cross-check principle principle in pediatric audiometry that the results of any single audiometric test cannot be considered valid without an independent verification, or cross-check, from another audiometric test

cross hearing the perception of sound in

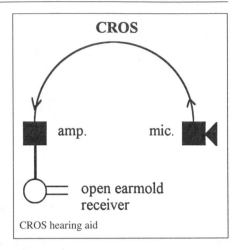

CROS hearing aid

one ear that has crossed over the head by bone-conducted transmission of a sound presented through an earphone to the opposite ear; SYN: contralateralization, crossover

crossed acoustic reflex acoustic reflex occurring in one ear as a result of stimulation of the other ear; SYN: contralateral acoustic reflex

crossed olivocochlear bundle COCB; group of efferent nerve fibers of the medial olivocochlear bundle, coursing from the periolivary nuclei near the medial superior olive, across the brainstem and along the vestibular nerve, to the outer hair cells of the contralateral cochlea

crossover the process in which sound presented to one ear through an earphone crosses the head via bone conduction and is perceived by the other ear; SYN: contralateralization, cross hearing

crossover frequency 1. in speech audiometry, the frequency above and below which is found equal information for accurate perception; 2. in hearing aids, the frequency that distinguishes two adjacent bands

crosstalk 1. spillover of a signal from one circuit to another; 2. in an audiometer, crosstalk occurs when the signal intended for exclusive routing to one earphone is also routed to the other

Crouzon syndrome congenital autosomal dominant disorder with manifestations related to premature fusion of the cranial sutures including ear canal atresia, commonly with sensorineural, conductive, or mixed hearing loss; SYN: craniofacial dysostosis

CRP corneoretinal potential; electrical potential generated by the voltage difference between the relatively positive cornea and the relatively negative retina

crura plural of crus

crura, stapes two struts that connect the head and neck of the stapes to the footplate

crus any anatomical structure resembling a leg; e.g., the incus has a short crus and a long crus, and the stapes has two crura connecting the head to the footplate

crus, common portion of the semicircular canal where the superior and posterior canals meet

cryoglobulinemia disorder characterized by markedly increased blood viscosity, with associated progressive hearing loss secondary to cochlear degeneration

cryptophthalmia congenital autosomal recessive eye disorder, characterized by absence of eyelids and by skin covering a rudimentary eye, with associated conductive hearing loss

crystal microphone early piezoelectric microphone in which mechanical stress was applied to generate electric current in crystals such as quartz and lithium sulfate

CSF cerebrospinal fluid; liquid filling the ventricles and the subarachnoid space surrounding the brain and spinal cord that supports and cushions the central nervous system against trauma and may serve to remove waste products of neuronal metabolism

CSOM chronic suppurative otitis media; persistent inflammation of the middle ear with infected effusion containing pus

CST Competing Sentence Test; test of dichotic processing of simple sentences

CT computed tomography; sectional radiographs of specified areas of the brain presented as a computer-generated image representing a synthesis of x-rays obtained from different directions on a given plane; SYN: computerized axial tomography

CTP caloric test position; conventional head position for caloric testing in which the patient lies in a supine position with the head angled at 30

cubic centimeter cc; unit of measure of volume; 1 cc equals 1 ml

cubic distortion product cochlear distortion that is the source of clinical DPOAEs, resulting from the interaction of two simultaneously presented pure tones at frequencies f_1 and f_2; c.d.p. is the cubic difference tone

that occurs at the frequency represented by $2f_1$-f_2

cue any verbal or nonverbal signal that communicates a message to the receiver

cue, acoustic segment of speech providing the necessary identifying information

cue, auditory verbal information provided to prompt a response as an aid to communication

cue, visual any gesture, posture, or facial expression that adds meaning to spoken language

cued discourse a speech audiometry technique involving multispeaker soundfield signal presentation in which the listener is asked to focus on the discourse presented from one loudspeaker to the exclusion of the others

cued speech speechreading accompanied by a system of hand positions near the mouth (cues) designed to discriminate between similar visual patterns

cupula gelatinous substance of the crista ampullaris in which the kinocilia of the vestibular hair cells are embedded

cupulolithiasis benign paroxysmal positional vertigo caused by inorganic deposits on the cupula of the posterior semicircular canal, which makes the cupula sensitive to gravitational force and thereby stimulable with changes in head position

curette instrument shaped like a loop, ring, or scoop used to remove new growths, abnormal tissue, or excessive cerumen

current rate of electron flow through an electrical circuit, measured in amperes

current, alternating ac; electric current that periodically changes its value or direction of flow

current, direct dc; electric current of a fixed value that flows continuously in one direction

current procedural terminology codes CPT codes; numeric codes assigned to diagnostic and treatment procedures, used primarily for billing and reimbursement purposes

curvilinear compression hearing aid compression in which the compression ratio increases as input level increases, providing dynamic-range compression for low-level and mid-level inputs and compression limiting for high-level input

custom earmold earmold made for a specific individual from an ear impression

custom hearing aid   ITE, ITC, or CIC hearing aid made for a specific individual from an ear impression

cutaneous   pertaining to the skin

cuticular plate   thickened membrane at the apex of each cochlear hair cell

CV   consonant vowel; syllable used in speech audiometric measures that consists of a consonant followed by a vowel

CVA   cerebrovascular accident; interruption of blood supply to the brain due to aneurysm, embolism, or clot, resulting in sudden loss of function related to the affected portion of the brain; COL: stroke

CVB   cisplatin, videsine, bleomycin; potentially ototoxic chemotherapy regimen used in the treatment of esophageal cancer

CVC   consonant-vowel-consonant; a word or syllable used in speech-recognition testing, consisting of a vowel or diphthong between two consonants; SYN: CNC

CVIII   Cranial Nerve VIII

cyanosis   bluish discoloration of the skin and mucous membranes due to reduced oxygen saturation of the blood

cycle   1. complete sinusoidal wave; 2. complete compression and rarefaction of a sound wave

cycles per second   cps; measurement of sound frequency in terms of the number of complete cycles of a sinusoid that occur within a second; SYN: Hz

cymba   superior, boat-shaped aspect of the concha bowl

cytoarchitecture   structural arrangement of cells typical of a region

cytocochleogram   graphic depiction of percentage loss of structures of the organ of Corti as a function of distance along the basilar membrane

cytodifferentiation   developmental separation or distinguishing of cells

cytogenesis   development of cells

cytomegalic inclusion disease   condition caused by the introduction of cytomegalovirus into cells and tissues of the body, which may result in progressive, fluctuating sensorineural hearing loss

cytomegalovirus   CMV; intrauterine prenatal or postnatal herpetoviral infection, usually transmitted in utero, which can cause central nervous system disorder, including brain damage, hearing loss, vision loss, and seizures

Cz   coronal (C) midline (z) electrode location, or vertex electrode, typically used for noninverting-electrode placement in auditory evoked potential testing, according to the 10–20 International Electrode System nomenclature

D

DAC digital-to-analog conversion; the process of turning numerical (digital) representation of a waveform into a continuously varying (analog) signal

dactyl finger or toe

dactyl speech fingerspelling; manual communication

dactylology use of fingerspelling or, more broadly, manual communication

DAF delayed auditory feedback; condition in which a listener's speech is delayed by a controlled amount of time and delivered back to the listener's ears, interfering with the rate and fluency of the speech

DAI direct audio input; direct input of sound into a hearing aid by means of a hardwire connection between the hearing aid and an assistive listening devices or other sound source

damage risk criterion DRC; amount of exposure time to sound of a specified frequency and intensity that is associated with a defined risk of hearing loss

damped wave damped wave train

damped wave train progressive decrease in amplitude of an acoustic waveform over time

damper, acoustic a valve that provides smoothing of the frequency characteristics of an acoustic signal

damping decrease in amplitude of an acoustic waveform over time

daPa decaPascal; unit of pressure in which 1 daPa equals 10 Pascals

Darwinian ear a pinna in which the upper border is not rolled over to form the helix

Darwinian tubercle small projection or cartilage thickening on the upper portion of the helix

DAS dorsal acoustic stria; nerve fiber bundle that emanates from the dorsal cochlear nucleus and synapses in the contralateral lateral lemniscus and inferior colliculus, bypassing the superior olivary complex

DAT digital audio tape; type of magnetic tape used with tape recorder/player employing digital conversion of acoustic signals

day/night equivalent level in sound-exposure analysis, a description of the intru-

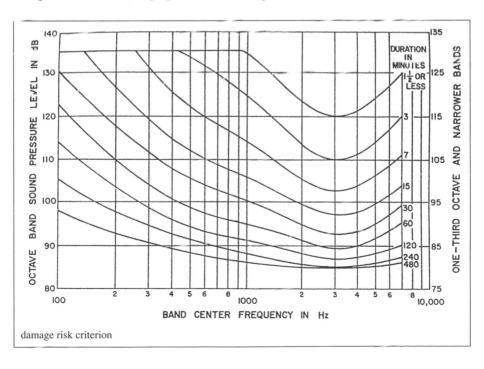

damage risk criterion

57

siveness of sound that differentiates between quieter hours of the night and busier hours of the day, attributing greater intrusiveness during quieter hours

dB decibel; one-tenth of a bel; unit of sound intensity, based on a logarithmic relationship of one intensity to a reference intensity

dB gain decibels of gain; the difference between the input SPL and the output SPL of an amplifier or hearing aid

dB HL decibels hearing level; decibel notation used on the audiogram that is referenced to audiometric zero

dB HTL decibels hearing threshold level; decibel notation used to refer to a patient's threshold of hearing sensitivity

dB nHL decibels normalized hearing level; decibel notation referenced to behavioral thresholds of a sample of normal-hearing persons, used most often to describe the intensity level of click stimuli used in evoked potential audiometry

dB SL decibels sensation level; decibel notation that refers to the number of decibels above a person's threshold for a given acoustic signal

dB SPL decibels sound pressure level; dB SPL equals 20 times the log of the ratio of an observed sound pressure level to the reference sound pressure level of 20 microPascals (or 0.0002 dynes/cm^2, 0.0002 microbar, 20 microNewtons/meter^2)

dBA decibels expressed in sound pressure level as measured on the A-weighted scale of a sound level meter filtering network, used in the measurement of environmental noise in the workplace

dBB decibels expressed in sound pressure level as measured on the B-weighted scale of a sound level meter filtering network

dBC decibels expressed in sound pressure level as measured on the C-weighted scale of a sound level meter filtering network

dBm decibels referenced to 1 milliwatt

dc direct current; electric current of a fixed value that flows continuously in one direction

DCA hearing aid digitally controlled analog hearing aid; hybrid hearing device in which microphone-amplifier-loudspeaker functions are analog, but their parameters are under digital control

DCN dorsal cochlear nucleus; dorsal portion of the cochlear nucleus that receives

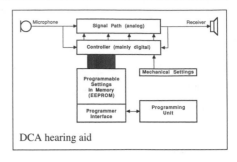

DCA hearing aid

nerve fibers from the posterior branch of Cranial Nerve VIII after it bifurcates

DCPN direction-changing positional nystagmus; abnormal nystagmus that changes direction either with head position changes or with head kept in the same position

DDx differential diagnosis; diagnosis of a disease or disorder in a patient from among two or more diseases or disorders with similar symptoms or findings

deaf having no or very limited functional hearing

deaf and dumb obsolete term denoting the condition of deafness accompanied by mutism; abandoned as being pejorative

deaf culture ideology, beliefs, and customs shared by many individuals with prelinguistic deafness

deaf mute obsolete term for an individual who is deaf and lacks speech; abandoned as being pejorative

deaf speech quality of speech common among persons with deafness

deafen to cause deafness

deafferentation loss of sensory nerve fibers from a specified portion of the body

deafness the condition of having no or very limited functional hearing

deafness, congenital reduced hearing sensitivity existing at or dating from birth, resulting from pre- or perinatal pathologic conditions

deafness, conversion nonorganic hearing loss resulting from the transformation of severe anxiety into the physical manifestation of deafness; SYN: hysterical deafness, psychogenic deafness

deafness, cortical central auditory disorder related to bilateral temporal lobe lesions, often characterized by difficulty in recognizing auditory signals or understanding speech despite normal or near-normal cochlear function; SYN: central deafness

deafness, familial   deafness occurring in members of the same family

deafness, hereditary   deafness of genetic origin

deafness, hysterical   rare psychogenic disorder of hearing, caused by conversion of emotional trauma to a physical manifestation

deafness, nerve   misnomer for sensorineural hearing loss

deafness, postlinguistic   deafness occurring after speech and language have developed

deafness, prelinguistic   deafness occurring prior to speech and language development

deafness, psychogenic   rare disorder characterized by apparent, but nonorganic, hearing loss resulting from psychological trauma

deafness, word   inexact term describing the inability to understand spoken language, as in fluent or receptive aphasia

deafness management quotient   DMQ; formula used to predict success in an oral education program, based on weighted factors related to residual hearing, central function, intellect, family support, and socioeconomics

Deafness Research Foundation   DRF; foundation that funds scientific research in hearing and deafness

decaPascal   daPa; unit of pressure in which 1 daPa equals 10 Pascals

decay   1. diminution of the physical properties of a stimulus; 2. diminution of perception or function

decay, reflex   perstimulatory reduction in the amplitude of an acoustic reflex in response to continuous stimulus presentation

decay, tone   perstimulatory adaptation, in which an audible sound becomes inaudible during prolonged stimulation

decay rate   speed with which amplitude of a sound diminishes

decibel   dB; one-tenth of a bel; unit of sound intensity, based on a logarithmic relationship of one intensity to a reference intensity

decibel meter   an electronic instrument designed to measure sound intensity in decibels in accordance with an accepted standard; SYN: sound level meter

decompression   surgical technique of removing bone surrounding nerve to relieve pressure due to edematous neural tissue or to a tumor that cannot be excised

deconvolution   decomposition or unfolding of a complex response or data set

decruitment   abnormally slow growth in loudness perception with increasing intensity, associated with retrocochlear pathology; ANT: recruitment

decussate   to cross over, as nerve fibers crossing from the cochlear nucleus to the contralateral superior olivary complex

decussation   the crossing over of homonomous nerve fiber bundles from one side of the brain to the other

deep   anatomical direction, referring to structures that are located near the center of the body; ANT: superficial

deep auricular artery   branch of the internal maxillary artery that divides into posterior and anterior branches to supply a large portion of the tympanic membrane

deep sedation   level of sedation in which patients are not easily aroused and may be unable to breathe independently

deformity   congenital or acquired deviation from the normal shape or size of a portion of the body

degeneration   deterioration of an anatomic structure resulting in diminution of function

degeneration, anterograde   neural degeneration forward along afferent pathways, secondary to deafferentation

degeneration, infantile cochleosaccular   idiopathic or viral selective degeneration in infancy of the cochlea and saccule with preservation of the utricle and cristae, resulting in unilateral or bilateral profound sensorineural hearing loss

degeneration, retrograde   neural degeneration backward along pathways

degenerative   pertaining to degeneration

degrees of freedom   df; in statistics, the number of data points that are free to vary if the statistic is known; e.g., if the mean of a set of 10 numbers is known, then 9 of the numbers are free to vary, because the 10th will be determinable from knowing the rest

Deiter cells   large cell bodies of the organ of Corti that rest on the basilar membrane and extend to, and cradle, the bases of the outer hair cells to provide support

delayed auditory feedback   DAF; condition in which a listener's speech is delayed by a controlled amount of time and delivered back to the listener's ears, interfering with the rate and fluency of the speech

delayed endolymphatic hydrops endolymphatic hydrops occurring in two phases, an initial profound hearing loss in one ear followed by development of episodic vertigo in the ipsilateral ear or fluctuating hearing loss and episodic vertigo in the previously normal hearing ear

delayed feedback audiometry DFA; the use of delayed auditory feedback in assessing the organicity of a suspected functional hearing loss; the delayed delivery of speech, if audible, interferes with fluency or rate of speech

delayed latency in auditory brainstem response measurement, an abnormal prolongation of the time between signal onset and major peaks of the response

delayed-onset auditory deprivation the apparent decline in word-recognition ability in the unaided ear of a person fitted with a monaural hearing aid, resulting from asymmetric stimulation; SYN: late-onset auditory deprivation

delayed response delayed latency

delayed speech and language general classification of speech and language skills as less well developed than expected for a child's age

delta rhythm or waves slow EEG waves of less than 4 Hz

dementia progressive deterioration of cognitive function

dementia, senile primary degenerative dementia occurring in old age, characterized by progressive cognitive deterioration, loss of memory, and emotional lability

demyelinating disease autoimmune disease process that causes scattered patches of demyelination of white matter throughout the central nervous system, resulting in retrocochlear disorder when the auditory nervous system is affected

demyelination, demyelinization destruction or loss of myelin sheath surrounding nerve fibers

dendrite afferent process of a neuron that conducts impulses toward the cell body

density the ratio of mass to volume

Denver Scale of Communication Function self-assessment inventory used to assess the impact of hearing loss on an individual's life

deoxyribonucleic acid DNA; large and complex molecules carrying genetic instructions

depolarization abrupt decrease in membrane electrical potential

deprivation, auditory diminution or absence of sensory opportunity for neural structures central to the end organ, due to a reduction in auditory stimulation resulting from hearing loss

dermal pertaining to the skin

dermatitis nonspecific skin condition that may affect the pinna, characterized by dryness, itching, crusting, and weeping

descending method audiometric technique used in establishing hearing sensitivity thresholds by varying signal intensity from audible to inaudible; ANT: ascending method

desired sensation level DSL; number of decibels above behavioral threshold required to amplify the long-term speech spectrum to a prescribed level across the frequency range

desired sensation level prescriptive procedure DSL prescriptive procedure; method of choosing gain and frequency response of a hearing aid so that the long-term spectrum of speech is amplified to the desired sensation levels, estimated across the frequency range from audiometric thresholds

desquamated epithelium cells shed from the outer layer of the skin or other membranes

detectability threshold detection threshold

detection threshold absolute threshold of hearing sensitivity

development natural progression from embryonic to adult life stages

developmental pertaining to development

developmental age age at which children acquire specific skills

developmental disability category of mentally or physically handicapping conditions that appear in infancy or early childhood and are related to abnormal development

dextral pertaining to the right side; ANT: sinistral

df degrees of freedom; in statistics, the number of data points that are free to vary if the statistic is known

DFA delayed feedback audiometry; the use of delayed auditory feedback in assessing the organicity of a suspected functional hearing loss; the delayed delivery of speech, if audible, interferes with fluency or rate of speech

DHAP   dexamethasone-cytarabine-cisplatin; potentially ototoxic chemotherapy regimen used in non-Hodgkin's lymphoma

DI   directivity index; quantification of the directional properties of a hearing aid microphone, expressed as the decibel improvement in signal-to-noise ratio over that expected for an omnidirectional microphone

diabetes mellitus   metabolic disorder caused by a deficiency of insulin, with chronic complications including neuropathy and generalized degenerative changes in blood vessels

diagnosis   Dx; determination of the nature of disease or disorder

diagnosis, differential   DDx; diagnosis of a disease or disorder in a patient from among two or more diseases or disorders with similar symptoms or findings

diagnosis-related groups   DRG; major diagnostic categories into which patients are classified for the purpose of determining reimbursement levels

diagnostic   pertaining to diagnosis

diagnostic audiometry   measurement of hearing to determine the nature and degree of hearing impairment

diagnostic test   a measure used to determine the nature of a disease or disorder

diagnostic therapy   treatment that, in its course, provides insight into the nature of a disease or disorder

diagnostician   an expert in making diagnoses

diaphragm   1. thin partition separating adjacent regions; 2. a thin plate in a microphone that vibrates in response to sound pressure waves or a thin plate in a loudspeaker that vibrates in response to applied voltage to create sound pressure waves

diastrophic dwarfism   autosomal dominant craniofacial disorder, characterized by marked shortness of stature, hand deformity, and severe clubfoot, which may include congenital sensorineural hearing loss

diathesis   genetic predisposition to a certain disease or disorder

dichotic   1. divided into two parts; 2. pertaining to different signals presented to or reaching each ear

dichotic amplification   seldom used fitting technique in which high-frequency emphasis amplification is fitted to the right ear and flat-frequency response to the left ear, in an effort to exploit the right-ear advantage

for processing speech; SYN: split-band amplification

dichotic CVs   speech audiometric test of central auditory function in which different consonant-vowel (CV) syllables are presented simultaneously to each ear

dichotic digits   speech audiometric test of central auditory function in which different numbers (from 1–10, excluding 7) are presented simultaneously to each ear

dichotic hearing aid fitting   dichotic amplification

dichotic listening   the task of perceiving different signals presented simultaneously to each ear

dichotic sentence identification test   DSI test; speech audiometric test of central auditory function in which different synthetic sentences are presented simultaneously to each ear

dichotomy   division into two parts or categories based on specified characteristics

dielectric   insulating material or substance that may transmit electricity by induction but not conduction

diencephalon   posterior part of the forebrain, including the thalamus, hypothalamus, epithalamus, and subthalamus, serving as a relay and integration center for sensory input to the cortex

difference limen   DL; the smallest difference that can be detected between two signals that vary in intensity, frequency, time, etc.; SYN: differential threshold, just-noticeable difference

difference limen for frequency   DLF; smallest difference in frequency of a signal that can be detected

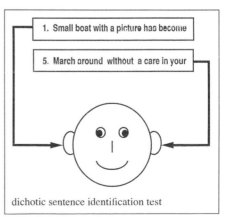

dichotic sentence identification test

difference limen for intensity DLI; smallest difference in intensity of a signal that can be detected

difference tone a distinctive tone perceived at a frequency equal to the difference between the frequencies of two stimulating tones

difference waveform in electrophysiologic measurement, the waveform that results from the subtraction of one waveform from a different waveform, such as monaural from binaural ABR waveforms

differential amplifier amplifier used in evoked potential measurement to eliminate extraneous noise; the voltage from one electrode's input is inverted and subtracted from another input, so that any electrical activity that is common to both electrodes is rejected

differential comparison probe-microphone technique in which the SPL at the reference microphone is subtracted from the SPL at the probe microphone at the time of measurement

differential diagnosis DDx; diagnosis of a disease or disorder in a patient from among two or more diseases or disorders with similar symptoms or findings

differential sensitivity the capacity of the auditory system to detect differences between auditory signals that differ in intensity, frequency, time; SYN: auditory acuity; COM: absolute sensitivity

differential threshold difference limen

differentiation, auditory auditory figure-ground discrimination

diffraction scattering or deflection of sound waves as they encounter edges, openings, or different media

diffuse not localized or definitely limited; spread about

diffuse field sound field containing many reflected waves of random incidence so that the average sound pressure obtained throughout the room is nearly uniform

DiGeorge syndrome congenital disorder characterized by agenesis of the thymus and parathyroid glands with anomalies of the cardiovascular and renal systems and craniofacial structures, including pinna malformation and atresia of the external auditory meatus

digital numeric representation of a signal as a discrete value at a discrete moment in time; ANT: analog

digital audio tape DAT; type of magnetic tape used with tape recorder/player employing digital conversion of acoustic signals

digital filter software algorithm that reduces selected frequencies of a signal

digital hearing aid hearing aid that processes a signal digitally; SYN: DSP hearing aid

digital signal processing DSP; manipulation by mathematical algorithms of a signal that has been converted from analog to digital form

digital signal processing hearing aid DSP hearing aid; hearing aid that converts output from the microphone from analog to digital form, uses software algorithms to manipulate gain characteristics, and converts the signal back to analog form for delivery to the loudspeaker

digital-to-analog conversion DAC; the process of turning numerical (digital) representation of a waveform into a continuously varying (analog) signal

digitally controlled analog hearing aid DCA hearing aid; hybrid hearing device in which microphone-amplifier-loudspeaker functions are analog, but their parameters are under digital control

dihydrostreptomycin aminoglycocide antibiotic, which can be ototoxic; characterized by a predilection for the auditory system and delayed-onset hearing loss following its administration

dilantin diphenyl hydantoin; anticonvulsant drug, which can have a teratogenic effect on the auditory system of the developing embryo when taken by the mother during pregnancy, resulting in congenital hearing loss

dilation; dilatation physiologic, pathologic, or artificial enlargement of a canal, cavity, or vessel

dimeric tympanic membrane thin area of the tympanic membrane, secondary to the healing of a perforation; consists of epidermis and mucous membrane

din background noise consisting of a mixture of discordant sounds

diode semiconductor that allows current flow in only one direction

diode, light-emitting LED; a small light on a device, often used to indicate that the device is on or activated

diotic 1. pertaining to both ears; 2. pertaining to identical signals presented to or reaching each ear

diotic listening the task of perceiving identical signals presented simultaneously to each ear

DIP switch dual in-line package switch; a row of integrated circuit switches that allows the same electronic instrument to be configured in different ways

diphasic referring to or occurring in two phases

diphenyl hydantoin dilantin; anticonvulsant drug, which can have a teratogenic effect on the auditory system of the developing embryo when taken by the mother during pregnancy, resulting in congenital hearing loss

diplacusis auditory condition in which the sense of pitch is distorted so that a pure tone is heard as two tones or as noise or buzzing; double hearing

diplacusis binauralis diplacusis in which identical sounds are perceived differently in each ear

diplacusis dysharmonica binaural diplacusis in which sound of identical frequency is perceived to be of a different pitch in each ear

diplacusis echoica diplacusis in which a single sound is perceived as being repeated in the affected ear

diplacusis monauralis diplacusis in which one sound is perceived as two different sounds in the same ear

diplopia double vision

direct audio input DAI; direct input of sound into a hearing aid by means of a hardwire connection between the hearing aid and an assistive listening devices or other sound source

direct current dc; electric current of a fixed value that flows continuously in one direction

direct relationship the condition in which the values of two sets of measures are positively correlated, so that the greater the magnitude of one, the greater the magnitude of the other; ANT: inverse relationship

direction-changing positional nystagmus, central DCPN, central; abnormal positional nystagmus in which nystagmus changes direction when the head is kept in the same position, characteristic of central pathology

direction-changing positional nystagmus, peripheral DCPN, peripheral; abnormal positional nystagmus in which nystagmus changes directions with changes in head position, characteristic of nonlocalized vestibular pathology

direction-fixed positional nystagmus abnormal positional nystagmus that beats in the same direction regardless of head position, characteristic of peripheral vestibular pathology

directional having the characteristic of being more sensitive to sound from a focused directional range; COM: omnidirectional

directional hearing ability to determine the direction from which a sound is approaching

directional hearing aid hearing instrument that contains a directional microphone

directional microphone microphone with a transducer that is more responsive to sound from a focused direction; in hearing aids, the microphone is designed to be more sensitive to sounds emanating from the front than from behind

directional preponderance DP; superiority in one direction or the other of the slow phase velocity of nystagmus; e.g., for caloric labyrinthine stimulation, right-beating nystagmus (RW+LC) is compared to left-beating nystagmus (RC+LW), where R=right, L=left, W=warm, and C=cool

directivity the tendency of a source to radiate, or of a microphone to receive, sound more efficiently in one direction

directivity factor effect of the direction from which acoustic waves reach a microphone

directivity index DI; quantification of the directional properties of a hearing aid microphone, expressed as the decibel improvement in signal-to-noise ratio over that expected for an omnidirectional microphone

directivity pattern, polar expression of the directional characteristics of a hearing aid microphone, usually displayed in a polar plot that depicts the relative amplitude output of a hearing aid as a function of angle of sound incidence

disability a limitation or loss in function

disability, developmental category of mentally or physically handicapping conditions that appear in infancy or early childhood and are related to abnormal development

disability, hearing functional limitations imposed by a hearing impairment

disability, learning LD; lack of skill in one or more areas of learning that is inconsistent with the person's intellectual capacity and is not the result of visual, hearing, motor, or emotional disorder

disarticulation 1. separation; 2. a break or disconnection of the ossicular chain

disarticulation, ossicular detachment or break in the bones of the ossicular chain

discomfort level intensity level at which sound is perceived to be uncomfortably loud; SYN: loudness discomfort level

disconjugate eye movement movement of eyes in different directions

discourse, connected running or continuous speech, as in a talker reading a story, used in speech audiometry primarily as background competition; SYN: continuous discourse

discrete separate and distinct; not continuous

discrete frequency audiometer audiometer in which pure-tone frequencies are separate and distinct; COM: sweep-frequency audiometer

discrimination in speech audiometry, generic term for word-recognition ability

discrimination, auditory perceptual process by which an individual distinguishes and differentiates among sounds or words

discrimination, frequency perceptual process by which an individual distinguishes test signals of different frequencies presented consecutively

discrimination, speech SD; old term for word recognition

discrimination, speech sound the ability to differentiate among speech sounds

discrimination loss the amount of loss in word-recognition ability, expressed as the difference between word-recognition score and 100%

discrimination score DS; early term for word-recognition score, expressed as the percentage of words correctly perceived and identified

disease pathologic entity characterized by a recognized cause, identifiable signs and symptoms, and/or consistent anatomic alteration

disequilibrium disturbance in balance function

disinhibition removal of inhibitory influences in the nervous system

disorder abnormality; disturbance of function

disorder, hearing disturbance of structure and/or function of hearing

disorder, retrocochlear hearing disorder resulting from a neoplasm or other lesion located on Cranial Nerve VIII or beyond in the auditory brainstem or cortex

dispense to prepare and distribute

dispensing audiologist an audiologist who dispenses hearing aids

dissonance a discordant, harsh combination of sounds

distal away from the center or point of origin; ANT: proximal

distance index index of the directional property of a hearing aid microphone, indicating how much further from a source the same signal-to-noise ratio can be maintained as compared to an omnidirectional microphone

distance receptor sensory organ that can perceive stimuli at some distance from the body

distinctive feature basic element of a phoneme, such as manner or place of articulation, that differentiates it from another phoneme

distorted speech test speech audiometric technique in which the acoustic characteristics of the speech targets have been distorted to reduce the extrinsic redundancy of the signal

distortion undesired product of an inexact, or nonlinear, reproduction of an acoustic waveform

distortion, amplitude inacurate reproduction of sound waves when the limits of an amplifier are exceeded and the output is no longer proportional to the input; SYN: harmonic distortion, nonlinear distortion

distortion, harmonic amplitude distortion of a signal in the form of additional harmonic components

distortion, intermodulation amplitude distortion of aperiodic signals by a hearing aid, resulting in the addition of frequencies in the output that were not present in the input

distortion, nonlinear reduction in fidelity of an amplified signal as a result of an output level that varies with input level

distortion, transient the inexact reproduction of a sound resulting from failure of an amplifier to process or follow sudden changes of voltage

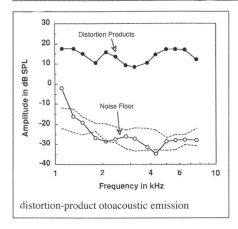

distortion-product otoacoustic emission

distortion product acoustic energy resulting from cochlear nonlinearity that occurs at frequencies that are a combination of two stimulating frequencies, created when two pure tones are presented simultaneously to the cochlea

distortion product, cubic cochlear distortion that is the source of clinical DPOAEs, resulting from the interaction of two simultaneously presented pure tones at frequencies f_1 and f_2; c.d.p. is the cubic difference tone that occurs at the frequency represented by $2f_1-f_2$

distortion-product evoked otoacoustic emission distortion-product otoacoustic emission

distortion-product otoacoustic emission DPOAE; otoacoustic emission, measured as the cubic distortion product that occurs at the frequency represented by $2f_1-f_2$, resulting from the simultaneous presentation of two pure tones (f_1 and f_2)

distortional bone conduction component of bone-conducted hearing created by alternating compressions and expansions of the bony labyrinth, resulting in fluid displacement in the membranous labyrinth; SYN: compressional bone conduction

diuretic drug that stimulates the flow of urine by inhibiting resorption of sodium and water; used in the treatment of hypertension and of edema from cardiac and renal disease

diuretic, loop class of agents, including ethacrynic acid, that promote the excretion of urine by inhibiting resorption of sodium and water in the kidneys; may be ototoxic in high doses

Dix-Hallpike maneuver rapid body maneuver performed during ENG testing in which the patient is seated with the head turned 45 degrees and then pulled backward rapidly until supine with the head hanging over the edge of the examining table

Dix-Hallpike test ENG subtest designed to determine if nystagmus can be elicited with the Dix-Hallpike maneuver

dizygotic pertaining to twins derived from two separate zygotes

dizziness general term used to describe various symptoms such as faintness, giddiness, light-headedness, or unsteadiness

DL difference limen; the smallest difference that can be detected between two signals that vary in intensity, frequency, time, etc.; SYN: differential threshold, just-noticeable difference

DLF difference limen for frequency; smallest difference in frequency of a signal that can be detected

DLI difference limen for intensity; smallest difference in intensity of a signal that can be detected

DMQ deafness management quotient; formula used to predict success in an oral education program, based on weighted factors related to residual hearing, central function, intellect, family support, and socioeconomics

DNA deoxyribonucleic acid; large and complex molecules carrying genetic instructions

DNE did not evaluate

DNT did not test

Doerfler-Stewart test test of the organicity of hearing loss in a patient suspected of having a functional overlay, involving the presentation of spondaic words in quiet and in the presence of noise

dominant hereditary hearing loss hearing loss due to transmission of a genetic characteristic or mutation in which only one gene of a pair must carry the characteristic in order to be expressed, and both sexes have an equal chance of being affected

dominant progressive hearing loss DPHL; genetic condition in which sensorineural hearing loss gradually worsens over a period of years, caused by dominant inheritance

Doppler effect a change in pitch when a sound source and a listener are in rapid motion away from or toward each other

Doppler shift magnitude of the pitch change when a sound source and listener are in rapid motion away from or toward each other

dorsal anatomical direction, referring to structures that are located toward the backbone; SYN: posterior; ANT: anterior

dorsal acoustic stria DAS; nerve fiber bundle that emanates from the dorsal cochlear nucleus and synapses in the contralateral lateral lemniscus and inferior colliculus, bypassing the superior olivary complex

dorsal cochlear nucleus DCN; dorsal portion of the cochlear nucleus that receives nerve fibers from the posterior branch of Cranial Nerve VIII after it bifurcates

dorsal nucleus of the lateral lemniscus LLD; one of three large fiber tracts, located along the lateralmost edge of the pons, consisting of ascending auditory fibers from the cochlear nucleus and superior olivary complex

dorsomedial inferior colliculus portion of the inferior colliculus receiving descending fibers from the cortex and fibers from the contralateral dorsomedial inferior colliculus

dosimeter, audio a body-worn instrument used to measure accumulated level and duration of noise to which a person is exposed over a specified time period

dosimetry the process of measuring accumulated level and duration of noise exposure over a specified time period

double-blind study an experiment in which neither the subjects nor the investigators are aware of group placement; e.g., whether a subject was placed in the group that received an experimental drug or the group that received a placebo

double hearing protection combination of earplug and earmuff hearing protection devices, used during very-high-level noise exposures

down-beating nystagmus 1. vertical nystagmus in which the fast phase is downward; 2. pathologic down-beating vertical nystagmus, characterized by increased nystagmus velocity on downward gaze, consistent with central vestibular pathology

Down syndrome congenital genetic abnormality, characterized by mental retardation and characteristic facial features, with high incidence of chronic otitis media and associated conductive, mixed, and sensorineural hearing loss

download to transfer data from one digital system to another, as in downloading fitting parameters from a database into a hearing aid

downward spread of masking the masking of a low-frequency sound by an intense level of high-frequency sound; SYN: remote masking

DP 1. directional preponderance; 2. distortion product

DPHL dominant progressive hearing loss; genetic condition in which sensorineural hearing loss gradually worsens over a period of years, caused by dominant inheritance

DPOAE distortion-product otoacoustic emission; otoacoustic emission, measured as the cubic distortion product that occurs at the frequency represented by $2f_1 - f_2$, resulting from the simultaneous presentation of two pure tones (f_1 and f_2)

DPT Demerol, Phenergan, and Thorazine; drug mixture used for sedation of children undergoing evoked potential audiometry

DRC damage risk criterion; amount of exposure time to sound of a specified frequency and intensity that is associated with a defined risk of hearing loss

DRF Deafness Research Foundation; foundation that funds scientific research in hearing and deafness

DRG diagnosis-related group; one of major diagnostic categories into which patients are classified for the purpose of determining reimbursement levels

dri-aid kit a package of products compiled into a kit that are used to reduce moisture in hearing aids

drum COL: tympanic membrane

DS discrimination score; early term for word-recognition score, expressed as the percentage of words correctly perceived and identified

DSI dichotic sentence identification test; speech audiometric test of central auditory function in which different synthetic sentences are presented simultaneously to each ear

DSL desired sensation level; number of decibels above behavioral threshold necessary to amplify the long-term speech spectrum to a prescribed level across the frequency range

DSP digital signal processing; manipula-

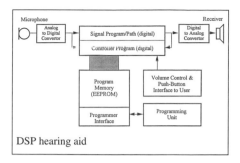

DSP hearing aid

tion by mathematical algorithms of a signal that has been converted from analog to digital form

DSP hearing aid   digital signal processing hearing aid that converts output from the microphone from analog to digital form, uses software algorithms to manipulate gain characteristics, and converts the signal back to analog form for delivery to the loudspeaker

dual in-line package switch   DIP switch; a row of integrated circuit switches that allows the same electronic instrument to be configured in different ways

dual-time-constant compression   output-limiting technique in some hearing aids in which the release time of a compression circuit varies as a function of the duration of the input signal

Duane retraction syndrome   autosomal dominant eye disorder, characterized by congenital paralysis of Cranial Nerve VI, with congenital sensorineural or conductive hearing loss

duct   tubular structure conducting any fluid

ductus reuniens   tube connecting the saccule to the scala media, carrying endolymph between the vestibular and auditory membranous labyrinths

dura mater   tough fibrous membrane that forms the outer envelope of the brain and spinal cord

duration   length of time

duty cycle   percentage of time that a signal is on out of the total duration of the signal plus intersignal interval

Dx   diagnosis; determination of the nature of disease or disorder

dynamic microphone   microphone consisting of a thin diaphragm that, as it moves, induces voltage in a coil in a magnetic field

dynamic platform posturography   quantitative assessment of the integrated function of the balance system for postural stability during quiet and perturbed stance; performed by a computer-based moving platform and motion transducers

dynamic range   1. amplitude range over which an electronic instrument operates; 2. the difference in decibels between a person's threshold of sensitivity and threshold of discomfort

dynamic-range compression   hearing aid compression algorithm with a low threshold of activation, designed to package signals between a listener's thresholds of sensitivity and discomfort level in a manner that matches loudness growth

dyne   unit of force, defined as the amount necessary to accelerate 1 gram a distance of 1 centimeter per second

dyne/cm^2   unit of force exerted on 1 square centimeter; the reference level for measuring decibels in sound pressure level is 0.0002 dynes/cm^2

dynorphin   endogenous opioid peptide found in the cochlea

dysacusia   disacusis

dysacusis   1. impairment in suprathreshold hearing ability; 2. ear pain or discomfort from exposure to sound

dysaudia   speech impairment secondary to hearing loss

dyschondroplasia   disorder in the development of early embryonic aggregation of cartilage cells, leading to deformities associated with arrested growth of the long bones; SYN: chondrodysplasia

dysfunction   abnormal functioning

dyslexia   impaired reading ability

dysmorphism   abnormality of shape

dysostosis   defective or incomplete ossification

dysphemia   communication disorder due to psychoneurosis

dysplasia   abnormal tissue development

dysplasia, Scheibe   developmental abnormality of the phylogenetically newer parts of the inner ear, specifically the cochlea and saccule, and sparing of the utricle and semicircular canals, with associated sensorineural hearing loss

E

E wave expectancy wave; event-related potential occurring between a warning stimulus and an imperative stimulus, associated with readiness to respond

E&E eyes and ears

EA educational age; grade-level-equivalent age of a student based on standardized achievement tests

EAA Educational Audiology Association; professional association of audiologists with a particular interest in the provision of audiologic services in the schools

EABR electrically evoked auditory brainstem response; ABR generated by electrical stimulation of the cochlea with either an extracochlear promontory electrode or a cochlear implant

EAC external auditory canal

EAM external auditory meatus; canal extending from the auricle to the tympanic membrane

EAP electrically evoked action potential; compound action potential generated by electrical stimulation of the cochlea with either an extracochlear promontory electrode or a cochlear implant

ear the organ of hearing, including the auricle, external auditory meatus, tympanic membrane, tympanic cavity and ossicles, and cochlear and vestibular labyrinth

ear, artificial standardized device used to couple the earphone of an audiometer to a sound level meter microphone for the purpose of calibrating an audiometer

ear, aviator's traumatic inflammation disorder of the middle ear caused by sudden changes in air pressure in the pneumatized spaces of the temporal bone on descent from high altitude; SYN: aerotitis media

ear, Aztec an auricle with no lobule; SYN: Cagot ear

ear, Blainville asymmetry in size or shape of the auricles

ear, boilermaker's early term for noise-induced hearing loss, after workers who were exposed to excessive noise levels for many years making or repairing boilers

ear, Cagot an auricle having no lobulus

ear, cauliflower thickening and malformation of the auricle following repeated trauma, commonly related to injury caused by the sport of wrestling

ear, Darwinian a pinna in which the upper border is not rolled over to form the helix

ear, external EE; outer ear consisting of the auricle, external auditory meatus, and lateral surface of the tympanic membrane

ear, far the aided ear in a test situation in which the signal is presented to the side of the head opposite the aided ear; ANT: near ear

ear, farmer's asymmetry in hearing sensitivity in farmers, apparently due to one ear being exposed to more tractor noise as they look back over their shoulder

ear, glue inflammation of the middle ear with thick, viscid, mucuslike effusion; SYN: mucoid otitis media

ear, inner structure comprising the sensory organs for hearing and balance, including the cochlea, vestibules, and semicircular canals

ear, middle portion of the hearing mechanism extending from the medial membrane of the tympanic membrane to the oval window of the cochlea, including the ossicles and middle ear cavity; serves as an impedance matching device of the outer and inner ears

ear, near the aided ear in a test situation in which the signal is presented to the same side of the head; ANT: far ear

ear, nontest in audiometry, the ear that is not intended to be the test ear, or the ear with masking

ear, outer peripheral-most portion of the auditory mechanism, consisting of the auricle, external auditory meatus, and lateral surface of the tympanic membrane; SYN: external ear

ear, scroll auricular deformity in which the rim is rolled forward and inward

ear, swimmer's colloquial term for diffuse red, pustular lesions surrounding hair follicles, usually due to gram-negative bacterial infection during hot, humid weather and often initiated by swimming; SYN: acute diffuse external otitis

ear advantage dominance of one ear over the other in processing information

ear bank a depository of temporal bones used for research and educational purposes

ear canal external auditory meatus

ear canal resonance enhancement of sound by passage through the external auditory meatus, typically centered near 3000 Hz

ear canal stenosis narrowed or constricted external auditory meatus

ear defenders ear protectors

ear effect, external EEE; influence of outer ear structures on the acoustic characteristics of sounds reaching the tympanic membrane

ear effect, ipsilateral phenomenon in which patients with left temporal lobe lesions score poorly on the right ear on dichotic measures as expected, but also score poorly on the left ear; this effect is not observed on the right ear in right temporal lobe lesions

ear impression cast made of the concha and ear canal for creating a customized earmold or hearing aid

ear inserts expandable cuff placed into the external auditory meatus to direct sound from an earphone into the ear canal

EAR plugs Etymotic Applied Research plugs; ear inserts made of an expandable material, designed to attenuate excessive noise levels

ear protection collective term for hearing protection devices, such as earplugs or muffs, used to attenuate excessive noise levels

ear protectors hearing protection devices, such as earplugs or muffs, used to attenuate excessive noise levels

ear trumpet early nonelectronic hearing instrument, often shaped like a trumpet, designed to amplify sound by collecting it through a large opening and directing it through a small passage to the ear canal

ear wax colloquial term for cerumen, the waxy secretion of the ceruminous glands in the external auditory meatus

earache pain in the ear; SYN: otalgia

eardrum thin, membranous vibrating tissue terminating the external auditory meatus and forming the major portion of the lateral wall of the middle ear cavity, onto which the malleus is attached; SYN: tympanic membrane

earhook portion of a behind-the-ear hearing aid that connects the case to the earmold tube and hooks over the ear

earhook, high-pass earhook containing a filter that attenuates hearing aid output below 2000 Hz to 3000 Hz

earhook, low-pass earhook on a behind-the-ear hearing aid, containing a filter that attenuates high frequencies and passes low frequencies

earlobe lower noncartilaginous portion of the external ear; SYN: lobule

Early Speech Perception test ESP test; test battery designed to assess the speech-perception ability of young children; includes a standard and low-verbal version with subtests for pattern perception, spondee identification, and word identification

earmold coupler formed to fit into the auricle that channels sound from the earhook of a hearing aid into the ear canal

earmold, canal type of earmold that uses only the canal portion of the ear impression with the helix and concha areas removed

earmold, canal-lock canal earmold with a fingerlike projection along the bottom of the concha to retain the earmold in place

earmold, continuous flow adapter CFA earmold; earmold with a constant interior tubing diameter designed to permit high-frequency amplification with a smooth frequency response

earmold, custom earmold made for a specific individual from an ear impression

earmold, extended-range type of non-occluding earmold with a large diameter bell canal, designed to extend high-frequency amplification

earmold, free-field type of nonoccluding earmold with a small bridge that holds the earmold tube to the concha ring and directs the tube into the ear canal

earmold, half-shell earmold consisting of a canal and thin shell, with a bowl extending only part of the way to the helix

earmold, hearing protection custom-made earmold designed to attenuate sound for protection against noise

earmold, Lybarger non-occluding earmold with a tube that has two diameters, creating a resonance above 4000 Hz

earmold, MCT minimal contact technology earmold; earmold designed to reduce the occlusion effect by limiting contact with the cartilaginous portion of the external auditory meatus and instead sealing around its perimeter at the medial tip

earmold, nonoccluding open earmold

earmold, open nonoccluding earmold with a small outside-diameter canal portion that allows unamplified low-frequency sound to pass around the mold and directs amplified sound through the canal portion tubing; used in high-frequency hearing loss and CROS fittings

earmold, resonator earmold in which the sound channel has been altered to enhance resonance in the high frequencies

earmold, shell debulked, but otherwise full-sized earmold used for high-gain hearing aids when an acoustic seal is essential

earmold, skeleton earmold in which the bowl has been cut out, leaving an outer concha rim, but retaining the portion that seals the external auditory meatus

earmold, standard conventional type of earmold with a bowl completely filling the concha

earmold, stock noncustomized earmold used mostly for demonstration or temporary use while a custom earmold is being made

earmold, tinnitus open style of earmold for use with a tinnitus masker

earmold, uplift specialized earmold for use by individuals with normal hearing and prolapsed ear canals, designed with a funnel-shaped bore for acoustic enhancement

earmold, wide-range earmold designed with the specific function of providing maximum acoustic enhancement at the higher frequencies around 5000 Hz

earmold acoustics the influence of an earmold's dimensions, such as bore length and diameter, on the spectral content of sound reaching the tympanic membrane

earmold block cotton or spongelike plug placed deeply in the external auditory meatus to protect the tympanic membrane from materials used in making earmold impressions

earmold bore hole in an earmold through which amplified sound is directed into the ear canal; SYN: sound bore

earmold impression cast made of the concha and ear canal for creating a customized earmold

earmold modification change in the structure of an earmold to alter the fit or the acoustic characteristics

earmold vent bore made in an earmold that permits the passage of sound and air particles into the otherwise blocked external auditory meatus, used for aeration of the canal and/or acoustic alteration

earmuffs circumaural hearing protection devices, consisting of rigid molded plastic earcups that seal around the ear via foam or fluid-filled cushions, designed to attenuate excessive noise levels

earphone transducer that converts electrical signals from an audiometer into sound delivered to the ear

earphone, circumaural headphone with cushions that encircle the pinna

earphone, insert earphone whose transducer is connected to the ear through a tube leading to an expandable cuff that is inserted into the external auditory meatus

earpiece early term for earmold, referring especially to the combined button receiver/earmold that was used with body-worn hearing aids

earplug hearing protection devices, made of any of various materials, that is placed into the external auditory meatus to attenuate excessive noise levels

earplug, hi-fi hearing protection device designed to attenuate sound equally across the frequency range to maintain high (hi) fidelity (fi) reproduction of sound, especially music

earplug, musician's hearing protection device designed to attenuate sound equally across the frequency range to maintain the fidelity of sound, especially music

echo a returned or reverberating sound

echo chamber room designed to produce high levels of reverberation

echoacousia subjective perception of repetition of a sound following its cessation

echoic pertaining to an echo

echolalia tendency of an individual to imitate speech sounds of another person without modification, occurring normally during speech development, but abnormally in adults with aphasia

echolocation determination of location of an object by detecting the deflections of an emitted sound off that object; used by bats naturally and by submarines for sonar detection

ECMO extracorporeal membrane oxygenation; therapeutic technique for augmenting ventilation in high-risk infants

ECochG, ECoG electrocochleography; method of recording transient AEPs from the cochlea and Cranial Nerve VIII, including the cochlear microphonic, summating potential, and compound action potential, with a promontory or ear-canal electrode

ectoderm outermost of the three primary embryonic layers

ectodermal dysplasia autosomal dominant facial-limb disorder, characterized by peculiar lobster-claw deformity of hands and feet, associated with small or malformed auricles, ossicular malformation, and conductive and sensorineural hearing loss

ectopic located other than in the normal place, as in ectopic salivary gland tissue in the middle ear

EDA electrodermal audiometry; method of determining hearing sensitivity in cases of suspected functional hearing loss by measuring psychogalvanic skin response to sound, following conditioning to the sound paired with a mild shock

edema abnormal accumulation of fluid in body tissue; swelling

edematous characterized by edema

education plan, individualized IEP; federally mandated, annually updated plan for the education of children with handicapping conditions

educational age EA; grade-level-equivalent age of a student based on standardized achievement tests

educational audiologist audiologist with a subspecialty interest in the hearing needs of school-age children in an academic setting

educational audiology audiology subspecialty devoted to the hearing needs of school-age children in an academic setting

Educational Audiology Association EAA; professional association of audiologists with a particular interest in the provision of audiologic services in the schools

Edward syndrome chromosomal abnormality, characterized by microcephaly, agenesis of bones of the extremities, congenital heart disease, craniofacial anomalies, and mental retardation, with associated outer, middle, and inner ear anomalies; SYN: trisomy 18 syndrome

EE external ear; outer ear consisting of the auricle, external auditory meatus, and lateral surface of the tympanic membrane

EEA electroencephalic audiometry; earliest use of electrophysiologic responses to predict hearing sensitivity, involving observation of changes in EEG patterns in response to auditory stimulation

EEE external ear effect; the influence of outer ear structures on the acoustic characteristics of sounds reaching the tympanic membrane

EEG electroencephalography; electroencephalogram

EENT eye, ear, nose, and throat; early term used to denote a physician with a specialty in diagnosis and treatment of diseases of the eye, ear, nose, and throat

EEPROM electrically erasable programmable read-only memory; computer memory used in many hearing devices for storing electroacoustic configurations

effective gain difference in decibels between hearing sensitivity thresholds with and without a hearing device; SYN: functional gain

effective masking EM; condition in which noise is just sufficient to mask a given signal when the signal and noise are presented to the same ear simultaneously

effective sound pressure level intensity level of sufficient magnitude to produce a specified response

effector peripheral tissue, such as a muscle or outer hair cell, that receives motor nerve impulses

efferent pertaining to the conduction of the descending nervous system tracts from central to peripheral; ANT: afferent

efferents, olivocochlear efferent fiber system of the olivocochlear bundles

effusion 1. escape of fluid into tissue or a cavity; 2. effused material

effusion, middle ear MEE; exudation of fluid from the membranous walls of the middle ear cavity, secondary to inflammation

effusion, mucoid thick, viscid, mucuslike fluid

effusion, purulent fluid containing pus

effusion, serous thin, watery, sterile fluid secreted by a mucous membrane

eighth cranial nerve eighth nerve

eighth nerve Cranial Nerve VIII, consisting of the auditory and vestibular nerves

eighth nerve tumor generic term referring to a neoplasm of Cranial Nerve VIII, most often a cochleovestibular Schwannoma; SYN: acoustic tumor

elastic reactance reduction of low-frequency vibrations due to stiffness of the vibrating object

elasticity restoring force of a material that causes components of the material to return to their original shape or location following displacement

electret microphone type of condenser microphone that uses a permanently charged material as the dielectric between the two polarized plates

electric response audiometry ERA; evoked response audiometry

electrical field area of electrical activity surrounding its source

electrical impedance opposition to the flow of electrical current, measured in ohms

electrical potential amount of available electromotive force

electrically evoked action potential EAP; compound action potential generated by electrical stimulation of the cochlea with either an extracochlear promontory electrode or a cochlear implant

electrically evoked auditory brainstem response EABR; auditory brainstem response generated by electrical stimulation of the cochlea with either an extracochlear promontory electrode or a cochlear implant

electrically evoked middle latency response EMLR; auditory middle latency response generated by electrical stimulation of the cochlea with either an extracochlear promontory electrode or a cochlear implant

electro-oculography EOG; electrical recording of corneoretinal potentials related to eye movement, used in electronystagmography testing

electroacoustic pertaining to the conversion of an electric signal to an acoustic signal or vice versa

electroacoustic analysis electronic measurement of various parameters of the acoustic output of a hearing aid

electrocardiographic response audiometry early electrophysiologic measure designed to predict hearing sensitivity by using an electrocardiogram to monitor changes in heart rate in response to sound stimulation; SYN: cardiac evoked response audiometry

electrocochleogram evoked potential recording obtained by electrocochleography

electrocochleography ECochG; method of recording transient auditory evoked potentials from the cochlea and Cranial Nerve VIII, including the cochlear microphonic, summating potential, and compound action potential, with a promontory or ear canal electrode

electrode specialized terminal or metal plate through which electrical energy is measured from or applied to the body

electrode, active 1. electrode that is attached to the positive-voltage, noninverting side of a differential amplifier; 2. vertex electrode in conventional auditory brainstem response recordings; COM: reference electrode, ground electrode

electrode, bipolar an electrode array with two poles that are active for recording or delivering electrical signals

electrode, common in electrophysiologic measurement, the electrode that attaches the patient to ground; SYN: ground electrode

electrode, ground in electrophysiologic measurement, the electrode that attaches the patient to ground; SYN: common electrode

electrode, inverting electrode that is attached to that side of a differential amplifier that inverts the input by 180; reference or earlobe electrode in conventional auditory brainstem response recordings

electrode, monopolar an electrode with one pole that is active for recording or delivering electrical signals

electrode, noninverting electrode that is attached to the positive-voltage side of a differential amplifier that does not invert the input; the active or vertex electrode in conventional auditory brainstem response recordings

electrode, reference inverting electrode attached to that side of a differential amplifier that inverts the input by 180°; earlobe electrode in conventional auditory brainstem response recordings; COM: active electrode

electrode, scalp noninvasive surface electrode attached to the scalp by conductive paste or gel

electrode, surface noninvasive electrode attached by conductive paste or gel to the skin

electrode, transtympanic needle electrode placed through the tympanic membrane onto the promontory of the middle ear cavity; used as a recording electrode in electrocochleography and stimulating electrode in promontory testing

electrode, vertex electrode that is placed at the top and center of the head; the noninverting or active electrode in conventional auditory brainstem response recordings; SYN: Cz electrode

electrode location location of electrode placement in auditory evoked potential testing, usually designated according to the 10–20 International Electrode System nomenclature, including left (A1) and right (A2) earlobes, vertex (Cz), and forehead (Fpz)

Electrode System, 10-20 International conventional system for describing electrode location on the scalp in evoked potential measurement, so named because each electrode is 10% or 20% of the distance between the nasion, the inion, and left and right pre-auricular points

electrodermal audiometry EDA; method of determining hearing sensitivity in cases of suspected functional hearing loss by measuring psychogalvanic skin response to sound, following conditioning to the sound paired with a mild shock

electroencephalic audiometry EEA; earliest use of electrophysiologic responses to predict hearing sensitivity, involving observation of changes in EEG patterns in response to auditory stimulation

electroencephalogram EEG; record obtained by electroencephalography

electroencephalograph instrument used to record electrical potentials of the brain from electrodes attached to the scalp

electroencephalography EEG; the recording of electrical potentials of the brain from scalp electrodes

electrolyte any solution that conducts electrical current and is decomposed by it

electromagnetic field area in which rapid periodic variation in an electrical field produces magnetic changes that can be transduced by induction coils, such as hearing aid telecoils

electromechanical transducer device, such as a bone vibrator, designed to convert electrical energy into mechanical energy

electromotility in hearing, changes in the length of outer hair cells in response to electrical stimulation

electromotive force pressure or potential difference producing the flow of an electrical current, measured in volts

electromyography EMG; recording of electrical activity generated by muscles

electronic erasable programmable read-only memory EEPROM; computer memory used in many hearing devices for storing electroacoustic configurations

electronystagmograph instrument designed to record eye movement during electronystagmography

electronystagmography ENG; method of measuring eye movements, especially nystagmus, via electro-oculography, to assess the integrity of the vestibular mechanism

electrophonic effect sensation of hearing resulting when an alternating electrical current is passed through the body

electrophysiologic response audiometry ERA; prediction of hearing sensitivity based on the recording of physiologic electrical potentials in response to auditory stimulation

electrostatic pertaining to static electricity

electrostatic microphone condenser microphone in which the variation of capacitance in response to sound level controls the electrical signal

elevated threshold absolute threshold that is poorer than normal and thus at a decibel level that is greater or elevated

elliptical recess small fossa in the vestibule containing the utricle

EM 1. effective masking; 2. environmental microphone

embolism occlusion or obstruction of a blood vessel by a transported clot or other mass

embolus a clot occluding a blood vessel

embryo an organism in its early, developing stage

embryonal rhabdomyosarcoma malignant neoplasm in young children, arising in many parts of the body including the middle ear, associated with bleeding from the ear or otorrhea

embryonic pertaining to an embryo or rudimentary stage of development

EMG electromyography; recording of electrical activity generated by muscles

eminence prominent portion on the surface of a bone

emission 1. a discharge; 2. otoacoustic emission from the cochlea

emission, otoacoustic OAE; low-level sound emitted by the cochlea, either spontaneously or as an echo or other sound evoked by an auditory stimulus, related to the function of the outer hair cells of the cochlea

EMLR electrically evoked middle latency response; auditory middle latency response generated by electrical stimulation of the cochlea with either an extracochlear promontory electrode or with a cochlear implant

empyema of mastoid type of acute mastoiditis, characterized by pus in the mastoid cavity

encephalic   pertaining to the brain

encephalitis   inflammation of the brain

encephalogram   the recording made by encephalography

encephalography   radiographic imaging of the brain

encephalomyelitis   acute inflammation of the brain and spinal cord

encephalon   brain

encephalopathy   any disorder of the brain

encoding   process of receiving and briefly registering information through the auditory system

end organ   1. terminal structure of a nerve fiber; 2. hair cells of the organ of Corti

end plate   complex ending of a motor nerve fiber at its junction with muscle tissue

endaural   within the ear, usually referring to the surface of the external auditory meatus

endemic   disease or condition that is continually prevalent in a region or among a group of people

endemic cretinism   type of congenital hypothyroidism resulting from failure of normal thyroid development during gestation, often accompanied by growth retardation, mental retardation, and mixed hearing loss

endocochlear potential   EP; electrical potential or voltage of endolymph in the scala media

endoderm   innermost of the three primary embryonic layers

endogenous   originating or produced within an organism or one of its parts

endogenous opiod peptides   neurotransmitters, such as enkephalins and dynorphins found in the cochlea, that have a variety of actions in the nervous system

endolymph   fluid in the scala media, having a high potassium and low sodium concentration, that bathes the gelatinous structures of the membranous labyrinth

endolymphatic duct   passageway in the vestibular aqueduct that carries endolymph between the endolymphatic sac and the utricle and saccule of the membranous labyrinth

endolymphatic fistula   unhealed rupture of the cochlear duct

endolymphatic hydrops   excessive accumulation of endolymph within the cochlear and vestibular labyrinths, resulting in fluctuating sensorineural hearing loss, vertigo, tinnitus, and a sensation of fullness

endolymphatic hydrops, contralateral delayed   endolymphatic hydrops occurring in two phases—an initial profound hearing loss in one ear followed by development of fluctuating hearing loss and episodic vertigo in the previously normal-hearing ear

endolymphatic hydrops, ipsilateral delayed   endolymphatic hydrops occurring in two phases—an initial profound hearing loss in one ear followed by development of episodic vertigo in the ear with the hearing loss

endolymphatic potential   electrical potential within the endolymphatic space and cells of approximately 70 millivolts to 90 millivolts positive relative to the perilymph

endolymphatic sac   saclike portion of the membranous labyrinth, connected via the endolymphatic duct, presumably responsible for absorption of endolymph

endolymphatic shunt   surgical technique designed to create a hole in the membranous labyrinth in order to relieve endolymphatic hydrops

endolymphatic space   middle of three channels of the cochlear duct that is filled with endolymph and contains the organ of Corti; SYN: scala media

endomastoiditis   inflammation of the interior of the mastoid cavity

endorphine   any of the opioidlike polypeptide neurotransmitters found in the brain

endosalpingitis   inflammation of the lining of the eustachian tube

endoscope   instrument designed to examine the interior of a canal or internal organ

endoscopy   examination with an endoscope of the interior of a canal or internal organ

endothelium   layer of squamous cells that line internal cavities of the body

ENG   electronystagmography; a method of measuring eye movements, especially nystagmus, via electro-oculography, to assess the integrity of the vestibular mechanism

Engelmann syndrome   autosomal dominant skeletal disorder associated with progressive sensorineural, mixed, or conductive hearing loss

engineering noise control   reduction of noise exposure by controlling workplace noise at the source by quieting the noise-generating machinery; COM: administrative noise control

enkephalin endogenous opiod peptide neurotransmitter found in the cochlea

ENT ear, nose, and throat

ENT physician ear, nose, and throat physician; medical specialist in the diagnosis and treatment of diseases of the ear, nose, and throat; SYN: otorhinolaryngologist, otolaryngologist

entoderm endoderm

envelope in acoustics, representation of a waveform as the smooth curve joining the peaks of the oscillatory function

environmental microphone EM; the microphone on a hearing aid that transduces airborne sound

EOAE evoked otoacoustic emission; otoacoustic emission that occurs in response to acoustic stimulation; COM: spontaneous otoacoustic emission

EOG electro-oculography; electrical recording of corneoretinal potentials related to eye movement used in electronystagmography testing

EP 1. endocochlear potential; 2. evoked potential

epicanthal fold vertical fold of skin extending from the root of the nose to the inner angle of the eye

epidemic parotitis contagious systemic viral disease, characterized by painful enlargement of parotid glands, fever, headache, and malaise, associated with sudden, permanent, profound unilateral sensorineural hearing loss; SYN: mumps, parotiditis

epidemiology study of disease in a population and the factors influencing its presence

epidermoid cholesteatoma or other cystic tumor arising from aberrant skin cells

epidermoid carcinoma cancerous neoplasms of the auricle, external auditory canal, middle ear, and/or mastoid

epidermoid cyst early term for cholesteatoma, describing a tumorlike mass of squamous epithelium and cholesterol in the middle ear

epineurium connective tissue encapsulating a nerve trunk

epiphenomenon unusual secondary consequence or symptom not necessarily associated with the circumstances it accompanies

episodic appearing in acute, repeated occurrences

epithelia, sensory in the ear, groups of sensory and supporting cells of the organ of Corti in the cochlea, the cristae ampullares

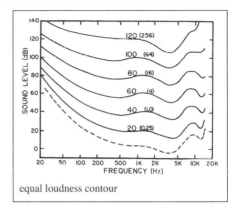

equal loudness contour

in the semicircular canals, and the maculae in the utricle and saccule

epithelial pertaining to epithelium

epithelium avascular cellular layer covering skin and mucous membrane

epitympanic above the tympanic membrane

epitympanic recess portion of the middle ear cavity located above the tympanic membrane; SYN: attic

epitympanum attic of the middle ear cavity

equal loudness contour loudness level curve representing sound pressure levels required to produce a given loudness across the frequency range for normal hearing at various phon levels

equalization in probe-microphone measures, the process of making the output sound pressure level equal across frequency in a soundfield

equilibrium the condition of being evenly balanced

equipotentiality capacity for developing to the same extent in the same way

equivalent input noise level magnitude of internal noise generated by a hearing aid

equivalent level Leq; equivalent sound level

equivalent level, day/night in sound-exposure analysis, a description of the intrusiveness of sound that differentiates between quieter hours of the night and busier hours of the day, attributing greater intrusiveness during quieter hours

equivalent sound level Leq; measurement of a time-varying sound, expressed as a time-weighted energy average, representing the total sound energy over a given time period as if the sound were unvarying; SYN: equivalent level

equivalent volume in immittance measurement, the translation of changes in probe-tone SPL into volume changes, so that an increase in SPL would appear as a decrease in equivalent volume of a cavity and a decrease in SPL would appear as an increase in equivalent volume

ER-3A insert earphones Etymotic Research insert earphones used in audiometry

ERA electric, electrophysiologic, or evoked response audiometry

erg unit of energy equal to the amount of work done by 1 dyne acting through a distance of 1 centimeter

erosive having the property of eroding or wearing away

ERP event-related potential; evoked potential elicited by an endogenous response to an external event, such as the P3 or CNV

erysipelas acute inflammatory disease of the skin, which can affect the external ear

erythema inflammatory redness of skin due to capillary dilatation

erythroblastosis fetalis abnormally large amount of bilirubin in the blood at birth, which is a risk factor for sensorineural hearing loss; SYN: hyperbilirubinemia

erythromycin lactobionate antibiotic agent, used to treat gram-positive bacterial infections, which may cause transient reversible sensorineural hearing loss in therapeutic doses

ESP Early Speech Perception test; test battery designed to assess the speech-perception ability of young children; includes a standard and low-verbal version with subtests for pattern perception, spondee identification, and word identification

ET eustachian tube; passageway leading from the nasopharynx to the middle ear, which opens to equalize middle ear air pressure

et al. [L. *et alii*] and others

ETD eustachian tube dysfunction; failure of the eustachian tube to open, usually due to edema in the nasopharynx

ethacrynic acid ototoxic loop diuretic, used in the treatment of edema caused by cardiac or renal disease and as an antihypertensive agent, which can cause reversible or permanent sensorineural hearing loss

etiologic pertaining to the cause of a disease or condition

etiology the study of the causes of a disease or condition

eust. eustachian

eustachian salpingitis inflammation of the eustachian tube

eustachian tube ET; passageway leading from the nasopharynx to the anterior wall of the middle ear, which opens to equalize middle ear air pressure; SYN: auditory tube

eustachian tube, patulous abnormally patent eustachian tube, resulting in sensation of stuffiness, autophony, tinnitus, and audible respiratory noises

eustachian tube dysfunction ETD; failure of the eustachian tube to open, usually due to edema in the nasopharynx

evaluation diagnostic assessment to describe nature and degree of a disorder

evaluation, hearing aid HAE; process of choosing suitable hearing aid amplification for an individual, based on measurement of acoustic properties of the amplification and perceptual response to the amplified sound

event, frequent in event-related potential measurement, the stimulus that occurs more often

event, rare in event-related potential measurement, the target stimulus that occurs less often

event-related potential ERP; evoked potential elicited by an endogenous response to an external event, such as the P3 or CNV

evoked otoacoustic emission EOAE; otoacoustic emission that occurs in response to acoustic stimulation; COM: spontaneous otoacoustic emission

evoked potential EP; electrical activity of the brain in response to sensory stimulation

evoked potential, auditory AEP; electrophysiologic response to sound, usually distinguished according to latency, including ECoG, ABR, MLR, LVR, SSEP, P3

evoked potential, somatosensory SEP; evoked electrical activity of the brain created by stimulation of the somatosensory system, usually by electrical stimulation over a peripheral nerve or the spinal cord

evoked potential, steady-state SSEP; auditory evoked potential in which the response waveform approximates the pattern of periodic stimulation, such as the stimulus rate or rate of stimulus modulation, e.g., 40-Hz response

evoked potential, transient auditory evoked potential of brief duration, occurring in response to a stimulus and ending prior to the next stimulus presentation; examples are the ECochG, ABR, AMLR, LLAEP; COM: steady-state evoked potential

evoked potentials, multimodality MEP; collective term referring to the sensory evoked potentials, including auditory, visual, and somatosensory electrophysiologic measures

evoked response audiometry ERA; electrophysiologic prediction of hearing sensitivity

evoked response audiometry, brainstem BERA; brainstem response audiometry

evoked response audiometry, cardiac CERA; electrophysiologic technique for predicting hearing sensitivity by measuring changes in heart rate in response to auditory stimulation

evoked response audiometry, cortical CERA; electrophysiologic technique for predicting hearing sensitivity by measuring late-latency auditory evoked responses to auditory stimulation

EWOK either way, okay; hearing aid circuit that automatically senses the polarity of a battery and reverses it if the battery has been inserted incorrectly

exacerbation an increase in the severity of a condition

exceedance level measurement of the impact on an acoustic environment of industrial noise, expressed as the percentage of time during which the sound in a particular environment exceeds a specified criterion

excise to remove a part or a foreign body by cutting

excitation pattern pattern of neural activity, as a function of characteristic frequency across neurons, evoked by sound of a specified frequency and intensity

exogenous originating outside the organism; ANT: endogenous

exostosis rounded hard bony nodule, usually bilateral and multiple, growing from the osseous portion of the external auditory meatus, caused by extended exposure to cold water; often found in divers or surfers

expansion in hearing aid circuitry, the in-

creasing of range of variation of the output in comparison to the input; ANT: compression

expectancy wave E wave; event-related potential occurring between a warning stimulus and an imperative stimulus, associated with readiness to respond

exponent numeric symbol expressing the number of times that a base is to be used as a factor

exposure, noise level and duration of noise to which an individual is subjected

exposure limits, permissible the highest intensity level in decibels to which an employee can be exposed for a specified duration of time and still meet occupational safety guidelines

extended high-frequency audiometer an audiometer that generates frequencies in excess of 8000 Hz

extended-range earmold type of non-occluding earmold with a large diameter bell canal, designed to extend high-frequency amplification

extended receiver tubing extension of the receiver tubing beyond a hearing aid casing to reduce feedback and to prevent cerumen accumulation

external outside, toward the outside

external acoustic meatus external auditory meatus

external auditory canal EAC; external auditory meatus

external auditory meatus EAM; canal extending from the auricle to the tympanic membrane

external canal external auditory meatus

external ear EE; outer ear consisting of the auricle, external auditory meatus, and lateral surface of the tympanic membrane

external ear effect EEE; influence of outer ear structures on the acoustic characteristics of sounds reaching the tympanic membrane

external noise noise source in a hearing aid resulting from anything before the microphone portion of the instrument; ANT: internal noise

external otitis inflammation of the lining of the external auditory meatus

external otitis, acute circumscribed reddened, pustular lesion surrounding a hair follicle, usually due to staphylococci infection during hot, humid weather; SYN: furunculosis

external otitis, acute diffuse diffuse reddened, pustular lesions surrounding hair follicles, usually due to gram-negative bacterial infection during hot, humid weather and often initiated by swimming; COL: swimmer's ear

external otitis, chronic diffuse inflammation of the external auditory meatus, characterized by itching and a persistent or recurring scaling or weeping dermatitis, caused by bacterial infection

external otitis, malignant severe bacterial inflammation of the temporal bone, beginning as a focal area of ulceration in the external auditory meatus, which may spread through the tympanic membrane to the middle ear and soft tissue of the mastoid space

external otitis media misnomer for external otitis

external radiating arterioles branch of the main cochlear artery that divides to form capillary networks supplying the scala vestibuli, Reissner's membrane, stria vascularis, spiral prominence, and spiral ligament

external vent type of earmold vent characterized by an external channel that runs along the length of the canal portion into the body of the mold

extirpation surgical removal

extra-axial outside the brainstem; ANT: intra-axial

extra-axial tumor lesion that originates outside the brainstem, e.g., cochleovestibular Schwannoma

extracorporeal membrane oxygenation ECMO; therapeutic technique for augmenting ventilation in high-risk infants

extraneous noise ambient or unwanted noise

extraocular muscles muscles located around the eye, including the lateral, medial, superior, and inferior rectus

extratympanic manometry early technique for measuring pressure changes in the external auditory meatus to monitor the acoustic stapedial reflex

extrinsic originating outside; ANT: intrinsic

extrinsic redundancy in speech audiometry, the abundance of information present in the speech signal; ANT: intrinsic redundancy

exudate fluid discharge

eye speed, vestibular VES; measure of nystagmus expressed as the speed of the slow phase: SYN: slow-phase velocity

eyeglass hearing aid early style of hearing aid built into one or both earpieces of eyeglass frames

F

f frequency

F statistic ratio of estimates of variance, such as analysis of variance and multiple regression analysis

f_0 fundamental frequency; principal or lowest component frequency of pattern repetition in the acoustic spectrum of a speech sound

$f_0/f_1/f_2$ **processing** cochlear implant processing strategy designed to extract frequency and amplitude estimates of f_1 and f_2 from a speech signal and deliver them to an electrode corresponding to each frequency band at a pulse rate equal to f_0

f_1 formant 1 or first formant; first frequency region above f_0 of prominent energy in the acoustic spectrum of a speech sound

f_2 formant 2 or second formant; second frequency region above f_0 of prominent energy in the acoustic spectrum of a speech sound

f_3 formant 3 or third formant; third frequency region above f_0 of prominent energy in the acoustic spectrum of a speech sound

FAAA Fellow of the American Academy of Audiology

faceplate portion of a custom hearing aid that faces outward, usually containing the battery door, microphone port, and volume control

facial canal channel of bone on the medial wall of the middle ear cavity through which the facial nerve passes; SYN: fallopian canal

facial diplegia bilateral facial paralysis

facial-hypoglossal anastomosis surgical procedure used to reinnervate the facial nerve following paralysis

facial nerve Cranial Nerve VII; cranial nerve that provides efferent innervation to the facial muscles and afferent innervation from the soft palate and tongue

facial nerve monitoring intraoperative EMG monitoring of facial nerve function, used to provide a warning if the facial nerve is stimulated during surgery

facial nerve palsy facial paralysis or paresis

facial nerve paralysis facial paralysis

facial numbness peculiar sensation of the face due to impaired cutaneous perception, associated with facial nerve disorder

facial palsy facial paralysis or paresis

facial palsy, infrachordal facial nerve paralysis or paresis caused by a lesion located inferior to the chorda tympani branch, not affecting taste, lacrimation, or the stapedial reflex

facial palsy, infrastapedial facial nerve paralysis or paresis due to a lesion located between the chorda tympanic branch and the stapedius muscle nerve, affecting taste, but not affecting the stapedial reflex or lacrimation

facial palsy, suprageniculate facial nerve paralysis or paresis due to a lesion located between the geniculate ganglion and motor nucleus, affecting taste, lacrimation, and the stapedial reflex

facial palsy, suprastapedial facial nerve paralysis or paresis due to a lesion located between the stapedius muscle nerve and the geniculate ganglion, affecting taste and the stapedial reflex, but not lacrimation

facial paralysis loss of voluntary movement of the face due to facial nerve disorder

facial paresis partial or incomplete loss of voluntary movement of the face due to facial nerve disorder

facial weakness paresis of the face due to facial nerve disorder

FACP Fellow of the American College of Physicians

FACS Fellow of the American College of Surgeons

factors, frequency utilization factors

factors, risk health, environmental, and lifestyle factors that enhance the likelihood of having or developing a specified disease or disorder

factors, utilization epidemiologic factors of a defined population that influence use of healthcare services

fading-numbers test obsolete group hearing test in which pairs of one-digit numbers were presented at successively lower intensity levels, via phonograph

failure-of-fixation test caloric stimulation ENG subtest, performed approximately 90 seconds after irrigation, in which nystagmus is measured with eyes closed and with eyes open and fixated; results are expressed as fixation index

faint-speech test early word-recognition

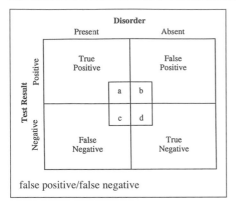

false positive/false negative

method of presenting monosyllabic targets at from 5 dB SPL to 15 dB SL

fall time time required for a gated signal to decrease to a specified percentage of its maximum amplitude; ANT: rise time

fallopian aqueduct facial canal

fallopian canal facial canal

false-alarm rate percentage of time that a diagnostic test is positive when no disorder exists; ANT: hit rate

false fundus membrane formed across the ear canal lateral to the tympanic membrane following chronic inflammation

false negative FN; F_{neg}; test outcome indicating the absence of a disease or condition when, in fact, that disease or condition exists

false-negative response in audiometry, failure to respond to an audible stimulus presentation

false paracusis apparent hearing improvement in noisy surroundings due to others speaking louder; SYN: paracusis willisi

false positive FP; F_{pos}; test outcome indicating the presence of a disease or condition when, in fact, that disease or condition is not present

false-positive response in audiometry, response to a nonexistent or inaudible stimulus presentation

familial deafness deafness occurring in members of the same family

familial goiter form of congenital hypothyroidism caused by defects in thyroid biosynthesis; may be accompanied by sensorineural hearing loss, as in the case of Pendred syndrome

family service plan, individualized IFSP; federally mandated, annually updated plan for the education of preschool children

with handicapping conditions and their families

FAP fluorouracil, adriamycin, platinol (cisplatin); potentially ototoxic chemotherapy regimen used in the treatment of esophageal cancer

far ear the aided ear in a test situation in which the signal is presented to the side of the head opposite the aided ear; ANT: near ear

far field in an audiometric test booth, the area that is far enough from the sound source for the inverse square law to prevail

far field recording measurement of evoked potentials from electrodes on the scalp at a distance from the source

farad unit of electrical capacity

farmer's ear asymmetry in hearing sensitivity in farmers, apparently due to one ear being exposed to more tractor noise as they look back over their shoulder

fascia fibrous tissue that envelops the body beneath the skin, encloses muscles, and separates their layers

fascia temporalis tissue covering the temporal muscle

fasciculus band or bundle of nerve or muscle fibers

fast Fourier transformation FFT; rapid algorithm for determining the Fourier transform, or the spectrum of frequency components of a waveform

fast phase component of nystagmus that represents the saccadic system of eye movement control required to reposition a visual target on the retinal fovea; ANT: slow phase

fasting blood glucose blood test to determine disorders of blood sugar (glucose) metabolism, such as severe diabetes

fatigue, auditory a reduction in responsiveness of the auditory sensory receptors following exposure to prolonged or intense acoustic stimulation; SYN: temporary threshold shift

fatigue, perstimulatory auditory adaptation, or the reduction in loudness or audibility of sound, during prolonged stimulation

fatigue, poststimulatory temporary change in hearing sensitivity following exposure to sound; SYN: temporary threshold shift

FBL fitting by loudness; fitting strategy for hearing aids with dynamic-range compression, based on measures of loudness growth, prediction of loudness growth, or assumption of average loudness growth

FCC Federal Communication Commission; U.S. government agency whose responsibilities include regulating radio waves over which FM systems broadcast

FCE fluorouracil-cisplatin-etoposide; potentially ototoxic chemotherapy regimen used in treatment of gastric cancer

FDA Food and Drug Administration; U.S. government agency whose responsibilities include regulating medical devices such as hearing aids

FDC fluorouracil-doxorubicin-cisplatin; potentially ototoxic chemotherapy regimen used in treatment of gastric cancer

FDL frequency difference limen; smallest difference in frequency of a signal that can be detected

Fechner's law law of psychophysics that describes the direct proportionality between the magnitude of loudness and acoustic sound pressure level in decibels

Federal Communication Commission FCC; U.S. government agency whose responsibilities include regulating radio waves over which FM systems broadcast

fee-for-service traditional healthcare payment system in which reimbursement is made to a provider for each service provided

feedback, acoustic sound produced when an amplification system goes into oscillation, produced by amplified sound from the receiver reaching the microphone and being re-amplified; e.g., hearing aid squeal

feedback, auditory perception of one's own vocalizations

feedback, internal in a hearing aid, abnormal acoustic feedback occurring within the instrument's casing

Fehr corneal dystrophy autosomal recessive eye disorder associated with progressive sensorineural hearing loss of delayed onset; SYN: Harboyan syndrome

feigned deafness functional or exaggerated hearing loss

fence upper or lower boundary

fence, low lowest dB level designated to be substantial enough to be considered a hearing loss, usually expressed as the pure-tone average of thresholds obtained at 500 Hz, 1000 Hz, and 2000 Hz

fenestra anatomical aperture or small opening

fenestra cochleae fenestra rotunda

fenestra ovalis opening in the labyrinthine wall of the middle ear space, leading into the scala vestibuli of the cochlea, into which the footplate of the stapes fits; SYN: oval window, fenestra vestibuli; COM: vestibular window

fenestra rotunda round opening on the medial wall of the middle ear leading into the cochlea covered by the round window membrane; SYN: round window, cochlear window, cochlear fenestra

fenestra tympanica fenestra rotunda

fenestra vestibuli fenestra ovalis

fenestration an opening

fenestration operation early surgical procedure in which an opening in the otic capsule was created in cases of otosclerosis

Feré effect change in electrical resistance of the skin in response to an external stimulus

fetal of or pertaining to the fetus

fetal alcohol syndrome syndrome in children of women who abuse alcohol during pregnancy, characterized by low birthweight, failure to thrive, and mental retardation, associated with recurrent otitis media and sensorineural hearing loss

FFR 1. fixed frequency response; 2. frequency following response

FFS failure of fixation suppression; failure of visual fixation to suppress nystagmus in ENG measurement

FFT fast Fourier transformation; rapid algorithm for determining the Fourier transform, or spectrum of frequency components of a waveform

FG functional gain; difference in decibels between aided and unaided hearing sensitivity thresholds

FHL functional hearing loss; hearing loss that is exaggerated or feigned

fiber threadlike structure

fiber, nerve axon or dendrite of a neuron

fiber of Corti anatomic structures that form the tunnel of Corti

fibrocartilage elastic cartilage of predominantly white fibrous tissue, which constitutes the main structure of the pinna

fibrocystic sclerosis proliferation of fibrous tissue and cyst formation, which can obliterate the pneumatized spaces of the temporal bone

fibroma benign neoplasm developed from fibrous connective tissue

fibroproliferation, tympanic membrane proliferation of fibrous tissue growth in the submucosal and subcutaneous layers of the tympanic membrane, resulting from chronic inflammation, causing thickening and stiffness

fibroproliferative external otitis chronic diffuse outer ear bacterial inflammation, characterized by narrowing of the lumen of the canal

fibrosis proliferation of fibrous tissue

fibrotic drum tympanic membrane with reduced function due to the formation of fibrous tissue

fidelity, high faithful reproduction of sound with minimal distortion

field in acoustics, the area over which sound waves are distributed

field reference point in probe-microphone measurements, the location of the sound inlet of the reference microphone during equalization or measurement

fifth cranial nerve Cranial Nerve V; trigeminal nerve that provides motor innervation to the muscles of mastication and sensory innervation from the front of the head

Fig6 algorithm for fitting nonlinear hearing aids that have wide-dynamic-range compression, in which fitting curves are calculated for low, moderate, and high-level sounds based on a patient's audiometric thresholds

figure-ground perception of one aspect of a sensory input as the foreground or figure and all other aspects as the background or ground

figure-ground, auditory relation of relevant acoustic information to competing background noise

filter in acoustics, a device that differentially enhances and attenuates certain frequencies, thereby modifying the spectrum of the signal

filter, active filter circuit in which the response varies with gain of the amplifier

filter, adaptive high-frequency nonlinear automatic signal processing circuit in a hearing aid in which gain at high frequencies decreases as input level increases; SYN: BILL

filter, adaptive low-frequency nonlinear automatic signal processing circuit in a hearing aid in which gain at low frequencies decreases as input level increases; SYN: TILL

filter, anti-aliasing low-pass filter designed to reduce aliasing distortion that can occur in the conversion of a signal from analog to digital form

filter, band-pass an electronic filter that allows a specified band of frequencies to pass, while reducing or eliminating frequencies above and below the band

filter, digital software algorithm that reduces selected frequencies of a signal

filter, high-cut SYN: low-pass filter; high-frequency filter; ANT: high-pass filter

filter, high-frequency low-pass filter, attenuating the higher frequencies

filter, high-pass bandpass filter that attenuates low frequencies and allows high frequencies to pass; SYN: low-frequency filter; ANT: low-pass filter

filter, low-cut SYN: high-pass filter; low-frequency filter; ANT: low-pass filter

filter, low-frequency high-pass filter, attenuating the lower frequencies

filter, low-pass bandpass filter that attenuates high frequencies and allows low frequencies to pass; SYN: high-frequency filter; ANT: high-pass filter

filter, narrow-band an electronic filter that allows a specified band of frequencies to pass through while reducing or eliminating frequencies above and below the band; SYN: band-pass filter

filter, notch filtering network that removes a discrete portion of the frequency range, used in evoked potential measurement to remove 60-Hz noise and in hearing aids to limit amplification in a discrete frequency region of better hearing

filter, octave filter in which the upper bandpass limit is twice the frequency of the lower limit

filter, passband an electronic filter that allows a specified band of frequencies to pass, while reducing or eliminating frequencies above and below the band; SYN: band-pass filter

filter, passive filter circuit in which the response is constant, regardless of amplifier gain

filter, sintered small container of partially fused metal particles that can be controlled to provide attenuation of specific frequency ranges

filter, switched capacitor integrated circuit filter system that permits a variety of filtering characteristics, including low-pass, high-pass, band-pass, and notched

filter, third-octave filter that passes a frequency band with a width of one-third octave

filter skirt rate of attenuation of a filter, expressed in dB per octave

filtered speech test test of word recognition in which the target words have been low-pass filtered at around 800 Hz in an effort to reduce the extrinsic redundancy of the signal

FIM functional independence measures; collective assessment of an individual's capacity to function independently

fingerspelling form of manual communication in which each letter of the alphabet is represented by a different position or movement of the fingers

first-order neuron nerve fiber carrying information from a sensory end organ to the point of its first synaptic connection; in the auditory system, first-order neurons emanate from the cochlear hair cells and terminate at the cochlear nucleus

fissure cleft or slit

fistula an abnormal passage formed within the body by disease, surgery, injury, or other defect

fistula, endolymphatic unhealed rupture of the cochlear duct

fistula, perilymphatic abnormal passageway between the perilymphatic space and the middle ear, resulting in the leak of perilymph at the oval or round window; caused by congenital defects or trauma

fistula, round window passageway between the perilymphatic space and the middle ear occurring at the round window, caused by congenital defects or trauma; results in leak of perilymph

fistula auris congenita congenital fistula of the auricle

fistula test diagnostic test, designed to detect labyrinthine fistulae, in which the air pressure in the external auditory meatus is changed to determine if nystagmus can be elicited

fistulize to surgically create a passage in a structure

fitting 1. the process of selecting hearing aid characteristics; 2. the characteristics of a hearing aid that represent the end result of the hearing aid selection process

fitting, prescriptive strategy for fitting hearing aids by the calculation of a desired gain and frequency response, based on any

of a number of formulas that incorporate pure-tone audiometric thresholds and may incorporate uncomfortable loudness information

fitting, reverse curve hearing aid gain and frequency response shaped to fit a rising hearing loss configuration in which low-frequency hearing sensitivity is poorer than high-frequency sensitivity

fitting by loudness FBL; fitting strategies for hearing aids with dynamic-range compression, based on measures of loudness growth, prediction of loudness growth, or assumption of average loudness growth

fitting range range of hearing loss for which a specific hearing aid circuit, configuration, earmold, etc. is appropriate

Fitzgerald Key early aural rehabilitation technique for teaching grammar and syntax by providing visible sentence patterns and symbols to represent the various parts of speech

5-dB rule hearing conservation rule stating that intensity level of sound can be increased by 5 dB for every 50% reduction in the duration of exposure to that sound

fixation firm attachment; held in a fixed position

fixation, stapes immobilization of the stapes at the oval window, often due to new bony growth resulting from ototsclerosis

fixation index index used in failure-of-fixation caloric measurement, expressed as the ratio of slow-phase velocity of nystagmus with eyes open to slow-phase velocity with eyes closed

fixation suppression in ENG assessment, reduction or elimination of nystagmus by visual fixation

fixed-frequency audiometry the use of Békésy or automatic audiometry to track sensitivity threshold at a single, fixed frequency; COM: sweep-frequency audiometry

fixed-frequency response FFR; subgroup of automatic signal processing techniques that includes compression limiting and wide-dynamic-range compression, wherein gain is automatically increased or decreased in response to input, regardless of input frequency

flaccid limp or weak; lacking in stiffness

flaccid portion refers to flaccid section of the tympanic membrane; SYN: pars flaccida, Shrapnell's membrane

flat audiogram audiogram configuration

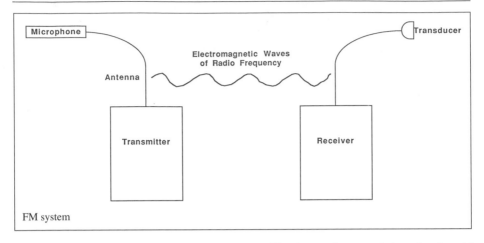

FM system

in which hearing sensitivity is similar across the audiometric frequency range

flat response flat-frequency response; amplification that is equal across a given frequency range

flat-spectrum noise noise with equal energy content across a continuous band of frequencies

Fletcher-Munson curves equal loudness contours

fluctuating hearing loss loss of hearing sensitivity, characterized by aperiodic change in degree

flutter-fusion the perception of an interrupted signal as being continuous when the rate of interruption exceeds a fusion threshold

flux discharge of energy or material

FM frequency modulation; the process of creating a complex signal by sinusoidally varying the frequency of a carrier wave; COM: amplitude modulation

FM amplification system FM system

FM auditory trainer classroom amplification system in which a remote microphone/transmitter worn by the teacher sends signals via FM to a receiver worn by the student

FM boot small bootlike device containing an FM receiver that attaches to the bottom of a behind-the-ear hearing aid

FM system an assistive listening device, designed to enhance signal-to-noise ratio, in which a remote microphone/transmitter worn by a speaker sends signals via FM to a receiver worn by a listener

FM system, coupled personal FM amplification receiver coupled to a hearing aid telecoil by a neckloop

FM system, personal a wearable assistive listening device consisting of a remote microphone/transmitter worn by a speaker that sends signals via FM to a receiver worn by a listener; designed to enhance the signal-to-noise ratio

FN 1. facial nerve; 2. false negative

F$_{neg}$ false negative; test outcome indicating the absence of a disease or condition when, in fact, that disease or condition exists

focal capillary hyperplasia proliferation of small blood vessels within the trunk of Cranial Nerve VIII in the internal auditory meatus, resulting in an enlargement of the nerve trunk

focal CROS subtype of CROS hearing aid arrangement in which a tube is used to channel sound from the concha of the unaided ear into a microphone on the same side

FOG full-on gain; hearing aid setting that produces maximum acoustic output

foil one of a set of targeted words, sentences, or other stimulus choices available in a multiple-choice format

Food and Drug Administration FDA; U.S. government agency whose responsibilities include regulating medical devices such as hearing aids

footplate base of the stapes that fits in the oval window

footplate fixation disorder in which the stapes footplate is fixed to bone surrounding the oval window

foramen   natural opening through bone

foramen, stylomastoid   opening in the temporal bone through which the facial nerve and stylomastoid artery pass

forced-choice paradigm   psychophysical procedure in which the subject is forced to choose one condition or item from among two or more

forensic audiology   audiology subspecialty devoted to legal proceedings related to hearing loss and noise matters

fork, tuning   a two-pronged metal fork that, when struck, produces a specific tonal frequency

formant   region of prominent energy in the acoustic spectrum of a speech sound

formant 1 f_1; first frequency region above f_0 of prominent energy in the acoustic spectrum of a speech sound

formant 2 f_2; second frequency region above f_0 of prominent energy in the acoustic spectrum of a speech sound

formant 3 f_3; third frequency region above f_0 of prominent energy in the acoustic spectrum of a speech sound

formant frequencies   frequency regions at which acoustic energy of speech is concentrated, usually designated f_0, f_1, f_2, etc.

formant transition   period of rapid frequency change in a formant

forward masking   form of temporal masking in which a noise preceding a tone acts to mask that tone, even though the sounds are not presented simultaneously

fossa   a groove, depression, or hollow

fossa incudis   recess in the middle ear that forms the depression into which the short crus of the incus is fitted

Fourier analysis   Fourier transform

Fourier series   graphic representation of a Fourier transform

Fourier transform   mathematical algorithm for decomposing a waveform into its amplitude and phase components, providing the amplitude of specific frequency components that make up a complex waveform; SYN: Fourier analysis

FP   false positive

F_{pos}   false positive; test outcome indicating the presence of a disease or condition when, in fact, that disease or condition is not present

Fpz   frontoproximal (Fp) midline (z) electrode location, or forehead electrode, typically used for ground-electrode placement in auditory evoked potential testing, according to the 10–20 International Electrode System nomenclature

fracture   fx; breaking of a bone or cartilage

fracture, longitudinal   linear break that courses longitudinally through the temporal bone, often tearing the tympanic membrane and disrupting the ossicles, typically caused by a blow to the parietal or temporal regions of the skull

fracture, transverse   a break that traverses the temporal bone perpendicular to the long axis of the petrous pyramid; usually caused by a blow to the occipital region of the skull, resulting in extensive destruction of the membranous labyrinth

free field   a sound field undisturbed by the effects of boundaries or objects, e.g., an anechoic chamber

free-field earmold   type of nonoccluding earmold with a small bridge that holds the earmold tube to the concha ring and directs the tube into the ear canal

free-field-to-eardrum transfer function   effects of the torso, head, and external ear on an acoustic signal as it is transferred from the free field to the tympanic membrane

fremitus   vibration felt by placing the hand on the chest or other part of the body during vocalization

Frenzel glasses   Frenzel lenses; glasses with specialized lenses that suppress optical fixation; used for observing eye movement during caloric vestibular testing

frequencies, reference test   frequencies of 1000 Hz, 1600 Hz, and 2500 Hz at which reference test gain is established

frequencies, speech   audiometric frequencies at which a substantial amount of speech energy occurs, conventionally considered to be 500 Hz, 1000 Hz, and 2000 Hz

frequency   the number of times a repetitive event occurs in a specified time period; e.g., for a sine wave, the number of periods occurring in 1 second, expressed as cycles per seconds or Hertz (Hz)

frequency, basic   fundamental frequency

frequency, center   frequency at the center of a bandwidth

frequency, characteristic   CF; the frequency to which an auditory nerve fiber is most sensitive

frequency, crossover   1. in speech audiometry, the frequency above and below which is found equal information for accurate perception; 2. in hearing aids, the frequency that distinguishes two adjacent bands

frequency, fundamental f_0; principal or lowest component frequency of pattern repetition in the acoustic spectrum of a speech sound

frequency, high HF; nonspecific term referring to frequencies above approximately 2000 Hz

frequency, low LF; nonspecific term referring to frequencies below around 1000 Hz

frequency, mid nonspecific term referring to frequencies around 1000 Hz to 2000 Hz

frequency, natural frequency at which a secured mass will vibrate most readily when set into free vibration; SYN: resonant frequency

frequency, Nyquist frequency equal to one-half of the analog-to-digital sampling rate, determining the highest frequency that can be sampled without distortion from aliasing

frequency, resonant frequency at which a secured mass will vibrate most readily when set into free vibration; SYN: natural frequency

frequency analyzer a sound level meter with bandpass filters used to determine the level of each frequency band of a complex sound; SYN: spectrum analyzer

frequency control potentiometer or other controlling device on a hearing aid that changes the frequency response; SYN: tone control

frequency-dependent compression hearing aid compression whose activation threshold varies by frequency

frequency difference limen FDL; difference limen for intensity; smallest difference in frequency of a signal that can be detected

frequency discrimination ability to distinguish test signals of different frequencies presented consecutively

frequency factors epidemiologic factors of a defined population that influence use of healthcare services; SYN: utilization factors

frequency following response FFR; short-latency auditory evoked potential of the same frequency as the low-frequency tone burst used to elicit the response

frequency formant frequency region at which acoustic energy of speech is concentrated

frequency-independent compression hearing aid compression whose activation threshold is the same at all frequencies

frequency-modulated tone sinusoidal signal whose frequency varies at a fixed rate; SYN: warble tone

frequency modulation FM; the process of creating a complex signal by sinusoidally varying the frequency of a carrier wave; COM: amplitude modulation

frequency range, audible range of frequencies that can be heard, which, in young humans, is from approximately 15 Hz to 20,000 Hz

frequency range, HAIC standard developed by HAIC to describe the range of frequencies of a hearing aid response

frequency resolution the ability to distinguish among sounds of different frequencies presented simultaneously

frequency-resolving power the capacity of a system to separate or differentiate among frequencies

frequency response output characteristics of a hearing aid, expressed as gain as a function of frequency

frequency response, adaptive hearing aid circuitry technique in which frequency response changes as input level changes

frequency response, fixed FFR; subgroup of automatic signal processing techniques, including compression limiting and wide-dynamic-range compression, wherein gain is automatically increased or decreased in response to input, regardless of input frequency

frequency response, flat amplification that is equal across a given frequency range

frequency response, level-dependent LDFR; automatic signal processing that alters the frequency response of a hearing aid as a function of input level

frequency selectivity the ability to discriminate among sounds of different frequencies in the presence of competing masking or other frequencies

frequency shaping the process of deriving selective amplification of some frequencies over others to match the configuration of a hearing loss

frequency theory theory of pitch perception that explains low-frequency processing based on the frequency of neural impulses in the auditory nerve

frequency transposer circuitry that converts frequency components of a waveform from one range into another range

frequency transposition hearing aid hearing device designed to transpose higher frequency energy into lower frequency amplification, designed for use in patients with corner audiograms

frequent event in event-related potential measurement, the stimulus that occurs more often; ANT: rare event

fricative speech sound generated by friction of air through a restricted opening, such as [f], and [s]

Friedrich ataxia autosomal recessive nervous system disorder characterized by progressive spinocerebellar ataxia, associated with progressive sensorineural hearing loss of delayed onset

front-end noise source of noise located in the microphone, pre-amplifier, or volume control of a hearing aid

front routing of signals FROS; eyeglass hearing aid in which the microphone is placed near the front of the glasses and routed back to the amplifier at the ear

frontal plane anatomic plane of reference that divides a structure into anterior (front) and posterior (back) portions; SYN: coronal plane

FROS front routing of signals; eyeglass hearing aid in which the microphone is placed near the front of the glasses and routed back to the amplifier at the ear

Fsp algorithm used to estimate the likelihood of the presence of an auditory evoked potential, based on the F distribution of the variance of the averaged evoked potential divided by the variance of a single point (sp) in time across successive samples

FTLB full-term live birth

FTNB full-term newborn

FTND full-term normal delivery

FTNSD full-term normal spontaneous delivery

FU follow up

full-dynamic-range compression wide-dynamic-range compression

full-on gain FOG; hearing aid setting that produces maximum acoustic output

full-term descriptive of a pregnancy of normal length; not premature

function, input/output I/O function; curve that plots output intensity level as a function of input intensity level; used to describe the gain characteristics of an amplifier

function, performance-intensity PI function; graph of percentage-correct speech-recognition scores as a function of presentation level of the target signals

functional 1. pertaining to a function; 2. working appropriately; 3. not organic or caused by a structural defect

functional disorder dysfunction in the absence of any known organic cause

functional gain FG; difference in decibels between aided and unaided hearing sensitivity thresholds

functional hearing loss FHL; hearing loss that is exaggerated or feigned

functional independence measures FIM; collective assessment of an individual's capacity to function independently

functional overlay 1. exaggeration of an organic disorder; 2. non-organic consequence of an organic disorder

fundamental fundamental frequency, or the lowest frequency in a periodic wave

fundamental frequency f_0; principal or lowest component frequency of pattern repetition in the acoustic spectrum of a speech sound

furosemide ototoxic loop diuretic used in the treatment of edema or hypertension, which can cause sensorineural hearing loss secondary to degeneration of the stria vascularis; SYN: Lasix

furunculosis reddened, pustular lesion surrounding a hair follicle, usually due to staphylococci infection during hot, humid weather; SYN: acute circumscribed external otitis

fusiform cells spindle-shaped cell type within the dorsal cochlear nucleus

fusion, auditory process by which interrupted sound is perceived as continuous

fusion, binaural 1. phenomenon wherein different sounds presented to the two ears fuse into a single sound image somewhere in the head; 2. integration of simultaneous but different speech signals presented to the two ears

Fx fracture

G

G conductance; ease of energy flow associated with resistance; reciprocal of resistance

GABA gamma-aminobutyric acid; inhibitory neurotransmitter present throughout the auditory system

GAD glutamic acid decarboxylase; amino acid neurotransmitter, which synthesizes GABA and is concentrated in the dorsal cochlear nucleus

gain 1. in hearing aids, the amount in dB by which the output level exceeds the input level; 2. in evoked potentials, the amount of amplification of the input EEG activity; 3. in rotary chair testing, the ratio of peak eye velocity to peak chair velocity

gain, acoustic 1. increase in sound output; 2. in a hearing aid, the difference in dB between the input to the microphone and the output of the receiver

gain, effective difference in dB between hearing sensitivity thresholds with and without a hearing device; SYN: functional gain

gain, full-on FOG; hearing aid setting that produces maximum acoustic output

gain, functional FG; difference in dB between aided and unaided hearing sensitivity thresholds

gain, HAIC standard developed by HAIC describing average hearing aid gain, calculated as the average of gain at 500 Hz, 1000 Hz, and 2000 Hz

gain, HFA full-on high-frequency average full-on gain; an ANSI hearing aid specification, derived by calculating the HFA output to a 50-dB-SPL or 60-dB-SPL input with the hearing aid adjusted to its full-on gain setting

gain, insertion hearing aid gain, defined as the difference in gain with and without a hearing aid

gain, peak acoustic amount of gain at a point along the frequency response of a hearing aid at which gain is maximal

gain, prescribed gain and frequency response of a hearing aid determined by any of several prescriptive formulas

gain, real-ear nonspecific term referring generally to the gain of a hearing aid at the tympanic membrane, measured as the difference between the SPL in the ear canal and the SPL at the field reference point for a specified sound field

gain, real-ear aided REAG; measurement of the difference, in dB as a function of frequency, between the SPL in the ear canal and the SPL at a field reference point for a specified sound field with the hearing aid in place and turned on

gain, real-ear insertion REIG; probe-microphone measurement of the difference, in dB as a function of frequency, between the real-ear unaided gain and the real-ear aided gain at the same point near the tympanic membrane

gain, real-ear occluded REOG; probe-microphone measurement of the difference, in dB as a function of frequency, between the SPL in the ear canal and the SPL at a field reference point for a specified sound field with a hearing aid in place and turned off

gain, real-ear unaided REUG; probe-microphone measurement of the difference, in dB as a function of frequency, between the SPL in an unoccluded ear canal and the SPL at the field reference point for a specified sound field

gain, reference test ANSI standard gain level with a 60-dB-SPL input and the volume control of the hearing aid adjusted so that the gain at the reference test frequencies is 17 dB less than that at SSPL-90

gain, reserve the remaining gain in a hearing aid; the difference between use gain and the gain at which feedback occurs

gain, unity gain of 1 dB of output for every 1 dB of input

gain, use amount of gain provided by a hearing aid with the volume control adjusted to the setting at which it is typically worn

gain control manual or automatic control designed to adjust the output level of a hearing instrument; SYN: volume control

gain control, automatic AGC; nonlinear hearing aid compression circuitry designed to automatically change gain as signal level changes or limit output when signal level reaches a specified criterion; SYN: automatic volume control

gain control, preset secondary gain control in a hearing aid, which is inaccessible to the wearer, that can be manipulated by the fitter to limit the range of amplification available to the wearer

gain prefitting the use of probe-microphone measurement prior to ordering a custom hearing device to provide individual corrections to the desired coupler values for gain and output

gain selection prescriptive and other approaches for specifying gain and frequency response of a hearing aid

gain target, prescriptive the desired gain and frequency response of a hearing aid, generated by a formula, against which the actual output of a hearing aid is compared

galvanic pertaining to an electric current

galvanic skin response GSR; change in skin resistance as a result of an emotional response to a stimulus; SYN: psychogalvanic skin response

galvanic skin response audiometry method of determining hearing sensitivity in cases of suspected functional hearing loss by measuring psychogalvanic skin response to sound, following conditioning to the sound paired with a mild shock; SYN: electrodermal audiometry

gamete 1. any germ cell; 2. one of two cells undergoing conjugation

gamma-aminobutyric acid GABA; inhibitory neurotransmitter present throughout the auditory system

ganglia masses of cell bodies in the peripheral nervous system

ganglia, acousticovestibular embryologic precursor to the vestibular and auditory ganglia

ganglia, auditory cell bodies of the auditory nerve fibers, clustered in the modiolus; SYN: spiral ganglia

ganglia, basal large subcortical nuclei of the cerebrum, including the caudate and lentiform nuclei of the corpus striatum and the amygdaloid nuclear complex

ganglia, geniculate cell bodies of the sensory branch of Cranial Nerve VII

ganglia, Scarpa's two adjacent cell-body masses of the peripheral vestibular neurons, located in the internal auditory canal, associated with the superior and inferior divisions of the vestibular nerve portion of Cranial Nerve VIII; SYN: vestibular ganglia

ganglia, spiral cell bodies of the auditory nerve fibers, clustered in the modiolus; SYN: auditory ganglia

ganglia, vestibular two adjacent cell-body masses of the peripheral vestibular neurons, located in the internal auditory canal, associated with the superior and inferior divisions of the vestibular nerve portion of Cranial Nerve VIII; SYN: Scarpa's ganglia

gap detection test of temporal processing, designed to assess the shortest pause that a subject can perceive between test signals

garamycin gentamicin

gated signal signal that is turned on and off in a specified manner

Gault's reflex eyeblink or twitch at the canthus caused by a sudden loud sound; SYN: auropalpebral reflex

gaussian noise noise with equal energy at all frequencies; SYN: white noise

gaze to look steadily in one direction for a period of time

gaze nystagmus nystagmus that occurs during horizontal gaze to one or both sides of midline

gaze nystagmus, bilateral horizontal nystagmus that beats to the right on right gaze and beats to the left on left gaze

gaze nystagmus, bilateral unequal nystagmus that is present in both gaze directions, but of different magnitude in one direction, consistent with central nervous system pathology

gaze testing component of ENG measurement in which eye movement is assessed as a patient fixates on a visual target at a specified location to the right and left of midline

GCS Glasgow coma score; method for grading depth of coma and severity of brain injury, based on eye opening, verbal response, and motor response

Gelfoam proprietary name for a thin absorbable gelatinous sponge used to repair membranous defects

Gelle test tuning fork test, designed to assess ossicular mobility, involving application of the fork to the mastoid while air pressure is adjusted in the external meatus; if perception does not change, the hearing loss is considered to be conductive in nature

gene the functional unit of heredity, composed of DNA

general anesthesia deepest level of sedation, characterized by total loss of sensation and consciousness

generator 1. device for converting mechanical energy into electrical energy; 2. source of electrical activity in the brain

genetic pertaining to heredity

genetic counseling advising of potential parents as to the probability of inherited disorders and conditions in their offspring

genetic hearing loss hearing loss related to heredity

genetics the study of heredity

geniculate thalamic nuclei of the visual (lateral) and auditory (medial) central nervous systems

geniculate, medial MG; auditory nucleus of the thalamus, divided into central and surrounding pericentral nuclei, that receives primary ascending fibers from the inferior colliculus and sends fibers, via the auditory radiations, to the auditory cortex

geniculate ganglion cluster of cell bodies of the sensory branch of Cranial Nerve VII

genotype the genetic constitution of an individual

gent. gentamicin

gentamicin; gentamycin gent.; ototoxic aminoglycoside antibiotic, used in the treatment of gram-negative infections

genu a structure of angular shape

geotropic nystagmus positional nystagmus that changes direction in relation to gravity, right beating when the right ear is down and left beating when the left ear is down

geriatric pertaining to the aging process

geriatrics branch of medicine concerned with pathologic aspects of aging

German measles mild viral infection, characterized by fever and a transient eruption or rash on the skin resembling measles; when occurring in pregnancy, may result in abnormalities in the fetus, including sensorineural hearing loss; SYN: rubella

gerontology scientific study of the process of aging

gestational age age since conception, measured in weeks and days from the first day of the last normal menstrual period

GFW battery Goldman-Fristoe-Woodcock auditory skills test battery

GIFROC frequency response that is added to a prescribed 2-cc coupler response to predict real-ear insertion response; inverse of CORFIG

Glasgow coma score GCS; method for grading depth of coma and severity of brain injury, based on eye opening, verbal response, and motor response

glia non-neuronal supporting tissues of the nervous system; SYN: neuroglia

glioblastoma rapidly growing and malignant tumor composed of undifferentiated glial cells

glioma any neoplasm derived from neuroglia

glomus jugulare glomus tumor arising on the jugular bulb or hypotympanum

glomus tumor small neoplasm of paraganglionic tissue with a rich vascular supply located near or within the jugular bulb

glomus tympanicum glomus tumor arising in the mesotympanum, with associated conductive hearing loss and pulsatile tinnitus

glossopharyngeal nerve Cranial Nerve IX; cranial nerve that provides efferent innervation to pharyngeal muscles and the parotid gland and afferent innervation from the auricle, eustachian tube, and posterior one-third of the tongue

glucocorticoids steroidlike compound with an anti-inflammatory effect, which, in large doses, has been associated with ototoxicity

glucose tolerance test test of blood sugar (glucose) metabolism wherein a fasting patient is given large amounts of glucose, and blood levels are monitored to determine the speed of metabolism

glue ear inflammation of the middle ear with thick, viscid, mucuslike effusion; SYN: mucoid otitis media

glutamic acid decarboxylase GAD; amino acid neurotransmitter, concentrated in the dorsal cochlear nucleus, which synthesizes GABA

glycerol test diagnostic test for Ménière's disease in which auditory function, including pure-tone sensitivity, word recognition, and ECochG SP/AP amplitude ratio, is assessed before and after ingestion of the diuretic glycerol

GME graduate medical education

goiter, familial form of congenital hypothyroidism caused by defects in thyroid biosynthesis; may be accompanied by sensorineural hearing loss, as in the case of Pendred syndrome

goiter, stippled epiphysis, and high protein-bound iodine congenital metabolic syndrome, characterized by thyroid overactivity, associated with profound sensorineural hearing loss

gold standard   outcome or condition that is designated as the criterion against which the test characteristics of all other measures are compared; a "truth" against which to compare sensitivity and specificity of diagnostic measures

Goldenhar syndrome   congenital musculoskeletal anomalies including microtia and atresia of the external auditory meatus; SYN: oculoauriculovertebral dysplasia

Goldman-Fristoe-Woodcock auditory skills battery   GFW battery; diagnostic measure of auditory skills, including auditory selective attention, discrimination, memory, and sound-symbol tests

Gradenigo syndrome   disorder characterized by the triad of paralysis of the external rectus muscle, pain behind the eye, and persistent otitis media and mastoiditis

granular myringitis   focal or diffuse replacement of the dermis of the tympanic membrane with granulation tissue

granulation tissue   minute connective tissue projections formed on inflamed tissue surface

granuloma   nodular inflammatory tumor-like mass

granuloma, cholesterol   circumscribed mass, formed in reaction to cholesterol deposits occurring in fluid-filled cells that are usually pneumatized; found in either the tym-

panomastoid compartment or the petrous apex, resulting in conductive or retrocochlear disorder

GRE   graduate record examination

greater epithelial ridge   inner portion of Kölliker's organ, consisting of a thickened, stratified embryonic epithelium from which the inner hair cells and supporting cells of the organ of Corti differentiate

greater superficial pretrosal nerve   branch of Cranial Nerve VII from which the nerve to the stapedius muscle arises

grommet tube   ventilation or pressure-equalization tube

ground electrode   in electrophysiologic measurement, the electrode that attaches the patient to ground; SYN: common electrode

group audiometry   simultaneous hearing testing of several patients, usually by means of a network of automated audiometers

GSR   galvanic skin response; change in skin resistance as a result of an emotional response to a stimulus; SYN: psychogalvanic skin response

guanine   one of four chemical bases that make up the genetic alphabet

gusher   spontaneous or surgically induced profuse flow of perilymphatic fluid from the oval window; SYN: perilymphatic gusher

gyrus; pl. gyri   prominent rounded elevation of the cerebral cortex

H

H & P history and physical; preliminary examination in medical assessment

H₀ null hypothesis; in statistics, the hypothesis that no difference exists between two or more sets of data

HA hearing aid; any electronic device designed to amplify and deliver sound to the ear, consisting of a microphone, amplifier, and receiver

HA-1 coupler standard 2-cc coupler used to connect a hearing aid to an electroacoustic analyzer; the HA-1 device allows direct coupling of an earmold or an in-the-ear hearing aid, with putty used to seal the earmold or shell into the device

HA-2 coupler standard 2-cc coupler used to connect a hearing aid to an electroacoustic analyzer; the HA-2 device has an earmold simulator and is used for testing earphones with nubs, such as an external receiver of a body aid

HA-3 coupler standard 2-cc coupler used to connect a hearing aid to an electroacoustic analyzer; the HA-3 device is used for testing modular ITE hearing aids, earphones, and insert receivers that do not have nubs

HA-4 coupler standard 2-cc coupler used to connect a hearing aid to an electroacoustic analyzer; the HA-4 device is a modification of the HA-2 with entrance tubing for use with postauricular or eyeglass hearing aids

habenulae perforata small openings in the edge of the osseous spiral lamina through which the peripheral nerve fibers of Cranial Nerve VIII pass as they course from the hair cells to the spiral ganglion

habilitation program or treatment designed to develop abilities or skills

habilitation, aural treatment of persons with congenital hearing impairment to improve the efficacy of overall oral/aural communication ability, including the use of hearing aids, auditory training, speech and language therapy, speechreading, manual communication

habituation 1. process of becoming accustomed; 2. process by which the nervous system inhibits responsiveness during repeated stimulation

HAE hearing aid evaluation; process of choosing suitable hearing aid amplification for an individual, based on measurement of acoustic properties of the amplification and perceptual response to the amplified sound

HAIC Hearing Aid Industry Conference; organization of hearing instrument manufacturers and other companies in the hearing industry; predecessor to the Hearing Industries Association

HAIC frequency range standard developed by HAIC to describe the range of frequencies of a hearing aid response

HAIC gain standard developed by HAIC describing average hearing aid gain, calculated as the average of gain at 500 Hz, 1000 Hz, and 2000 Hz

hair cells HC; sensory cells of the organ of Corti to which nerve endings from Cranial Nerve VIII are attached, so named because of the hairlike stereocilia that project from the apical end

hair cells, inner IHC; sensory hair cells arranged in a single row in the organ of Corti to which the primary afferent nerve endings of Cranial Nerve VIII are attached

hair cells, outer OHC; motile cells within the organ of Corti, which appear to be responsible for fine-tuning frequency resolution and potentiating the sensitivity of the inner hair cells

half-shell earmold earmold consisting of a canal and thin shell, with a bowl extending only part of the way to the helix

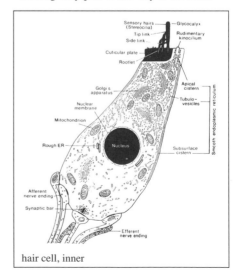

hair cell, inner

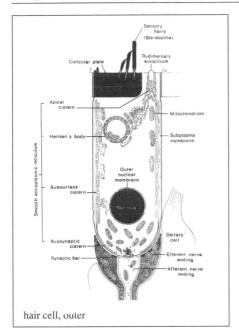

hair cell, outer

Hallgren syndrome recessive genetic disorder characterized by vestibulocerebellar ataxia, pigmentary retinal dystrophy, congenital sensorineural hearing loss, and cataract

hallucination, auditory apparent perception of sound that has no basis in external stimulation

hammer colloquial term for malleus

hand-hearing syndrome autosomal dominant disorder characterized by congenital hand abnormalities, including contracture of the digits and wasting of finger muscles, and sensorineural hearing loss

handicap the obstacles to psychosocial function resulting from a disability

handicap, hearing the obstacles to psychosocial function resulting from a hearing disability

handicapped having a handicap

HAPI Hearing Aid Performance Inventory; self-assessment questionnaire of a patient's perceived benefit from hearing aid use

Harboyan syndrome autosomal recessive eye disorder associated with progressive sensorineural hearing loss of delayed onset; SYN: Fehr corneal dystrophy

hard-of-hearing HOH; having a hearing impairment that is mild to severe; COM: deaf

hard peak clipping output-limiting technique in hearing aid amplification that removes the extremes of alternating current amplitude peaks at some predetermined level; COM: soft peak clipping

hard-wired attached by wire or cord

hard-wired auditory trainer early type of amplification device in which the listener's receiver was attached to a desk and the speaker's microphone was connected to an amplifier

harmonic component of a complex tone, the frequency of which is an integral multiple of the fundamental frequency

harmonic distortion amplitude distortion of a signal in the form of additional harmonic components

harmonic motion, simple continuous, symmetric, periodic back and forth movement of an object that has been set into motion

harmonic series full set of harmonics in periodic complex tones

Harvard PAL PB-50 word lists one of the first sets of monosyllabic word lists used in speech audiometry for word-recognition testing; developed at the psychoacoustics laboratory (PAL) at Harvard, word lists were designed to be phonetically balanced (PB)

Harvard Report classic 1946 report of research suggesting that individuals with hearing loss could be fitted most successfully with hearing aids incorporating a flat or gently sloping frequency response

HBP high blood pressure

HC hair cell; sensory cell of the organ of Corti to which nerve endings from Cranial Nerve VIII are attached, so named because of the hairlike stereocilia that project from the apical end

HCL highest comfortable level; the maximum level of gain at which loudness comfort can be achieved, used in the fitting of hearing aids to assist in determining output-limiting levels

HCP hearing conservation program; occupational program designed to quantify the nature and extent of hazardous noise exposure, monitor the effects of exposure on hearing, provide abatement of sound, and provide hearing protection when necessary

HD hearing device; hearing instrument

head baffle effect relative enhancement of high-frequency sound due to the acoustic diffraction of low-frequency sound by the auricle and head combining to form a wall or baffle

headphone transducer that converts electrical signals from an audiometer into sound delivered to the ear; SYN: earphone

headroom residual dynamic range of a hearing aid, expressed as the difference in dB SPL between a given output (such as gain at user settings) and the level of saturation of the device

headshadow effect attenuation of sound by the head in a free field, so that a sound approaching from one side of the head will be reduced in magnitude when it reaches the ear on the other side

headshake nystagmus test electro-oculographic recording of horizontal and vertical eye movement following the head being shaken or pivoted in time to a metronome for a fixed period of time

health information system HIS; computer database system designed specifically for healthcare institutions for information processing of patient demographic data, diagnosis, payer source, etc.

health maintenance organization HMO; managed care organization in which groups of professionals, along with a specified facility, provide enrollees with health care at fixed reimbursement rates

hear to perceive sound

hearing the perception of sound

hearing, normal hearing ability, including threshold of sensitivity and suprathreshold perception, that falls within a specified range of normal capacity

hearing, residual the remaining hearing ability in a person with hearing loss

hearing aid HA; any electronic device designed to amplify and deliver sound to the ear, consisting of a microphone, amplifier, and receiver

hearing aid, analog amplification device that uses conventional, continuously varying signal processing

hearing aid, behind-the-ear BTE hearing aid; a hearing aid that fits over the ear and is coupled to the ear canal via an earmold

hearing aid, BICROS bilateral contralateral routing of signals; a hearing aid system with one microphone contained in a hearing aid at each ear; the microphones lead to a single amplifier and receiver in the better hearing ear of a person with bilateral asymmetric hearing loss

hearing aid, BIFROS bilateral frontal routing of signals; hearing aid system with microphones placed in the front of eyeglass hearing aids

hearing aid, binaural CROS hearing aid system that separates the microphone from the receiver to reduce feedback; microphones are mounted in hearing aids on both sides of the head, and amplified signals are routed across the head to the opposite ear; SYN: criss-CROS

hearing aid, body-worn hearing aid with its components encased in a small box worn on the chest with a cord connected to a receiver worn on the ear, for use in cases of severe and profound hearing loss

hearing aid, bone-anchored surgically implanted bone-conduction receiver that interfaces with an external amplifier, designed to provide amplification for those with intractable middle ear disorder

hearing aid, bone-conduction hearing aid, used most often in patients with bilateral atresia, in which amplified signal is delivered to a bone vibrator placed on the mastoid, thereby bypassing the middle ear and stimulating the cochlea directly

hearing aid, BTE behind-the-ear hearing aid

hearing aid, canal hearing aid that fits mostly in the external auditory meatus with a small portion extending into the concha; SYN: in-the-canal hearing aid

hearing aid, carbon early hearing aid that used a carbon microphone

hearing aid, CIC completely-in-the-canal hearing aid

hearing aid, completely-in-the-canal CIC hearing aid; small amplification device, extending from 1 mm to 2 mm inside the meatal opening to near the tympanic membrane, that allows greater gain with less power due to the proximity of the receiver to the membrane

hearing aid, criss-CROS version of a CROS hearing aid designed for bilateral severe hearing loss in which the microphone on each side transmits its signal to the hearing aid in the opposite ear, thereby permitting substantial gain without feedback

hearing aid, CROS contralateral routing of signals; hearing aid designed for unilateral hearing loss, in which a microphone is placed on the poorer ear, and the signal is routed to a hearing aid on the better ear

hearing aid, CROS-plus modification

of a transcranial CROS arrangement in which a traditional CROS aid is fitted to the better ear and a power in-the-ear hearing aid is fitted to the unaidable ear

hearing aid, custom   ITE, ITC, or CIC hearing aid made for a specific individual from an ear impression

hearing aid, DCA   digitally controlled analog hearing aid

hearing aid, digital   hearing aid that processes a signal digitally; SYN: DSP hearing aid

hearing aid, digital signal processing   DSP hearing aid; hearing aid that converts output from the microphone from analog to digital form, uses software algorithms to manipulate gain characteristics, and converts the signal back to analog form for delivery to the loudspeaker

hearing aid, digitally-controlled analog   DCA hearing aid; hybrid hearing device in which microphone-amplifier-loudspeaker functions are analog, but their parameters are under digital control

hearing aid, directional   hearing instrument that contains a directional microphone

hearing aid, DSP   digital signal processing hearing aid

hearing aid, eyeglass   early style of hearing aid built into one or both earpieces of eyeglass frames

hearing aid, focal CROS   subtype of CROS hearing aid arrangement in which a tube is used to channel sound from the concha of the unaided ear into a microphone on the same side

hearing aid, frequency transposition   hearing device designed to transpose higher frequency energy into lower frequency amplification, designed for use in patients with corner audiograms

hearing aid, FROS   front routing of signals; eyeglass hearing aid in which the microphone is placed near the front of the glasses and routed back to the amplifier at the ear

hearing aid, high CROS   high-frequency contralateral routing of signals; conventional CROS hearing aid configuration, but with a high-frequency emphasis on the aided ear

hearing aid, implantable   any electronic device implanted in the mastoid cavity or middle ear space designed to amplify sound and deliver vibratory energy directly to the ossicles

hearing aid, in-the-canal   ITC hearing aid; canal hearing aid

hearing aid, in-the-ear   ITE hearing aid; custom hearing aid that fits entirely in the concha of the ear

hearing aid, IROS   ipsilateral routing of signals; monaural hearing aid designed for mild hearing loss, in which a high-frequency-emphasis hearing aid is coupled to the ear with an open earmold or tube fitting

hearing aid, ITC   in-the-canal hearing aid

hearing aid, ITE   in-the-ear hearing aid

hearing aid, master   electronic device that simulates a wide range of electroacoustic parameters of a hearing aid, used in the prefitting selection of hearing aid gain and frequency response

hearing aid, mini-CROS   CROS hearing aid with a short tube from the receiver on the good ear, designed to provide minimum gain to that ear

hearing aid, monaural   hearing aid worn on one ear only

hearing aid, multi-CROS   a CROS hearing aid system that can be changed to a CROS, BICROS, or conventional hearing aid configuration

hearing aid, multiple-memory   hearing aid that can be programmed to contain more than one frequency response for use under different listening conditions

hearing aid, nonlinear   hearing aid that incorporates compression circuitry producing nonlinear amplification

hearing aid, OTE   over-the-ear hearing aid

hearing aid, over-the-ear   OTE hearing aid; seldom-used term for a hearing aid that fits over the ear and is coupled to the ear canal via an earmold; SYN: postauricular hearing aid, BTE hearing aid

hearing aid, postauricular   a hearing aid that fits over the ear and is coupled to the ear canal via an earmold; SYN: behind-the-ear hearing aid, over-the-ear hearing aid

hearing aid, power CROS   monaural power hearing aid fitting that uses a contralateral routing of signals (CROS) strategy by placing the microphone on the opposite ear to reduce the potential for feedback

hearing aid, programmable   digitally controlled analog or digital signal processing hearing aid in which the parameters of the instrument are under computer control

hearing aid, pseudobinaural early, single body-worn hearing aid with Y-cord transmission to earmolds in both ears

hearing aid, quasi-digital early term for digitally controlled analog hearing aid

hearing aid, transcranial CROS contralateral routing of signal (CROS) strategy for unilateral hearing loss in which a high-gain in-the-ear hearing aid is fitted to the poor ear in an effort to transfer sound across the skull by bone conduction to the cochlea of the good ear

hearing aid, transpositional hearing aid that converts high-frequency acoustic energy into low-frequency signals for individuals with profound hearing loss who have measurable hearing only in the lower frequencies

hearing aid, vibrotactile device designed for profound hearing loss in which acoustic energy is converted to vibratory energy and delivered to the skin

hearing aid, Y-cord early body-worn hearing aid with the output of the amplifier directed to both ears by a Y-shaped cord

hearing aid acoustician European term for hearing aid dispenser

Hearing Aid Compatibility Act 1988 federal legislation mandating that telephones manufactured in or imported for use in the U.S. be hearing-aid compatible

hearing aid consultation process of counseling about the need for amplification and the types of devices available

hearing aid effect effect of the physical presence of a hearing aid on an observer's attitude toward the hearing aid wearer

hearing aid evaluation HAE; process of choosing suitable hearing aid amplification for an individual, based on measurement of acoustic properties of the amplification and perceptual response to the amplified sound

hearing aid evaluation, comparative hearing aid selection procedure in which aided speech-recognition ability is assessed with various amplification configurations or types in an effort to determine differences in aided performance

Hearing Aid Industry Conference HAIC; organization of hearing instrument manufacturers and other companies in the hearing industry; predecessor to the Hearing Industries Association

hearing aid orientation process of teaching a new hearing aid wearer proper use and application of amplification

Hearing Aid Performance Inventory HAPI; self-assessment questionnaire of a patient's perceived benefit from hearing aid use

hearing aid squeal shrill, high-pitched sound emitted from a hearing aid, resulting from acoustic feedback

hearing aid stethoscope stethoscope designed to auscultate a hearing instrument for the purpose of diagnostic listening

hearing conservation prevention or reduction of hearing impairment through a program of identification of risk, monitoring of hearing, protection from hazardous noise, and education

Hearing Conservation Amendment 1983 amendment to OSHA's Occupational Noise Exposure Regulation, designed to reduce or prevent noise-induced hearing loss and create occupational hearing conservation programs

hearing conservation program HCP; occupational safety and health program designed to quantify the nature and extent of hazardous noise exposure, monitor the effects of exposure on hearing, provide abatement of sound, and provide hearing protection when necessary

hearing conservation program, mobile hearing conservation service that uses a mobile test van to provide on-site industrial hearing screenings

hearing conservationist, occupational OHC; person who is certified by CAOHC to provide a comprehensive array of services related to hearing conservation

hearing device HD; hearing aid

hearing disability functional limitations resulting from a hearing impairment

hearing disorder disturbance of structure and/or function of hearing

hearing handicap obstacles to psychosocial function resulting from a hearing disability

Hearing Handicap Inventory HHI; self-assessment scale designed to yield information about an individual's perceived social and emotional consequences of hearing impairment

Hearing Handicap Inventory for Adults HHIA; modification of the HHIE designed to yield information about a non-elderly adult's perceived social and emotional consequences of hearing impairment

Hearing Handicap Inventory for the Elderly HHIE; modification of the HHI

Degree of hearing loss	dB range
Minimal hearing loss	10–25
Mild hearing loss	25–40
Moderate hearing loss	40–55
Moderately severe hearing loss	55–70
Severe hearing loss	70–90
Profound hearing loss	>90

hearing loss

designed to yield information about an elderly individual's perceived social and emotional consequences of hearing impairment

hearing impairment HI; abnormal or reduced function in hearing resulting from auditory disorder

hearing in noise test HINT; speech-audiometric measure of sentence-recognition ability in background noise

Hearing Industries Association HIA; trade association of manufacturers of hearing aids and other companies in the hearing industry

hearing instrument hearing aid

hearing level HL; the decibel level of sound referenced to audiometric zero, which is used on audiograms and audiometers, expressed as dB HL

hearing level, normalized nHL; the decibel level of a sound that lacks a standardized reference, referred to behaviorally determined normative levels, expressed as dB nHL

hearing loss HL; reduction in hearing sensitivity

hearing loss, acquired hearing loss that occurs after birth as a result of injury or disease; not congenital; SYN: adventitious hearing loss

hearing loss, adventitious loss of hearing sensitivity occurring after birth; ANT: congenital hearing loss

hearing loss, autoimmune auditory disorder characterized by bilateral, asymmetric, progressive, sensorineural hearing loss in patients who test positively for autoimmune disease

hearing loss, conductive reduction in hearing sensitivity, despite normal cochlear function, due to impaired sound transmission through the external auditory meatus, tympanic membrane, and ossicular chain

hearing loss, congenital reduced hearing sensitivity existing at or dating from birth, resulting from pre- or perinatal pathologic conditions

hearing loss, dominant hereditary hearing loss due to transmission of a genetic characteristic or mutation in which only one gene of a pair must carry the characteristic in order to be expressed, and both sexes have an equal chance of being affected

hearing loss, dominant progressive DPHL; genetic condition in which sensorineural hearing loss gradually worsens over a period of years, caused by dominant inheritance

hearing loss, fluctuating loss of hearing sensitivity characterized by aperiodic change in degree

hearing loss, functional FHL; hearing loss that is exaggerated or feigned

hearing loss, genetic hearing loss related to heredity

hearing loss, heredodegenerative hearing loss of genetic origin, with onset after birth

hearing loss, high-frequency nonspecific term referring to hearing sensitivity loss occurring at frequencies above approximately 2000 Hz

hearing loss, idiopathic hearing loss of unknown cause

hearing loss, low-frequency nonspecific term referring to hearing sensitivity loss occurring at frequencies below approximately 1000 Hz

hearing loss, mid-frequency nonspecific term referring to hearing sensitivity loss occurring at frequencies around 1000 Hz to 2000 Hz

hearing loss, mild loss of hearing sensitivity of 25 dB HL to 40 dB HL

hearing loss, mixed hearing loss with both a conductive and a sensorineural component

hearing loss, moderate loss of hearing sensitivity of 40 dB HL to 55 dB HL

hearing loss, moderately severe loss of hearing sensitivity of 55 dB HL to 70 dB HL

hearing loss, noise-induced NIHL; permanent sensorineural hearing loss caused by acoustic trauma from exposure to excessive sound levels

hearing loss, nonorganic apparent loss in hearing sensitivity in the absence of any organic pathologic change in structure; used to describe hearing loss that is feigned; SYN: functional hearing loss

hearing loss, nonsyndromic autosomal recessive or dominant genetic condition in which there are no other significant features besides hearing loss; SYN: recessive nonsyndromic hearing loss; ANT: syndromic hearing loss

hearing loss, occupational noise-induced hearing loss due to exposure to excessive sound levels on the job

hearing loss, organic hearing loss due to a pathologic process in the auditory system; ANT: functional hearing loss, nonorganic hearing loss

hearing loss, perceptive early term for sensorineural hearing loss

hearing loss, precipitous sensorineural hearing loss characterized by a steeply sloping audiometric configuration

hearing loss, profound loss of hearing sensitivity of greater than 90 dB HL

hearing loss, progressive adult-onset autosomal dominant nonsyndromic hearing loss with onset in adulthood, characterized by progressive, symmetric sensorineural hearing loss

hearing loss, recessive hereditary sensorineural most common inherited hearing loss, in which both parents are carriers of the gene but only 25% of offspring are affected; occurring in either nonsyndromic or syndromic form

hearing loss, sensorineural SNHL; cochlear or retrocochlear loss in hearing sensitivity due to disorders involving the cochlea and/or the auditory nerves fibers of Cranial Nerve VIII

hearing loss, severe loss of hearing sensitivity of 70 dB HL to 90 dB HL

hearing loss, ski-slope colloquial term referring to a hearing loss configuration characterized by normal hearing in the low frequencies and a precipitous loss in the high frequencies

hearing loss, sudden acute rapid-onset loss of hearing that is often idiopathic, unilateral, and substantial and that may or may not spontaneously resolve

hearing loss, symmetric hearing loss that is identical or nearly so in both ears

hearing loss, syndromic hearing loss that occurs as part of a constellation of other medical and physical disorders; ANT: nonsyndromic hearing loss

hearing loss, toxic loss in hearing sensitivity due to exposure to ototoxic drugs

hearing loss, transient temporary loss of hearing sensitivity

hearing loss, Type 1 type of hearing loss based on loudness growth, classified for the purpose of hearing aid fitting; caused by outer hair cell loss, and characterized by a loss of sensitivity for soft sound, but little or no hearing loss for loud sounds

hearing loss, Type II type of hearing loss based on loudness growth, classified for the purpose of hearing aid fitting; caused by outer hair cell loss and some inner hair cell loss, and characterized by a loss of hearing for soft sound and a loss of some loud speech cues

hearing loss, Type III type of hearing loss based on loudness growth, classified for the purpose of hearing aid fitting; caused by inner and outer hair cell loss, and characterized by a loss of sensitivity for soft and loud sounds

hearing loss, unilateral hearing sensitivity loss in one ear only

hearing loss, X-linked hereditary hearing loss due to a faulty gene located on the X chromosome, such as that found in Alport syndrome and Hunter syndrome

Hearing Performance Inventory HPI; self-assessment scale used to assess subjective impression of hearing performance in everyday communication situations

hearing protection broad category of devices and techniques designed to attenuate hazardous levels of noise

hearing protection, double combination of earplug and earmuff hearing protection devices, used during very-high-level noise exposures

hearing protection, insert any of various types of hearing protection devices that are placed into the external auditory meatus to attenuate excessive noise levels; SYN: earplugs

hearing protection device HPD; any of a number of devices used to attenuate excessive environmental noise to protect hearing, including those that block the ear canal or cover the external ear

hearing protection device, amplitude-sensitive nonlinear hearing protection device that provides little or no attenuation of low-intensity sound and significant attenuation of high-intensity sound

hearing protection device, nonlinear amplitude-sensitive hearing protection device that provides little or no attenuation of low-intensity sound and increasing attenuation of increasing sound intensity

hearing protection earmold custommade earmold designed to attenuate sound for protection against noise

hearing sensitivity capacity of the auditory system to detect a stimulus, most often described by audiometric pure-tone thresholds

hearing threshold absolute threshold of hearing sensitivity, or the lowest intensity level at which sound is perceived

hearing threshold level HTL; an individual's threshold, or the number of dB by which an individual's hearing threshold exceeds the normal threshold, expressed as dB HTL

heart-rate audiometry HRA; electrophysiologic technique for predicting hearing sensitivity by measuring heart-rate changes in response to auditory stimulation; SYN: cardiac evoked response audiometry

HEENT head, eyes, ears, nose, and throat

helicotrema passage at the apical end of the cochlea, connecting the scala tympani and the scala vestibuli

helix prominent ridge of the auricle, beginning just superior to the opening of the external auditory meatus and coursing around most of the edge of the auricle

Helmholtz resonator early device for studying acoustics, which had variously sized cavities with a protruding tube for insertion in the ear; designed for observation and measurement of the resonant effects of the shape and size of the cavities

hemiataxia ataxia affecting one side of the body

hemifacial microsomia craniofacial disorder, including eye and facial malformation, with preauricular tags, pinna malformation, microtia, and atresia

hemotympanum presence of blood in the middle ear

Hennebert's sign nystagmus produced by pressure applied to a sealed external auditory meatus, occurring in cases of labyrinthine fistula

Hensen's cells supporting cells of the organ of Corti to which the outer edge of the tectorial membrane is attached

hereditary genetically determined

hereditary deafness hearing loss or deafness of genetic origin

heredity results of genetic transmission of characteristics from one's ancestors

heredodegenerative hearing loss hearing loss of genetic origin, with onset after birth

hermetic seal airtight seal

herpes zoster infection caused by varicella-zoster virus with a vesicular eruption along the course of a nerve due to inflammation of ganglia, resulting from a latent virus

herpes zoster oticus HZO; herpes zoster infection that lingers in the ganglia and can be activated by systemic disease, resulting in vesicular eruptions of the auricle, facial nerve palsy, and sensorineural hearing loss; SYN: Ramsey-Hunt syndrome

Herrmann syndrome autosomal dominant nervous system disorder beginning in late childhood or early adolescence, with photomyoclonus and progressive sensorineural hearing loss, followed by diabetes mellitus and progressive dementia

hertz Hz; unit of measure of frequency, representing number of cycles per second; after physicist Heinrich Hertz

Heschl's gyrus transverse temporal gyrus that contains the auditory area of the cerebral cortex

heterolateral pertaining to the opposite side of the body; SYN: contralateral

heterophasic of different phases; out of phase; ANT: homophasic

heterotopia displacement of tissue from its normal location, as in salivary gland tissue in the middle ear

heterozygous characterized by different genes in a gene pair; ANT: homozygous

HF high frequency; nonspecific term referring to frequencies above approximately 2000 Hz

HFA high-frequency average; an ANSI hearing aid specification, expressed as the average of decibel response values at 1000 Hz, 1600 Hz, and 2500 Hz

HFA full-on gain high-frequency average full-on gain; an ANSI hearing aid specification, derived by calculating the HFA output to a 50-dB-SPL or 60-dB-SPL input with the hearing aid adjusted to its full-on gain setting

HFA SSPL90 high-frequency average saturation sound pressure level; an ANSI hearing aid specification, derived by calculating the HFA output to a 90-dB-SPL input with the hearing aid adjusted to its full-on gain setting

HHI Hearing Handicap Inventory; self-assessment scale designed to yield information about an individual's perceived social and emotional consequences of hearing impairment

HHIA Hearing Handicap Inventory for Adults; modification of the HHIE designed to yield information about a non-elderly adult's perceived social and emotional consequences of hearing impairment

HHIE Hearing Handicap Inventory for the Elderly; self-assessment scale designed to yield information about an elderly individual's perceived social and emotional consequences of hearing impairment

HI hearing impairment; abnormal or reduced function in hearing resulting from auditory disorder

hi-fi earplugs hearing protection devices designed to attenuate sound equally across the frequency range to maintain high (hi) fidelity (fi) reproduction of sound, especially music

HI-PRO proprietary computer interface module, designed as an industry standard, that is used to couple a programmable hearing aid to a computer

HIA Hearing Industries Association; trade association of manufacturers of hearing aids and other companies in the hearing industry

high CROS; HICROS high-frequency contralateral routing of signals; conventional CROS hearing aid configuration, but with a high-frequency emphasis on the aided ear

high-cut filter SYN: low-pass filter; high-frequency filter; ANT: high-pass filter

high fidelity faithful reproduction of sound with minimal distortion

high frequency HF; nonspecific term referring to frequencies above approximately 2000 Hz

high-frequency audiometer audiometer with a frequency range extended beyond 8000 Hz

high-frequency average HFA; an ANSI hearing aid specification, expressed as the average of decibel response values at 1000 Hz, 1600 Hz, and 2500 Hz

high-frequency average full-on gain HFA full-on gain; an ANSI hearing aid specification, derived by calculating the HFA output to a 50-dB-SPL or 60-dB-SPL input with the hearing aid adjusted to its full-on gain setting

high-frequency average saturation sound pressure level HFA SSPL90; an ANSI hearing aid specification, derived by calculating the HFA output to a 90-dB-SPL input with the hearing aid adjusted to its full-on gain setting

high-frequency filter low-pass filter, attenuating the higher frequencies

high-frequency hearing loss nonspecific term referring to hearing sensitivity loss occurring at frequencies above approximately 2000 Hz

high-level compression compression-limiting process of a hearing aid, characterized by a high threshold, high ratio, and long release time

high-level SISI early diagnostic test for retrocochlear disorder; modification of the SISI procedure administered at a high-intensity level at which those with normal hearing or cochlear hearing loss should perceive the small increments in intensity

high-pass earhook earhook containing a filter that attenuates hearing aid output below 2000 Hz to 3000 Hz

high-pass filter bandpass filter that attenuates low frequencies and allows high frequencies to pass; SYN: low-frequency filter; ANT: low-pass filter

high-risk register 1. record of names of infants who are at risk for hearing loss; 2. list of factors that put a child at risk for having or developing hearing loss

highest comfortable level HCL; the maximum level of output at which loudness comfort can be achieved, used in the fitting of hearing aids to assist in determining output-limiting levels

HINT hearing in noise test; speech-audiometric measure of sentence-recognition ability in background noise

HIS health information system; computer database system designed specifically for healthcare institutions for information processing of patient demographic data, diagnosis, payer source, etc.

histology the study of minute structures of cells and tissues as they relate to function

histopathology the study of disease-related changes in minute structures of cells and tissues

hit rate percentage of time that a diagnostic test is positive when a disorder exists; ANT: false-alarm rate

HIV human immunodeficiency virus; cytopathic retrovirus that causes AIDS and can result in infectious diseases of the middle ear and mastoid as well as peripheral and central auditory nervous system disorder; SYN: HTLV-III

HL 1. hearing level; 2. hearing loss

HML indices high, medium, low indices; method of expressing attenuation capabilities of hearing protection devices based on octave band measures

HMO health maintenance organization; managed care organization in which groups of professionals, along with a specified facility, provide enrollees with health care at fixed reimbursement rates

HNS head and neck surgery

HOH hard of hearing; HOH; having a hearing impairment that is mild to severe; COM: deaf

homeostasis state of equilibrium in the body

homogeneity the state of being homogeneous

homogeneity of audibility uniformity in terms of audibility throughout, as in lists of spondaic words used in speech threshold testing

homogeneous of uniform quality, composition, or structure throughout

homologous having a similarity of structure and origin, though not necessarily of function

homophasic of identical phase; in phase; ANT: heterophasic

homophenes words that appear the same on the lips

homozygous characterized by identical genes in a gene pair; ANT: heterozygous

horizontal ampulla bulging portion of the horizontal semicircular canal that contains the crista ampullaris

horizontal ampullar nerve nerve fiber bundle from the hair cells of the crista ampullaris of the horizontal semicircular canal that joins with similar bundles from the other semicircular canals, the utricle, and the saccule to form the vestibular branch of Cranial Nerve VIII

horizontal canal horizontal semicircular canal

horizontal plane anatomic plane of reference dividing the head into upper and lower portions; SYN: transverse section

horizontal semicircular canal one of three bony canals of the vestibular apparatus containing sensory epithelia that respond to angular motion; SYN: lateral semicircular canal

horizontal semicircular duct one of three membranous canals of the vestibular apparatus containing sensory epithelia that respond to angular motion; SYN: lateral semicircular duct

horn, Libby earmold horn, consisting of a smooth, tapered, one-piece sound tube of internal stepped-bore construction

horn bore tapered bore in an earmold that is widest in diameter at its medial aspect, designed to enhance high-frequency amplification

horn bore, reverse tapered bore in an earmold that is widest in diameter at its lateral aspect, designed to reduce high-frequency amplification

horn effect the change in frequency response of amplified sound by alteration of the diameter of an earmold bore at the entrance to or exit from an earmold; if the horn is placed at the exit or medial end of the earmold, high-frequency signals will be enhanced

HPD hearing protection device; any of a number of devices used to attenuate excessive environmental noise to protect hearing, including those that block the ear canal or cover the external ear

HPI Hearing Performance Inventory; self-assessment scale used to assess subjective impression of hearing performance in everyday communication situations

HRA heart-rate audiometry; electrophysiologic technique for predicting hearing sensitivity by measuring changes in heart rate in response to auditory stimulation; SYN: cardiac evoked response audiometry

HTL hearing threshold level; an individual's threshold, or the number of dB by which an individual's hearing threshold exceeds the normal threshold, expressed as dB HTL

HTLV-III human T-cell lymphotropic virus-III; SYN: HIV

human immunodeficiency virus HIV; cytopathic retrovirus that causes AIDS and can result in infectious diseases of the middle ear and mastoid as well as peripheral and central auditory nervous system disorder; SYN: HTLV-III

human T-cell lymphotropic virus-III HTLV-III; retrovirus that causes AIDS; SYN: HIV

Hunter syndrome mucopolysaccharidosis II; X-linked recessive disorder characterized by early onset and progression of growth failure, mental retardation, and other metabolic disorders, associated with conductive and sensorineural hearing loss

Hurler syndrome mucopolysaccharidosis I; autosomal recessive disorder characterized by early onset and severe progression of growth failure, mental retardation, and other metabolic disorders, associated with some degree of progressive hearing loss

Hx history

hybrid 1. anything of mixed origin; 2. in hearing aids, a device that has both analog and digital components

hydraulic operated by a fluid under pressure

hydrocephalus excessive accumulation of cerebrospinal fluid in the subarachnoid or subdural space

hydrops excessive accumulation of serous fluid in any of the tissues or cavities of the body

hydrops, cochlear excessive accumulation of endolymph within the cochlear labyrinth, resulting in fluctuating sensorineural hearing loss, tinnitus, and a sensation of fullness

hydrops, endolymphatic excessive accumulation of endolymph within the cochlear and vestibular labyrinths, resulting in fluctuating sensorineural hearing loss, vertigo, tinnitus, and a sensation of fullness

hydrops, labyrinthine excessive accumulation of endolymph within the membranous labyrinth; SYN: endolymphatic hydrops

hypacusis SYN: hypoacusis

hyperacusis abnormally sensitive hearing in which normally tolerable sounds are perceived as excessively loud

hyperbilirubinemia abnormally large amount of bilirubin (red bile pigment) in the blood at birth; risk factor for sensorineural hearing loss; SYN: erythroblastosis fetalis

hyperesthesia abnormally acute sensitivity to sensory stimuli

hypermetric saccades in ENG testing, condition in which the eyes overshoot the target during calibration, requiring additional saccades to bring them back to the target; ANT: hypometric saccades

hyperprolinemia II autosomal dominant metabolic disorder with late-onset progressive sensorineural hearing loss

hyper-recruitment excessive growth in

loudness perception with increasing intensity, so that loudness of a high-intensity tone in an impaired ear exceeds that in a normal ear; SYN: over-recruitment

hypertrophy increase in the bulk of a body part or organ

hyperuricemia endocrine-metabolic disorder with late-onset, progressive sensorineural hearing loss

hypoacusis a diminution in hearing sensitivity; SYN: hypacusis

hypochondriasis 1. morbid concern about one's health and exaggerated attention to any unusual bodily sensations; 2. false belief that one is suffering from a disease

hypogenesis embryonic underdevelopment

hypoglossal nerve Cranial Nerve XII; cranial nerve that provides efferent innervation to the muscles of the tongue

hypometric saccades in ENG testing, condition in which the eyes undershoot the target during calibration; ANT: hypermetric saccades

hypoplasia incomplete development or underdevelopment of tissue or an organ

hypothesis an assumption or supposition advanced as a guide to experimental investigation

hypothesis, null in statistics, the working hypothesis of the null or no difference between sets of data

hypothyroidism deficient production of thyroid hormone

hypotonia condition characterized by diminution of muscular tonicity

hypotympanic recess hypotympanum

hypotympanotomy surgical extirpation of small tumors in the lower tympanic cavity

hypotympanum floor of the middle ear space

hypoxia deficiency of oxygen in air, blood, or tissue

hysteresis the failure of coincidence of two associated phenomena

hysterical deafness rare psychogenic disorder of hearing caused by conversion of emotional trauma to a physical manifestation

Hz Hertz; unit of measure of frequency, representing cycles per second

HZO herpes zoster oticus; herpes zoster infection that lingers in the ganglia and can be activated by systemic disease, resulting in vesicular eruptions of the auricle, facial nerve palsy, and sensorineural hearing loss; SYN: Ramsey-Hunt syndrome

I

I tracing interrupted tracing; graph that results from threshold tracking in Békésy audiometry to an interrupted or pulsed tone at a fixed or swept frequency; ANT: continuous tracing

I/O function input/output function; curve that plots output intensity level as a function of input intensity level; used to describe the gain characteristics of an amplifier

IA interaural attenuation; reduction in the sound energy of a signal as it is transmitted by bone conduction from one side of the head to the opposite ear

IAC 1. internal auditory canal; 2. internal auditory meatus

IAM internal auditory meatus; an opening on the posterior surface of the petrous portion of the temporal bone through which the auditory and facial nerves pass

IAS intermediate acoustic stria; nerve bundle, the fibers of which emanate from the posterior ventral cochlear nucleus and synapse on the ipsilateral and contralateral periolivary nuclei and the contralateral lateral lemniscus

iatrogenic induced during or by treatment

IC 1. inferior colliculus; 2. integrated circuit

ICD International Classification of Diseases; classification system developed by the World Health Organization

ICD-9 codes codes representing ICD classifications of surgical, therapeutic, and diagnostic procedures

ICM ipsilateral competing message; in speech audiometry, noise or other competing signal that is delivered to the same ear as the target signal; ANT: CCM or contralateral competing message

ICN 1. intensive care nursery; 2. intermediate care nursery

icterus malignant jaundice that can result in sensorineural hearing loss

ICU intensive care unit; hospital unit designed to provide care for those needing extensive support and monitoring

IDE investigational device exemption; status granted by the U.S. Food and Drug Administration to permit clinical trials of new medical devices that have not yet been approved for clinical use

IDEA Individuals with Disabilities Education Act; U.S. public laws 94–142 and 99–457 mandating free and appropriate public education for all children, age 3 and older, who have handicapping conditions; also encourages services to infants and toddlers

identification audiometry testing designed to screen the hearing of large numbers of individuals, such as neonates and school age children, with the goal of identifying those who need more comprehensive audiologic assessment; SYN: screening audiometry

idiopathic of unknown cause

idiopathic hearing loss hearing loss of unknown cause

idiopathic nystagmus nonpathologic horizontal spontaneous nystagmus of unknown cause

IDL intensity difference limen; smallest difference in intensity of a signal that can be detected

IEP individualized educational plan; federally mandated, annually updated plan for the education of children with handicapping conditions

IFSP individualized family service plan; federally mandated, annually updated plan for the education of preschool children with handicapping conditions and their families

IHAFF Independent Hearing Aid Fitting Forum; group of audiologists who developed recommendations for the selection and fitting of nonlinear hearing aids

IHC inner hair cells; sensory hair cells arranged in a single row in the organ of Corti to which the primary afferent nerve endings of Cranial Nerve VIII are attached

IHS International Hearing Society; organization of hearing professionals, primarily hearing instrument specialists

IL intensity level; acoustic intensity in decibels; the IL of a sound is equal to 10 times the common log of the ratio of the measured acoustic intensity to a reference intensity

ILD interaural latency difference; the difference in latency of a component wave of an auditory evoked potential, usually ABR wave V, for right-ear versus left-ear stimulation, expressed in msec

IM intramuscularly; within the muscle, usually referring to a method of delivering drugs into the system

IMAC   ifosmadine-mesna-adriamycin-cis-platin; potentially ototoxic chemotherapy regimen used in the treatment of bony sarcoma

imaging, magnetic resonance   MRI; radiologic technique used to provide precise structural images; involves placing the body in a magnetic field and subjecting it to radiofrequency pulses, which result in imaged signals from excited hydrogen ions in body structures

iminoglycinuria   benign innate error of amino acid transport associated with hearing loss

immittance   encompassing term for energy flow through the middle ear, including admittance, compliance, conductance, impedance, reactance, resistance, and susceptance

immittance, static   measure of the contribution of the middle ear to acoustic impedance, calculated by subtracting the immittance measure of the external meatus, estimated by adding air pressure to decouple the middle ear, from the total immittance at its peak level

immittance audiometry   battery of immittance measurements, including static immittance, tympanometry, and acoustic reflex threshold determination, designed to assess middle ear function

immittance screening   rapid assessment of middle ear function by tympanometry

immunocytochemistry   study of cell structure by immunologic methods

immunodeficiency   condition of vulnerability to disease resulting from a defective immunologic mechanism

immunodeficiency panel   blood test designed to assess the quantity of immunoglobins, which protect the organism from viral and bacterial infections

impact noise   intermittent noise of short duration, usually produced by nonexplosive mechanical impact such as pile driving or riveting; distinguishable from impulse noise by longer rise times and longer duration

impacted cerumen   cerumen that causes blockage of the external auditory meatus

impairment   abnormal or reduced function

impairment, hearing   HI; abnormal or reduced function in hearing resulting from auditory disorder

impairment, sensory   abnormal functioning of one of the senses

impedance   Z; total opposition to energy flow or resistance to the absorption of energy, expressed in ohms

impedance, characteristic   impedance that occurs naturally based on a system's characteristics

impedance audiometry   immittance audiometry

impedance bridge   early instrument designed to carry out impedance audiometry, based on an electronic bridge circuit

impedance matching   the process of equalizing impedances of two devices or media

impedance matching device   structure or circuit designed to bridge an impedance mismatch; e.g., in the middle ear, where it provides a means of matching the low-impedance air pressure waves of sound to the high-impedance hydraulic system of the cochlea

impedance mismatch   condition in which two devices or media between which energy flows have different impedances

imperative signal   in measurement of the contingent negative variation evoked potential, the signal to which the listener must respond, which is preceded by the conditional signal

imperception, auditory   impairment in the recognition or interpretation of sound

implant   any device that has been surgically implanted; e.g., cochlear implant, implantable hearing aid, bone-anchored hearing aid

implant, auditory brainstem   ABI; electrode implanted at the juncture of Cranial Nerve VIII and the cochlear nucleus that receives signals from an external processor and sends electrical impulses directly to the brainstem

implant, cochlear   device that enables persons with profound hearing loss to perceive sound, consisting of an electrode array surgically implanted in the cochlea, which delivers electrical signals to CN VIII, and an external amplifier, which activates the electrode

implantable hearing aid   any electronic device implanted in the mastoid cavity or middle ear space designed to amplify sound and deliver vibratory energy directly to the ossicles

impression   ear impression; cast made of the concha and ear canal for creating a customized earmold or hearing aid

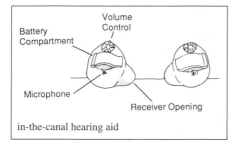

in-the-canal hearing aid

impulse   action potential of a nerve fiber

impulse noise   intermittent noise with an instantaneous rise time and short duration that creates a shock wave, usually produced by gunfire or explosion; distinguishable from impact noise by shorter rise time and duration

in phase   condition in which the pressure waves of two signals crest and trough at the same time; SYN: homophasic

in situ   in position; e.g., in the case of hearing aids, on the patient in position for use

in situ audiometry   assessment of hearing in which pure-tone thresholds and loudness discomfort levels are measured and expressed in ear canal SPL

in situ measurement   evaluation of hearing aid performance while the hearing aid is being worn

in-the-canal hearing aid   ITC hearing aid; custom hearing aid that fits mostly in the external auditory meatus with a small portion extending into the concha; SYN: canal hearing aid

in-the-ear hearing aid   ITE hearing aid; custom hearing aid that fits entirely in the concha of the ear

in utero   within uterus; not yet born

incidence   frequency of occurrence, expressed as the number of new cases of a disease or condition in a specified population over a specified time period

incident wave   sound wave moving away from the source onto a reflecting or refracting surface

inclusion cyst   firm cystic lesion found on the pinna, following incision or trauma

incudectomy   surgical removal of the incus

incudomalleolar joint   point of articulation of the incus and malleus

incudostapedial joint   point of articulation of the incus and stapes

incus   middle bone of the ossicular chain, located in the epitympanic recess; consists of a body and two crura, the shorter of which fits into the fossa incudis and the longer of which attaches to the head of the stapes; COL: anvil

incus, long process   long crus that connects the body of the incus to the lenticular process at the head of the stapes

incus, short crus   short leg of the incus that fits into the fossa incudis and serves as a pivotal point for the rocking motion of the ossicular chain

Independent Hearing Aid Fitting Forum   IHAFF; group of audiologists who developed recommendations for the selection and fitting of nonlinear hearing aids

indication   pointer as to the proper treatment of a condition

individualized education plan   IEP; federally mandated, annually updated plan for the education of children with handicapping conditions

individualized family service plan   IFSP; federally mandated, annually updated plan for the education of preschool children with handicapping conditions and their families

Individuals with Disabilities Education Act   IDEA; U.S. public laws 94–142 and 99–457, mandating free and appropriate public education for all children, age 3 and older who have handicapping conditions; also encourages services to infants and toddlers

induced nystagmus   nystagmus that occurs expectedly as a result of specific stimulation such as rotation and caloric stimulation; ANT: spontaneous nystagmus

induction   generation of an electric current or magnetic state by proximity to a different source of electricity or magnetism

induction, embryonic   1. the influence a substance exerts over future development of

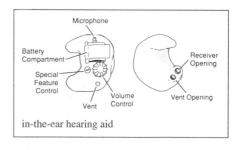

in-the-ear hearing aid

tissue; 2. the first of a series of embryologic processes, which in the auditory system includes formation of the otic placode and formation of the neural plate

induction coil conductor wound into a spiral to create a high concentration of material into which current flow is induced when a magnetic field enters its vicinity; in a hearing aid, the telecoil is the induction coil, and the telephone produces the magnetic field

induction loop continuous wire surrounding a room that conducts electrical energy from an amplifier, thereby creating a magnetic field; current flow from the loop is induced in the induction coil of a hearing aid telecoil

industrial audiometry assessment of hearing, including determination of baseline sensitivity and periodic monitoring, to determine the effects of industrial noise exposure on hearing sensitivity

industrial zone noise industrial noise emanating from within a circumscribed area surrounding the noise source

inertance inertia of the sound medium

inertia tendency of a body to remain in motion or to remain at rest

inertial bone conduction stimulation of the cochlea by the lag of the ossicular chain when the bones of the skull are set into motion by a bone vibrator; results in relative movement between the stapes and the oval window, which contributes to bone-conducted hearing

infantile cochleosaccular degeneration idiopathic or viral selective degeneration in infancy of the cochlea and saccule with preservation of the utricle and cristae, resulting in unilateral or bilateral profound sensorineural hearing loss

infantile meningogenic labyrinthitis inflammatory invasion of the labyrinth from the subarachnoid space via the cochlear aqueduct or internal auditory canal, secondary to meningitis, resulting in bilateral profound sensorineural hearing loss and impaired vestibular function

infarct localized area of ischemic necrosis resulting from infarction

infarction sudden insufficiency of blood supply due to occlusion of arterial supply or venous drainage

infection morbid state caused by invasion and multiplication of pathogenic microorganisms within the body

infectious able to be transmitted by infection

inferior anatomical direction, referring to structures that are located toward the bottom or lower surface; SYN: caudal; ANT: superior

inferior cerebellar artery large vessel arising from the basilar artery, a branch of which is the labyrinthine artery, which supplies the cochlea; SYN: anterior inferior cerebellar artery

inferior colliculus IC; central auditory nucleus of the midbrain; its central nucleus receives ascending input from the cochlear nucleus and superior olivary complex, and its pericentral nucleus receives descending input from the cortex

inferior colliculus, dorsomedial portion of the inferior colliculus receiving descending fibers from the cortex and fibers from the contralateral dorsomedial inferior colliculus

inferior colliculus, ventrolateral afferent portion of the central nucleus of the inferior colliculus that receives ascending input from the cochlear nucleus and superior olivary complex

inferior pontine syndrome vascular lesion of the pons involving several cranial nerves; symptoms include ipsilateral facial palsy, ipsilateral hearing loss, loss of taste from the anterior two-thirds of the tongue, and paralysis of lateral conjugate gaze movement

inferior tympanic artery branch of the ascending pharyngeal artery that supplies the mucosa and bone of the hypotympanum and promontory

inferior vestibular nerve division of the vestibular portion of Cranial Nerve VIII, consisting of neurons from the cristae of the posterior semicircular canal and the main portion of the macula of the saccule

inflammation tissue response to injury or destruction of cells, characterized by heat, swelling, pain, redness, and sometimes loss of function

infrachordal facial palsy facial nerve paralysis or paresis caused by a lesion located inferior to the chorda tympani branch, not affecting taste, lacrimation, or the stapedial reflex

infrared system assistive listening device consisting of a microphone/transmitter placed near the sound source of interest that broadcasts over infrared light waves to a receiver/amplifier, thereby enhancing the signal-to-noise ratio

infrasonic pertaining to sound frequencies below the range of human hearing; SYN: subsonic

infrastapedial facial palsy facial nerve paralysis or paresis due to a lesion located between the chorda tympanic branch and the stapedius muscle nerve, affecting taste, but not affecting the stapedial reflex or lacrimation

infrequent signal in recording the P3 event-related potential, the target signal to which the listener must attend, which occurs less often than the frequent signal; SYN: rare event

inherent natural to and characteristic of an organism; SYN: intrinsic, innate

inheritance, autosomal genetic inheritance related to non-sex-linked chromosomes

inheritance, autosomal dominant transmission of a genetic characteristic or mutation in which only one gene of a pair must carry the characteristic in order for it to be expressed and both sexes have an equal chance of being affected

inheritance, autosomal recessive transmission of a genetic characteristic or mutation in which both genes of a pair must share the characteristic in order for it to be expressed

inheritance, sex-linked inheritance in which the disordered gene is on the X chromosome; SYN: X-linked inheritance

inheritance, X-linked any genetic trait related to the X chromosome; transmitted by a mother to 50% of her sons, who will be affected, and 50% of her daughters, who will be carriers; transmitted by a father to 100% of his daughters

inhibit to restrain a process

inhibition reduction or arrest of a function

inhibition, residual temporary cessation of tinnitus following masking

inhibitor neurotransmitter that acts in an inhibitory manner

innate inborn; inherent; not acquired

inner ear structure comprising the sensory organs for hearing and balance, including the cochlea, vestibules, and semicircular canals

inner hair cells IHC; sensory hair cells arranged in a single row in the organ of Corti to which the primary afferent nerve endings of Cranial Nerve VIII are attached

inner pillars supporting pillars that stabilize the hair cells, extending from the basilar membrane to the top of the organ of Corti, forming the medial wall of the tunnel of Corti; ANT: outer pillars

inner rods inner pillars

inner spiral tunnel inner sulcus

inner sulcus a furrow within the organ of Corti, formed by the concave surface of the spiral limbus, the tectorial membrane, and the medial surface of the inner hair cells; SYN: spiral tunnel, inner spiral tunnel

inner supporting cells cells that constitute the inner sulcus

innervation distribution of nerve fibers to a structure

input 1. energy or information directed into a system; 2. to direct energy or information into a system

input compression process in which a hearing aid compresses a signal before it reaches the volume control, resulting in a constant dynamic range with a change in maximum output as gain is increased or decreased by the volume control; COM: output compression

input/output function I/O function; curve that plots output intensity level as a function of input intensity level; used to describe the gain characteristics of an amplifier

input-referred noise specification of front-end noise of a hearing instrument

input signal acoustic signal at the microphone of a hearing aid

insert earphone earphone whose transducer is connected to the ear through a tube leading to an expandable cuff that is inserted into the external auditory meatus; COM: circumaural earphone

insert hearing protection device any of various types of hearing protection devices that are placed into the external auditory meatus to attenuate excessive noise levels; SYN: earplugs

insertion gain hearing aid gain, defined as the difference in gain with and without a hearing aid

insertion gain, real-ear REIG; probe-microphone measurement of the difference, in dB as a function of frequency, between the real-ear unaided gain and the real-ear aided gain at the same point near the tympanic membrane

insertion loss difference in SPL at the tympanic membrane with the ear canal open

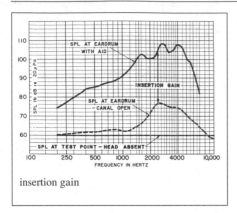

insertion gain

and with the ear canal occluded by an ear-mold or nonfunctioning hearing aid; the difference between the REUR and the REOR

insertion response, real-ear REIR; probe-microphone measurement of the difference, in dB as a function of frequency, between the real-ear unaided response and the real-ear aided response at the same point near the tympanic membrane

inspissation an increased thickness of fluid

integrated circuit IC; electronic circuit with its many interconnected elements formed on a single body of semiconductor material

integration, binaural fusion of simultaneous but different speech signals presented to the two ears; SYN: binaural fusion

intelligibility the extent to which speech can be understood

Intelligibility Rating Improvement Scale IRIS; patient estimation of the proportion of speech that can be understood in various listening situations

intensity, sound 1. sound power transmitted through a given area, expressed in watts/m^2; 2. generic term for any quantity relating to the amount or magnitude of sound

intensity difference limen IDL; smallest difference in intensity of a signal that can be detected

intensity level IL; acoustic intensity in dB, so that the IL of a sound is equal to 10 times the common log of the ratio of the measured acoustic intensity to a reference intensity

intensive care nursery ICN; hospital unit designed to provide care for newborns needing extensive support and monitoring

intensive care unit ICU; hospital unit designed to provide care for those needing extensive support and monitoring

intensive care unit, neonatal NICU; hospital unit designed to provide care for newborns needing greater than normal support and monitoring

intensive care unit, pediatric PICU; hospital unit designed to provide care for young children needing extensive support and monitoring

interaural between the ears

interaural attenuation IA; reduction in the sound energy of a signal as it is transmitted by bone conduction from one side of the head to the opposite ear

interaural latency difference ILD; the difference in latency of a component wave of an auditory evoked potential, usually ABR Wave V, for right-ear versus left-ear stimulation, expressed in msec

interface the point where two devices connect or otherwise come into contact

interference level, noise level at which noise masks the recognition of speech targets

interformant energy energy components of a speech signal that fall between the formant bands

interleave to overlap patterns of signals or responses

interleaved pulses processing early cochlear implant processing strategy in which trains of pulses, representing both speech features and waveform representation, were delivered to electrodes with temporal offsets to eliminate overlap across channels

intermediate acoustic stria IAS; nerve bundle, the fibers of which emanate from the posterior ventral cochlear nucleus and synapse on the ipsilateral and contralateral periolivary nuclei and the contralateral lateral lemniscus

intermediate care nursery ICN; hospital unit designed as a step-down facility for newborns leaving the intensive care unit prior to discharge

intermediate nucleus of the lateral lem-

$$\textbf{dB IL} = 10 \log \frac{\textbf{power}}{\textbf{power}_r}$$

intensity level

niscus LLI; one of three fiber tracts constituting auditory nuclei of the pons that serves as a relay for ascending auditory fibers from the PVCN and LSO in the hindbrain to the inferior colliculus

intermodulation distortion amplitude distortion of aperiodic signals by a hearing aid, resulting in the addition of frequencies in the output that were not present in the input

internal acoustic meatus internal auditory meatus

internal auditory artery blood vessel arising from the anterior inferior cerebellar artery and distributing to the dura and nerves of the internal auditory canal before dividing into the common cochlear artery and the anterior vestibular artery; SYN: labyrinthine artery

internal auditory canal IAC; internal auditory meatus

internal auditory meatus IAM; an opening on the posterior surface of the petrous portion of the temporal bone through which the auditory and facial nerves pass

internal carotid artery vessel providing the main blood supply to the cerebral hemisphere, located in the petrous apex region of the temporal bone; often encountered in temporal bone resection for tumor removal

internal ear inner ear

internal feedback in a hearing aid, abnormal acoustic feedback occurring within the instrument's casing

internal noise in a hearing aid, any sound not related to the input signal; e.g., circuit noise; ANT: external noise

internal radiating arterioles a group of arterioles constituting a branch of the main cochlear artery that divides to form capillary networks supplying the basilar membrane and hair cells

International Hearing Society IHS; organization of hearing professionals, primarily hearing instrument specialists; formerly National Hearing Aid Society

International Organization for Standardization ISO; association of specialists that determines standards for measuring instruments

international phonetic alphabet IPA; alphabet of symbols representing sounds of speech

interneurons neurons linking sensory and motor neurons

internuclear ophthalmoplegia eye movement disorder resulting from lesions of the medial longitudinal fasciculus

interpeak interval interpeak latency

interpeak latency difference in msec between the latencies of two peaks of an auditory evoked potential, such as the I to V interpeak latency of the auditory brainstem response; SYN: interpeak interval; interwave latency

interrupted speech test speech audiometric measure in which the extrinsic redundancy of the speech is reduced by rapid periodic interruption

interrupted tracing I tracing; graph that results from threshold tracking in Békésy audiometry to an interrupted or pulsed tone at a fixed or swept frequency; ANT: continuous tracing

interrupter switch the switch on an audiometer that interrupts or presents a test signal

interstice a small or narrow space between or within tissues or organs

interstimulus duration interstimulus interval

interstimulus interval ISI; the time between successive stimulus presentations

interstitial pertaining to interstices

interstitial fluid fluid found outside most cells of the body, with an ionic composition closely resembling that of perilymph

intersubject between or among subjects

intertragic incisure notch in the cartilage of the auricle, separating the tragus from the antitragus

interwave interval interpeak latency

intonation aspect of speech denoting changes in pitch, stress, and juncture

intonation contour the pattern of change in fundamental frequency of sound over time

intra-aural muscles stapedius and tensor tympani muscles of the middle ear

intra-aural reflex reflexive contraction of the intra-aural muscles in response to loud sound; stapedius muscle dominates the reflex in humans; SYN: acoustic reflex

intra-axial within the brainstem; ANT: extra-axial

intra-axial tumor tumor that originates within the brainstem

intracellular potential ionic potential within a cell

intractable tinnitus ringing that is resistant to treatment

intramuscular IM; within the muscle, usually referring to a method of delivering drugs into the system

intraoperative monitoring continuous assessment of integrity of cranial nerves during surgery; e.g., during acoustic tumor removal, Cranial Nerve VII is monitored because of proximity of the dissection, and Cranial Nerve VIII is monitored in an attempt to preserve hearing

intratympanic within the middle ear

intravenous IV; within the vein, usually referring to a method of delivering drugs into the system

intrinsic originating within; inherent; ANT: extrinsic

intrinsic redundancy in speech audiometry, the abundance of information present in the central auditory system due to the capacity inherent in its richly innervated pathways; ANT: extrinsic redundancy

inverse relationship the condition in which the values of two sets of measures are negatively correlated so that the greater the magnitude of one, the smaller the magnitude of the other; ANT: direct relationship

inverse square law principle describing how intensity changes as a function of the distance from the sound source; specifically, intensity varies inversely as the square of the distance from the source

inverting electrode electrode that is attached to that side of a differential amplifier that inverts the input by 180; reference or earlobe electrodes in conventional auditory brainstem response recordings; ANT: noninverting electrode

investigational device exemption IDE; status granted by the U.S. Food and Drug Administration to permit clinical trials of new medical devices that have not yet been approved for clinical use

ion atom or group of atoms charged with either positive or negative electricity, each traveling toward the pole with the opposite charge

ionic pertaining to ions

IPA international phonetic alphabet; alphabet of symbols representing sounds of speech

ipsilateral pertaining to or situated on the same side

ipsilateral acoustic reflex acoustic reflex occurring in one ear as a result of stimulation of the same ear; SYN: uncrossed acoustic reflex

ipsilateral competing message ICM; in speech audiometry, noise or other competing signal that is delivered to the same ear as the target signal; ANT: contralateral competing message

ipsilateral delayed endolymphatic hydrops endolymphatic hydrops occurring in two phases—an initial profound hearing loss in one ear, followed by development of episodic vertigo in the ear with the hearing loss

ipsilateral ear effect phenomenon in which patients with left temporal lobe lesions score poorly on the right ear on dichotic measures as expected, but also score poorly on the left ear; this effect is not observed on the right ear in right temporal lobe lesions

ipsilateral routing of signals IROS; method of monaural hearing aid fitting for mild hearing loss, in which a high-frequency-emphasis hearing aid is coupled to the ear with an open earmold or tube fitting; COM: CROS

IRIS Intelligibility Rating Improvement Scale; patient estimation of the proportion of speech that can be understood in various listening situations

IROS ipsilateral routing of signals

irradiation injury delayed-onset, progressive atrophy of the membranous labyrinth, particularly the spiral and annular ligaments, secondary to x-ray irradiation

irrigation, caloric process of introducing warm and cool water into the ear canal for caloric testing of vestibular function

irrigation, closed-loop method of warm or cool stimulation of the vestibular system in which water is delivered into a balloon-like catheter in the ear canal

irrigation, open-loop method of warm or cool stimulation of the vestibular system in which water is delivered directly into the ear canal

ischemia localized shortage of blood due to obstruction of blood supply

ISI interstimulus interval; the time between successive stimulus presentations

ISO International Organization for Standardization; association of specialists that determines standards for measuring instruments, after the Greek *isos,* meaning equal or similar

isometric of equal dimensions

isotretinoin accutane; retinoic acid drug prescribed for cystic acne; can have a teratogenic effect on the auditory system of the developing embryo when taken by the mother during pregnancy, resulting in congenital hearing loss

ITC hearing aid in-the-canal hearing aid; custom hearing aid that fits mostly in the external auditory meatus with a small portion extending into the concha; SYN: canal hearing aid

ITE hearing aid in-the-ear hearing aid; custom hearing aid that fits entirely in the concha of the ear

iterative repetitive; containing repetition; repetitious; repeating

IV intravenous; within the vein, usually referring to a method of delivering drugs into the system

J

J joule

Jacobson's nerve nerve arising from Cranial Nerve IX, providing the main sensory fibers to the mucosa of the mesotympanum and eustachian tube; SYN: tympanic nerve

jaundice disorder characterized by yellowish staining of tissue with bile pigments (bilirubin), which are excessive in the serum; in its severe form, it has been associated with sensorineural hearing loss; SYN: icterus

JCAHO Joint Commission on Accreditation of Healthcare Organizations; voluntary organization that provides support and accreditation to its member organizations, which are hospitals and other healthcare facilities; formerly JCAH

JCIH Joint Committee on Infant Hearing; organization formed to promote infant hearing healthcare with representation from AAA, AAO, AAP, ASHA, and others

jerk nystagmus general term for reciprocating movement of the eyes with different velocities in the two directions, including horizontal, vertical, oblique, or rotatory nystagmus

Jervell and Lange-Nielsen syndrome autosomal recessive cardiovascular disorder accompanied by congenital bilateral profound sensorineural hearing loss

Jewett waves waves or peaks of the auditory brainstem response, first described by Don Jewett as seven vertex-positive peaks occurring within 10 msec of stimulus onset, labeled as Waves I, II, III. . . . VII

jitter slight variance in a response or signal from event to event or cycle to cycle

JND just noticeable difference

joule J; unit of energy, expressed as the energy expended by an ampere flowing against 1 ohm for 1 sec; equal to 1 Newton/meter

jugular bulb bulbous protrusion of the sigmoid sinus at the beginning of the internal jugular vein, located in the floor of the hypotympanum

jugular fossa depression holding the jugular vein in the floor of the hypotympanum

jugular wall inferior wall or floor of the middle ear cavity

juncture in speech, suprasegmental cue that enables differentiation among messages by the manner in which syllables are joined in contextual speech

just noticeable difference JND; the smallest change in a stimulus that is detectable; SYN: difference limen

K

k   kilo; one thousand

K+   potassium; chemical found in low concentration in perilymph and high concentration in endolymph

K-AMP   hearing aid circuit with TILL processing designed by Killion (K) to provide substantial gain for low-intensity sound, reduced gain for moderate-level sound, no gain for high-intensity sound, and compression limiting for the highest-level sound

kanamycin   aminoglycocide antibiotic that resembles neomycin and has a selective ototoxicity to outer hair cells of the organ of Corti and the striolae of the utricle

karyotype   chromosomal characteristics of an individual

kc   kilocycle; 1000 cycles/sec; SYN: kHz

Kearns-Sayre syndrome   autosomal dominant disorder, characterized by cardiac abnormalities, progressive ophthalmoplegia, myopathies, neuropathies, and hearing loss

keloid   excessive scar tissue formation on the lobule, in the form of a shiny, firm mass, following trauma, surgery, or, often, ear piercing

KEMAR   Knowles electronics mannequin for acoustic research; model used in the measurement of hearing aid performance that simulates the acoustic properties of an average adult head and torso

keratin   protein substance present in cuticular structures

keratoma   horny tumor

keratopachyderma and digital constrictions   autosomal dominant disorder characterized by hyperkeratosis, ringlike furrows on fingers and toes, and congenital progressive sensorineural hearing loss

keratosis obturans   rapidly forming keratin-mass tumor, often mixed with cerumen, caused by abnormal migration of the skin in the external auditory meatus

kernicterus   form of severe neonatal jaundice associated with sensorineural hearing loss

kg   kilogram

kHz   kilohertz; 1000 Hz

kilocycle   kc; 1000 cycles per second; SYN: kHz

kilogram   kg; 1000 grams; unit of mass

kinesthesia   the sensory perception of position and movement of the body

kinocilium; pl. kinocilia   motile cilium embedded in the cupula of the cristae ampullares of the semicircular canals

Klippel-Feil syndrome   craniofacial disorder, characterized by short neck of limited mobility and eye disorders, including abducens nerve palsy; associated with severe to profound sensorineural hearing loss

kneepoint   1. point on an input-output function at which the slope changes from unity; 2. in hearing aids, the intensity level at which compression is activated; SYN: compression threshold

Knowles electronics mannequin for acoustic research   KEMAR

knuckle pads and leukonychia   autosomal dominant disorder, characterized by calluslike thickening of finger and toe joints and progressive whitening of finger and toenails; associated with conductive or sensorineural hearing loss

Kobrak minimal caloric test   early test of vestibular function in which the external auditory meatus was irrigated with cool water or ice water injected with a syringe and nystagmus was observed using Frenzel glasses

Kölliker's organ   thickened, stratified embryonic epithelium from which the inner and outer hair cells differentiate

Krabbe disease   autosomal recessive leukodystrophy with neonatal onset, characterized by progressive loss of muscle control, optic atrophy, tonic spasms, and sensorineural hearing loss

L

labial pertaining to the lips

labyrinth the inner ear, so named because of the intricate maze of connecting pathways in the petrous portion of each temporal bone, consisting of the canals within the bone and fluid-filled sacs and channels within the canals

labyrinth, bony osseous labyrinth

labyrinth, membranous soft-tissue, fluid-filled channels within the osseous labyrinth that contain the end organ structures for hearing and vestibular function

labyrinth, osseous intricate maze of connecting channels in the petrous portion of each temporal bone that contains the membranous labyrinth

labyrinthectomy surgical excision of the labyrinth

labyrinthine pertaining to the labyrinth

labyrinthine artery blood vessel arising from the anterior inferior cerebellar artery and distributing to the dura and nerves of the internal auditory canal before dividing into the common cochlear artery and the anterior vestibular artery; SYN: internal auditory artery

labyrinthine hydrops excessive accumulation of endolymph within the membranous labyrinth; SYN: endolymphatic hydrops

labyrinthine wall medial surface of the tympanic cavity, containing the promontory of the cochlea and the round and oval windows

labyrinthitis inflammation of the labyrinth, affecting hearing, balance, or both

labyrinthitis, acute inflammation of the labyrinth resulting in acute vertigo, vegetative symptoms, sensorineural hearing loss, and tinnitus

labyrinthitis, acute suppurative acute inflammation of the labyrinth with infected effusion containing pus

labyrinthitis, bacterial inflammation of the membranous labyrinth due to bacterial invasion

labyrinthitis, circumscribed inflammation of the labyrinth restricted to a defined, limited area

labyrinthitis, infantile meningogenic inflammatory invasion of the labyrinth from the subarachnoid space via the cochlear aqueduct or internal auditory canal, sec-ondary to meningitis, resulting in bilateral profound sensorineural hearing loss and impaired vestibular function

labyrinthitis, otogenic suppurative inflammation of the labyrinth caused by bacterial invasion from the middle ear into the vestibule, resulting in severe vertigo and hearing loss

labyrinthitis, serous inflammation of the labyrinth caused by otogenic or meningogenic bacterial toxins or contamination during surgery; SYN: toxic labyrinthitis

labyrinthitis, subclinical infantile meningogenic labyrinthitis secondary to subclinical bacterial or viral meningitis in a young infant, resulting in mild to profound loss of auditory and vestibular function

labyrinthitis, suppurative inflammation of the labyrinth caused by bacterial invasion of the cochlea by contiguous areas of the temporal bone, resulting in severe vertigo and hearing loss

labyrinthitis, syphilitic acquired or congenital labyrinthitis, secondary to syphilis, that results in progressive, fluctuating sensorineural hearing loss due to endolymphatic hydrops and degenerative changes in sensory and neural structures

labyrinthitis, toxic inflammation of the labyrinth caused by degradation of the tissue fluid environment in the inner ear due to bacterial toxins or contamination of perilymph during surgery; SYN: serous labyrinthitis

labyrinthitis, viral inflammation of the labyrinth due to viral infections, including mumps, measles, rubella, and herpes zoster oticus

labyrinthitis ossificans ossification within the cochlea, usually most severe in the basal turn of the scala tympani near the round window, often secondary to meningitis

laddergram a graph, resembling a ladder, that represents equal loudness levels of the two ears at various intensity levels, obtained via the alternating binaural loudness balance (ABLB) test

LAER late auditory evoked response; long-latency auditory evoked response

lag brief delay

lagena one of three sections of the membranous labyrinth of lower vertebrates that is the equivalent of the cochlea in mammals

lalognosis the understanding of speech

lamina thin plate or flat layer

lamina, reticular delicate netlike structure forming the continuous surface of the organ of Corti, comprising the phalangeal processes, tops of the pillars, and cuticular plates of the inner and outer hair cells

lamina, spiral shelf of bone arising from the modiolar side of the cochlea, consisting of two thin plates of bones between which course the nerve fibers from the auditory nerve to and from the hair cells

lamina basilaris cochleae basilar membrane of the cochlea upon which lies the organ of Corti

language complex system of symbols for communication

language, sign form of manual communication in which words and concepts are represented by hand positions and movements

language lateralization the propensity for spoken language to be processed in the left hemisphere of the brain

large vestibular aqueduct syndrome congenital disorder, often associated with Mondini dysplasia, resulting from faulty embryogenesis of the endolymphatic duct and sac, leading to endolymphatic hydrops with childhood-onset, bilateral, progressive sensorineural hearing loss

lasix ototoxic loop diuretic used in the treatment of edema or hypertension, which can cause sensorineural hearing loss secondary to degeneration of the stria vascularis; SYN: furosemide

late auditory evoked response LAER; long-latency auditory evoked response

late cortical response long-latency auditory evoked response

late-onset auditory deprivation the apparent decline in word-recognition ability in the unaided ear of a person fitted with one hearing aid, resulting from asymmetric stimulation

late vertex response LVR; long-latency auditory evoked response

latency time interval between two events, as a stimulus and a response

latency, absolute in auditory brainstem response analysis, the time in msec from signal onset to a waveform peak

latency, acoustic reflex time interval between the presentation of an acoustic stimulus and detection of an acoustic reflex

latency, delayed in auditory brainstem

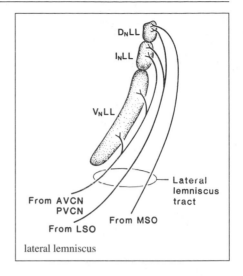

lateral lemniscus

response measurement, an abnormal prolongation of the time between signal onset and major peaks of the response

latency, interaural the difference in latency of a component wave of an auditory evoked potential, usually ABR Wave V, for right versus left ear stimulation, expressed in msec

latency, interpeak difference in msec between the latencies of two peaks of an auditory evoked potential, such as the I to V interpeak latency of the auditory brainstem response; SYN: interpeak interval; interwave latency

latent not manifest, but having the potential to be

lateral anatomical direction, referring to structures that are located away from the midline or toward the side; ANT: medial

lateral ampulla vestibular end organ of the lateral semicircular canal

lateral inferior pontine syndrome vascular lesion of the inferior pons, with symptoms that include facial palsy, loss of taste from the anterior two-thirds of the tongue, analgesia of the face, paralysis of lateral conjugate gaze movements, and hearing loss

lateral lemniscus LL; large fiber tract or bundle, formed by dorsal, intermediate, and ventral nuclei and consisting of ascending auditory fibers from the CN and SOC, that runs along the lateral edge of the pons and carries information to the inferior colliculus

lateral lemniscus, dorsal nucleus LLD; one of three fiber tracts, constituting auditory nuclei of the pons, that serves as a relay for ascending auditory fibers from the DCN, LSO, and MSO in the hindbrain to the inferior colliculus

lateral lemniscus, intermediate nucleus LLI; one of three fiber tracts, constituting auditory nuclei of the pons, that serves as a relay for ascending auditory fibers from the PVCN and LSO in the hindbrain to the inferior colliculus

lateral lemniscus, ventral nucleus LLV; one of three fiber tracts, constituting auditory nuclei of the pons, that serves as a relay for ascending auditory fibers from the AVCN, LSO, and MSO in the hindbrain to the inferior colliculus

lateral line organ organ found on the skin of lower vertebrates that contains the organ of hearing and the organ of balance

lateral malleolar ligament one of several ligaments responsible for maintaining the position of the ossicles, extending from the neck of the malleus to the bony wall near the notch of Rivinus

lateral olivocochlear bundle efferent pathway of nerve fibers emanating from the periolivary nuclei surrounding the LSO, coursing through the ipsilateral internal auditory meatus along the vestibular nerve, and terminating on afferent dendrites at the bases of inner hair cells

lateral rectus muscle muscle responsible for horizontal eye movement away from the midline

lateral semicircular canal one of three bony canals of the vestibular apparatus containing sensory epithelia that respond to angular motion; SYN: horizontal semicircular canal

lateral semicircular duct one of three membranous canals of the vestibular apparatus containing sensory epithelia that respond to angular motion; SYN: horizontal semicircular duct

lateral sinus largest of the venous sinuses, responsible for collecting blood from most of the head and neck

lateral superior olive LSO; one of the primary nuclei of the superior olivary complex, located in the hindbrain, receiving primary ascending projections directly from the ipsilateral AVCN and indirectly from the contralateral AVCN via the ipsilateral MTB

laterality preferential tendency to use the organs on one side of the body

lateralization 1. perception of a sound being located in one ear rather than the other in response to a signal delivered by a bone vibrator placed on the forehead; 2. identification of the apparent location within the head of a fused sound

lateralization, language the propensity for spoken language to be processed in the left hemisphere of the brain

lateralize to become perceived in one ear rather than the other

Laurence-Moon-Biedl-Bardet syndrome recessive eye disorder, characterized by retinitis pigmentosa, hypogenitalism, mental retardation, and progressive sensorineural hearing loss

lavalier microphone small microphone hung around the neck

LD learning disability; lack of skill in one or more areas of learning that is inconsistent with the person's intellectual capacity and is not the result of visual, hearing, motor, or emotional disorder

LDFR level-dependent frequency response; automatic signal processing that alters the frequency response of a hearing aid as a function of input level

LDL loudness discomfort level; intensity level at which sound is perceived to be uncomfortably loud, determined under earphones and expressed in dB HL or with probe microphone in dB SPL; SYN: uncomfortable loudness level

learning disability LD; lack of skill in one or more areas of learning that is inconsistent with the person's intellectual capacity and is not the result of visual, hearing, motor, or emotional disorder

LED light-emitting diode; a small light on a device, often used to indicate that the device is on or activated

left-beating nystagmus horizontal nystagmus in which the fast phase is toward the left

lemniscus fiber tract or bundle within the central nervous system

lemniscus, lateral LL; large fiber tract or bundle, formed by dorsal, intermediate, and ventral nuclei and consisting of ascending auditory fibers from the CN and SOC, that runs along the lateral edge of the pons and carries information to the inferior colliculus

lengthened-off-time test LOT test; early subtest of Békésy audiometry, in which the off time of interrupted signals was lengthened to enhance the separation of continuous and interrupted tracings in patients showing Type V patterns, consistent with functional hearing loss

lenticular process knob at the end of the long process of the incus, which has a lens-shaped end into which the head of the stapes fits

Leq equivalent sound level; measurement of a time-varying sound, expressed as a time-weighted energy average, representing the total sound energy experienced over a given time period as if the sound were unvarying

Leri-Weill disease autosomal dominant craniofacial-skeletal disorder, characterized by deformity of the radius and ulna bones, with conductive hearing loss due to outer ear and middle ear deformity; SYN: dyschondrosteosis; Madelung deformity

Lermoyez syndrome atypical form of Ménière's disease in which fluctuations of hearing and vertiginous episodes are inversely related, so that hearing improves before, during, and immediately after a vertiginous attack

lesion structural or functional pathologic change in body tissue

lesion, space-occupying neoplasm that exerts its influence by growing and impinging on neural tissues, as opposed to a lesion caused by trauma, ischemia, or inflammation

lesser epithelial ridge inner portion of Kölliker's organ; a thickened, stratified embryonic epithelium, from which the basilar membrane and outer hair cells differentiate

lesser superficial petrosal nerve part of the sensory nerve system of the ear formed by the joining of the tympanic nerve and the caroticotympanic nerve

Leudet tinnitus objective tinnitus, characterized by spasmodic dry clicking and caused by reflex spasm of the tensor palati muscle of the eustachian tube

leukemia disease characterized by hyperproduction of white blood cells that are deposited in spaces around organs where they are not ordinarily found, including intense infiltration of the petrous apex, tympanic membrane, perilymphatic spaces, etc.

leukodystrophy congenital, early-onset, rapidly progressive, fatal demyelinating disorder of the central nervous system, associated with auditory disorder

levator veli palatini along with the tensor veli palatini, one of two muscles of the nasopharynx responsible for opening the end of the eustachian tube by medial displacement of the cartilage; innervated by the pharyngeal plexus

level magnitude of sound

level, action level of noise exposure that requires a worker to be enrolled in an occupational hearing conservation program; defined by OSHA as 85 dBA for a time-weighted average of 8 hours

level, annoyance intensity level at which noise is judged subjectively to be disturbing or a nuisance

level, comfort comfortable loudness level

level, discomfort intensity level at which sound is perceived to be uncomfortably loud

level, equivalent sound Leq; measurement of a time-varying sound, expressed as a time-weighted energy average, representing the total sound energy over a given time period as if the sound were unvarying; SYN: equivalent level

level, exceedance description of the impact on an acoustic environmental of industrial noise, expressed as the percentage of time during which the sound in a particular environment exceeds a specified criterion

level, hearing HL; the decibel level of sound referenced to audiometric zero that is used on audiograms and audiometers, expressed as dB HL

level, hearing threshold HTL; an individual's threshold, or the number of dB by which an individual's hearing threshold exceeds the normal threshold, expressed as dB HTL

level, highest comfortable HCL; the maximum level of output at which loudness comfort can be achieved, used in the fitting of hearing aids to assist in determining output-limiting levels

level, intensity IL; acoustic intensity in dB, so that the IL of a sound is equal to 10 times the common log of the ratio of the measured acoustic intensity to a reference intensity

level, loudness quantity of loudness, usually expressed in phons or sones

level, loudness discomfort LDL; intensity level at which sound is perceived to be uncomfortably loud, determined under earphones and expressed in dB HL or with probe microphone in dB SPL; used as a target to set the RESR of a hearing aid

level, minimal response lowest level to which a child will respond behaviorally to sound

level, noise interference level at which noise masks the recognition of speech targets

level, noise pollution community noise level, expressed as the sum of the equivalent continuous sound level and an estimate of the increase of annoyance attributable to fluctuations of the sound levels

level, noise-emission standard measure of intensity of environmental or industrial noise, expressed as the decibel level at a specified distance and direction from a noise source in an open environment

level, normalized hearing nHL; the decibel level of a sound that lacks a standardized reference, referred to behaviorally determined normative levels, expressed as dB nHL

level, overall sound pressure total sound energy throughout the frequency range, measured without any frequency weighting

level, peak equivalent sound pressure pe SPL: decibel level of a 1000-Hz tone at an amplitude equivalent to the peak of a transient signal; used to express the intensity level of click stimuli used in auditory evoked potential testing

level, perceived noise expression in dB of the annoyance or unacceptability of loud sound, based on subjective ratings of noisiness; used primarily to assess the perception related to single-event aircraft flyover noise

level, saturation sound pressure maximum output generated by the receiver of a hearing aid, expressed as the root mean square sound pressure level

level, sensation SL; the intensity level of a sound in dB above an individual's threshold; usually used to refer to the intensity level of a signal presentation or a response above a specified threshold, such as puretone threshold or acoustic reflex threshold

level, sound pressure SPL; magnitude or quantity of sound energy relative to a reference pressure, 0.0002 dynes/cm^2 or 20 μPa

level, speech-interference SIL; masking or interference effect of noise on the intelligibility of speech communication, originally expressed as the articulation index and later as sound pressure levels in various octave bands

level, tolerance threshold of discomfort

level, uncomfortable UL; level at which sound is judged to be uncomfortably loud by a listener

level-dependent frequency response LDFR; automatic signal processing that alters the frequency response of a hearing aid as a function of input level

lexical pertaining to the lexicon

lexicon all of the linguistic signs, words, and morphemes in a given language

LF low frequency or frequencies; nonspecific term referring to frequencies below around 1000 Hz

LGOB loudness growth by octave bands; psychophysical technique in which loudness level is determined for various frequency bands, used as a fitting-by-loudness strategy for wide-dynamic-range-compression hearing aids

Libby horn earmold horn, consisting of a smooth, tapered, one-piece sound tube of internal stepped-bore construction

ligament band of fibrous tissue connecting or supporting bones, cartilage, or other structures

ligament, annular ring-shaped ligament that which holds the footplate of the stapes in the oval window

ligament, anterior malleolar one of several ligaments responsible for maintaining the position of the ossicles, extending from the anterior process of the malleus to the anterior wall of the middle ear cavity

ligament, auricular any of several ligaments that attach the auricle to the temporal bone

ligament, lateral malleolar one of several ligaments responsible for maintaining the position of the ossicles, extending from the neck of the malleus to the bony wall near the notch of Rivinus

ligament, posterior incudal one of several ligaments responsible for maintaining the position of the ossicles, extending from the short process of the incus to the posterior wall of the middle ear cavity

ligament, spiral band of connective tissue that affixes the basilar membrane to the outer bony wall, against which lies the stria vascularis within the scala media

ligament, superior malleolar one of several ligaments responsible for maintaining the position of the ossicles, extending from the head of the malleus to tegmen tympani

ligaments, malleolar bands of fibrous tissues suspending and supporting the malleus in the middle ear cavity; includes the superior, anterior, anterior suspensory, and lateral ligaments

light-emitting diode LED; a small light on a device, often used to indicate that the device is on or activated

light reflex bright triangular reflection on the surface of the tympanic membrane of the illumination used during otoscopic examination; SYN: cone of light

limen threshold

liminal pertaining to a threshold

limit end of any continuum

limited-range audiometer audiometer limited in frequency range and in function, used mostly in identification audiometry

limiting compression method of limiting maximum output of a hearing aid with compression circuitry

limits, method of psychophysical procedure for determining absolute or differential threshold in which the stimuli are presented at levels well above or below threshold and changed in small increments until the boundary of sensation is reached

line spectrum graphic representation of the frequency content of a signal in which vertical lines are plotted for frequency bands as a function of magnitude of energy in each band

linear pertaining to a line function

linear amplification hearing aid amplification in which the gain is the same for all input levels until the maximum output is reached

linear compression in hearing aids, amplifier gain that is linear at input levels that exceed the compression kneepoint

linear scale measurement scale in which each increment is equal to the next; COM: logarithmic scale

linearity of attenuation condition in which a change in an attenuator setting results in a comparable change in output

Ling five-sound test pediatric speech-detection measure consisting of five sounds chosen to represent the frequency range of speech—[u], [a], [i], [ʃ], [s]

lipofuscin fatty pigment granules that accumulate in the apical cytoplasm of hair cells and in supporting cells of the cochlear and vestibular end organs in the aging ear

lipoma common form of benign neoplasm composed of mature fat cells, not commonly found in the central nervous system, but reported occasionally as a tumor of the cerebellopontine angle

lipreading the process of understanding speech by careful observation of lip movement; SYN: speechreading

listening the voluntary direction of attention to a sound source

listening, dichotic the task of perceiving different signals presented simultaneously to each ear

listening, diotic the task of perceiving identical signals presented simultaneously to each ear

listening, selective focused attention on a particular sound source

listening check regular informal assessment of the output of a hearing aid or audiometer to insure its proper functioning

live-voice testing outdated speech audiometric technique in which speech signals are presented via a microphone with controlled vocal output; SYN: monitored live voice

LL lateral lemniscus; large fiber tract, formed by dorsal, intermediate, and ventral nuclei and consisting of ascending auditory fibers from the CN and SOC, that runs along the lateral edge of the pons and carries information to the inferior colliculus

LLAER long-latency auditory evoked response; auditory evoked potential, having two main waveform peaks—a vertex negative peak at approximately 90 msec following signal presentation and a vertex positive peak at approximately 180 msec following signal presentation; SYN: ALR

LLD dorsal nucleus of the lateral lemniscus; one of three fiber tracts, constituting auditory nuclei of the pons, that serves as a relay for ascending auditory fibers from the DCN, LSO, and MSO in the hindbrain to the inferior colliculus

LLI intermediate nucleus of the lateral lemniscus; one of three fiber tracts, constituting auditory nuclei of the pons, that serves as a relay for ascending auditory fibers from the PVCN and LSO in the hindbrain to the inferior colliculus

LLR   late-latency response; long-latency auditory evoked potential

LLV   ventral nucleus of the lateral lemniscus; one of three fiber tracts, constituting auditory nuclei of the pons, that serves as a relay for ascending auditory fibers from the AVCN, LSO, and MSO in the hindbrain to the inferior colliculus

lobectomy   surgical excision of a lobe of any organ or gland

lobster-claw syndrome   autosomal dominant facial-limb disorder, characterized by lobster-claw deformity of hands and feet, associated with small or malformed auricles, ossicular malformation, and conductive and sensorineural hearing loss; SYN: ectodermal dysplasia

lobule   inferior fleshy aspect of the auricle; SYN: earlobe

localization   identification of the azimuth of a sound source

localization, median plane   perception of a fused sound as being centered in the middle of the head

localization, vertical   identification of the direction of a sound source in the vertical plane

localized   1. limited to a definite area; 2. identified in terms of location

locus; pl. loci   a place

log   logarithm

logarithm   the exponent expressing the power to which a fixed number, the base, must be raised to produce a given number

logarithmic scale   measurement scale, such as the decibel scale, that is based on exponents of a base number; COM; linear scale

logon   a tone burst with a Gaussian-shaped envelope

Lombard effect   unconscious tendency to raise the level of vocal output above a background of noise

Lombard test   screening test of hearing loss organicity, designed to take advantage of the Lombard effect; involves introducing white noise into the ears while a patient talks and monitoring the intensity of vocal output to assess whether it changes

long arm 18 deletion syndrome   genetic imbalance syndrome involving partial deletion of the long arm of the 18th chromosome, characterized by mental retardation, microcephaly, short stature, retinal changes, and conductive hearing loss due to external and middle ear anomalies

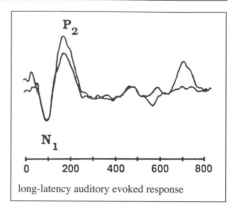

long-latency auditory evoked response

long-latency auditory evoked response   LLAER; auditory evoked potential, having two main waveform peaks—a vertex negative peak at approximately 90 msec following signal presentation and a vertex positive peak at approximately 180 msec following signal presentation; SYN: ALR

long process of the incus   long crus that connects the body of the incus to the lenticular process at the head of the stapes

long-term average speech spectrum   long-term speech spectrum

long-term memory   aspect of the information-processing function of the central nervous system that receives, modifies, and stores information on a permanent basis for later retrieval

long-term speech spectrum   LTSS; overall level and frequency composition of speech energy that represents everyday speech

longitudinal fracture   linear break that courses longitudinally through the temporal bone, often tearing the tympanic membrane and disrupting the ossicles, typically caused by a blow to the parietal or temporal regions of the skull; ANT: transverse fracture

longitudinal wave   type of pressure wave movement, such as a sound wave, in which particle movement is parallel to the wave movement; ANT: transverse wave

loop, induction   continuous wire surrounding a room that conducts electrical energy from an amplifier, thereby creating a magnetic field; current flow from the loop is induced in the induction coil of a hearing aid telecoil

loop, magnetic   continuous wire surrounding a room that conducts electrical energy from an amplifier, thereby creating a magnetic field; current flow from the loop is induced in the induction coil of a hearing aid telecoil or other receiver; SYN: induction loop

loop amplification system assistive listening device in which a microphone/amplifier delivers signals to a loop of wire encircling a room; the signals are received by the telecoil of a hearing aid via magnetic induction

loop diuretic class of agents, including ethacrynic acid, that promote the excretion of urine by inhibiting resorption of sodium and water in the kidneys; may be ototoxic in high doses

loop-induction auditory trainer loop amplification system in which an auditory training unit receives signals via magnetic induction through its telecoil from a loop of wire encircling a room that is sending signals generated by a microphone and amplifier

LOT test lengthened off-time test; early subtest of Békésy audiometry, in which the off-time of interrupted signals was lengthened to enhance the separation of continuous and interrupted tracings in patients showing Type V or functional patterns

loudness perception or psychological impression of the intensity of sound

loudness, critical bandwidth for range of frequencies over which complete loudness summation occurs and beyond which no further loudness growth occurs

loudness, fitting by FBL; fitting strategy for hearing aids with dynamic-range compression, based on measures of loudness growth, prediction of loudness growth, or assumption of average loudness growth

loudness balance test, alternate binaural ABLB; auditory test designed to measure loudness growth or recruitment in the impaired ear of a patient with unilateral hearing loss

loudness balance test, monaural MLB; test of loudness recruitment that compares loudness growth at a frequency at which the patient has normal hearing to loudness growth at a frequency at which the patient has hearing loss in the same ear

loudness balancing matching the loudness of two sounds, as between ears in the alternating binaural loudness balance test

loudness comfort level intensity level of a signal that is perceived as comfortably loud

loudness contours equal loudness contours; loudness level curves representing the sound pressure levels required to produce a given loudness across the frequency range for normal hearing at various phon levels

loudness discomfort level LDL; intensity level at which sound is perceived to be uncomfortably loud, determined under earphones and expressed in dB HL or with probe microphone in dB SPL; used as a target to set the RESR of a hearing aid

loudness growth by octave band test LGOB; psychophysical technique in which loudness level is determined for various frequency bands, used as a fitting-by-loudness strategy for wide-dynamic-range-compression hearing aids

loudness level quantity of loudness, usually expressed in phons or sones

loudness level, comfortable intensity level of a signal that is perceived as comfortably loud

loudness level, preferred signal level at which speech is rated as most comfortable

loudness level, uncomfortable ULL; UCL; intensity level at which sound is perceived to be uncomfortably loud; SYN: loudness discomfort level

loudness recruitment exaggeration of nonlinearity of loudness growth due to sensorineural hearing loss, wherein loudness grows rapidly at intensity levels just above threshold but may grow normally at high intensity levels

loudness summation the addition of loudness by the expansion of bandwidth even when overall sound pressure level remains the same

loudspeaker transducer that converts electrical energy into acoustic energy

loudspeaker azimuth direction of a loudspeaker, measured in angular degrees in the horizontal plane, in relationship to the listener

low-cut filter SYN: high-pass filter; low-frequency filter; ANT: low-pass filter

low fence lowest dB level designated to be substantial enough to be considered a hearing loss, usually expressed as the pure-tone average of thresholds obtained at 500 Hz, 1000 Hz, and 2000 Hz

low frequency LF; nonspecific term referring to frequencies below around 1000 Hz

low-frequency filter   high-pass filter, attenuating the lower frequencies

low-frequency hearing loss   nonspecific term referring to hearing sensitivity loss occurring at frequencies below approximately 1000 Hz

low-frequency sinusoidal harmonic acceleration testing   testing of vestibular function in which nystagmus is assessed following controlled, sinusoidal rotation in a rotating chair, designed for maximal stimulation of the horizontal semicircular canals

low-level compression   hearing aid compression circuitry that is activated in response to low intensity input, such as wide-dynamic-range compression

low-pass earhook   earhook on a behind-the-ear hearing aid, containing a filter that attenuates high frequencies and passes low frequencies

low-pass filter   bandpass filter that attenuates high frequencies and allows low frequencies to pass; SYN: high-frequency filter; ANT: high-pass filter

low-pass filtered speech test   LPFS test; word-recognition measure, consisting of monosyllabic words that have been bandpass filtered above approximately 800 Hz

low-redundancy speech test   any speech audiometric measure incorporating signals that have been altered to reduce their informational content, through, for example, bandpass filtering or time compression

LPFS test   low-pass filtered speech test

LSO   lateral superior olive; one of the primary nuclei of the superior olivary complex, located in the hindbrain, receiving primary ascending projections directly from the ipsilateral AVCN and indirectly from the contralateral AVCN via the ipsilateral MTB

LTSS   long-term speech spectrum; overall level and frequency composition of speech energy that represents everyday speech

lucidity   mental clarity

lucite   earmold material made of a fine grade dental acrylic, polymethyl methacrylate

lues   plague or pestilence, referring specifically to syphilis

luetic   pertaining to syphilis

lumen   space in the interior of a tubular structure

lupus pernio   cutaneous epithelioid granulomas on the ears and hands

lupus vulgaris   cutaneous tuberculosis characterized by nodular lesions on the nose and ears

Lybarger earmold   non-occluding earmold with a tube that has two diameters, creating a resonance above 4000 Hz

lymphokinesis   movement of endolymph in the semicircular canals

lymphomatoid granulomatosis   necrotizing infiltrative lesion of the blood, occurring in patients with immunodeficiency, that can affect the auditory nervous system in extreme cases

M

M1 left (1) mastoid (M) electrode location, typically used for inverting-electrode placement in auditory evoked potential testing, according to the 10–20 International Electrode System nomenclature

M2 right (2) mastoid (M) electrode location, typically used for inverting-electrode placement in auditory evoked potential testing, according to the 10–20 International Electrode System nomenclature

MA mental age; intellectual age, as measured on standardized tests

MAC battery minimum auditory capabilities battery; group of tests designed to assess auditory perception of persons with profound hearing loss

macrocephaly abnormal enlargement of the cranium; SYN. megacephaly; megalocephaly

macrotia congenital excessive enlargement of the auricle

macula; pl. maculae sensory epithelium within the utricle and saccule

macula, basilar cluster of cells in the embryonic otic vesicle that develops into the basilar membrane

macula sacculi neuroepithelial sensory area in the anterior wall of the saccule

macula utriculi neuroepithelial sensory area in the lateral wall of the utricle

Madelung deformity autosomal dominant craniofacial-skeletal disorder, characterized by deformity of the radius and ulna bones, with conductive hearing loss due to ossicular deformity and microtia; SYN: dyschondrosteosis; Leri-Weill disease

MAF minimum audible field; binaural threshold of sensitivity to sound presented in a sound field via loudspeaker placed at 0 azimuth; COM: minimum audible pressure

magnetic induction generation of an electric current or magnetic state by proximity to a different source of electricity or magnetism

magnetic loop continuous wire surrounding a room that conducts electrical energy from an amplifier, thereby creating a magnetic field; current flow from the loop is induced in the induction coil of a hearing aid telecoil or other receiver; SYN: induction loop

magnetic resonance imaging MRI; diagnostic technique used to provide precise structural images; involves placing the body in a magnetic field and subjecting it to radiofrequency pulses, which result in imaged signals from excited hydrogen ions in body structures

magnetoencephalography MEG; noninvasive technique, using scalp recordings, designed to measure spontaneous or sensory-evoked changes in magnetic fields of the cortex

magnitude greatness, particularly of size

magnitude estimation psychophysical procedure in which the patient is required to make direct numerical estimations of the sensory magnitudes produced by various stimuli

magnitude production psychophysical procedure in which the patient is required to adjust the level of a stimulus to correspond with a numerical value attributed to its magnitude

main cochlear artery branch of the common cochlear artery that supplies the apical three-fourths of the cochlea, including the modiolus

mainstreaming in education, the reassignment of children with disabilities from specialized classrooms into the regular school environment

MAIS Meaningful Auditory Integration Scale; assessment scale, completed by parents of children with hearing impairment, that assesses the effectiveness of hearing aids or cochlear implants

malformed low-set ears syndrome craniofacial disorder, characterized by deformed low-set ears and possible mental retardation, associated with conductive hearing loss commensurate with degree of auricular malformation

malignant 1. resistant to treatment; of progressive severity; 2. pertaining to a neoplasm that is locally invasive and destructive; cancerous

malignant aural adenoma rare malignant glandular tumor of the external auditory canal and middle ear, which is accompanied by hearing loss, otorrhea, pain, and cranial nerve palsies

malignant external otitis severe bacterial inflammation of the temporal bone, beginning as a focal area of ulceration in the external auditory meatus, which may spread through the tympanic membrane to the middle ear and soft tissue of the mastoid space

malignant otosclerosis severe active otosclerosis involving the oval window, round window, and most of the bony labyrinth, resulting in a mixed hearing loss which eventually progresses to severe or profound levels

malignant sclerosteosis skeletal bone sclerosing disorder present at birth and fatal at an early age, characterized by optic atrophy, retarded growth, fractures, hearing loss, mental retardation, and facial palsy

malinger to feign or exaggerate an illness or impairment such as hearing loss

malingering deliberately feigning or exaggerating an illness or impairment such as hearing loss

malleoincudal joint point of articulation of the malleus and incus

malleolar fold ridges in the tympanic membrane at its attachment to the malleus

malleolar ligaments bands of fibrous tissues suspending and supporting the malleus in the middle ear cavity; includes the superior, anterior, anterior suspensory, and lateral ligaments

malleolar stripe whitish streak on the tympanic membrane, viewed on otoscopic examination; caused by a reflection of the manubrium of the malleus

malleus largest and lateralmost bone of the ossicular chain, articulated on one end to the tympanic membrane and on the other to the incus; COL: hammer

malleus ankylosis stiffness or fixation of the malleus at its abutment to the tegmen tympani

managed care any healthcare or healthcare reimbursement plan or process in which an organization intercedes between patient and provider to make decisions about the nature and manner of services to be provided

managed care organization MCO; health management organization (HMO), preferred provider organization (PPO), insurance company, or other organization that participates in managed care

mandibulofacial dysostosis disorder of embryonic development, resulting in ocular anomalies, defects of the mandible, palate, teeth, and auricle, with associated conductive hearing loss commensurate with the degree of auricular malformation

manometer an instrument for measuring the pressure of gas and liquid

manometry measurement of the pressure of gas or liquid; used in early instrumentation for assessing middle ear function to detect changes in air pressure in the external auditory meatus secondary to stapedius muscle contraction

manual alphabet finger positions and hand movements used in fingerspelling to represent letters of the alphabet

manual audiometry any type of standard hearing measurement in which the examiner controls the stimulus presentation; ANT: automatic audiometry

manual communication method of communicating that involves the use of fingerspelling, gestures, and sign language

manual volume control in hearing aids, any type of control in which the user manipulates the intensity level of the signal; ANT: automatic volume control

manubrium handle of the malleus that extends from the head of the malleus, just below the middle of the tympanic membrane, to the umbo, at the upper part of the pars tensa

MAP minimum audible pressure; monaural threshold of sensitivity to sound presented via earphones; COM: minimum audible field

MAP mitomycin C, adriamycin, platinol (cisplatin); potentially ototoxic chemotherapy regimen used in the treatment of head and neck cancer

map, cochlear implant representation of the threshold and suprathreshold parameters for each electrode or electrode combination in an individual cochlear implant user's speech-coding program

mapping, topographic brain electrophysiologic technique designed to measure distribution of electrical activity across the scalp, in which voltages from ongoing EEG or AEPs are measured at multiple electrodes and represented as different colors in a map of the brain's activity

Marfan syndrome autosomal dominant craniofacial-skeletal disorder, characterized by arachnodactyly, scoliosis, joint hypermobility, and cardiac anomalies, with associated conductive, mixed, or sensorineural hearing loss

marginal cells one of three cell types of the stria vascularis, located on the endolymphatic surface

marginal perforation hole at the edge or margin of the tympanic membrane

Marshall syndrome autosomal dominant disorder, characterized by severe myopia, cataracts, and a malformed nose, with congenital progressive sensorineural hearing loss; SYN: saddle nose and myopia

mask in audiometry, to introduce sound to one ear while testing the other in an effort to eliminate any influence of contralateralization of sound from the test ear to the non-test ear

masked in audiometry, the condition in which an effective level of masking noise has been introduced into one ear while hearing sensitivity is being assessed in the other

masked aided threshold correction correction applied to the measurement of functional gain to account for the masking influence of amplified room noise or circuit noise on aided behavioral thresholds

masked threshold pure-tone or speech audiometric threshold obtained in one ear while the other ear was effectively masked

masker in audiometry, the noise signal used to mask the non-test ear

masker, tinnitus electronic hearing aid device that generates and emits broad-band or narrow-band noise at low levels, designed to mask the presence of tinnitus

masker response, real-ear REMR; probe-microphone measurement of tinnitus masker output

masking 1. use of noise to eliminate the participation of one ear while testing the other; 2. amount or process by which the threshold for one sound is raised by the presence of another sound; 3. noise that interferes with the audibility of another sound

masking, backward the masking of a sound by another sound that occurs milliseconds later

masking, central elevation in hearing sensitivity of the test ear, on the order of 5 dB, as a result of introducing masking noise in the non-test ear, presumably due to the influence of masking noise on central auditory function

masking, comodulation paradigm to measure release from masking by comparing perception of a stimulus in modulated noise to that in unmodulated noise

masking, contralateral the contralateralization of masking noise from the nontest

ear to test ear once it exceeds interaural attenuation; SYN: overmasking

masking, critical bandwidth for in masking pure tones, the frequency range of the masking noise, centered around the pure tone, over which effective masking occurs and beyond which no further masking effect occurs

masking, downward spread of the masking of a low-frequency sound by an intense level of high-frequency sound; SYN: remote masking

masking, effective EM; condition in which noise is just sufficient to mask a given signal when the signal and noise are presented to the same ear simultaneously

masking, forward form of temporal masking in which a noise preceding a tone acts to mask that tone, even though the sounds are not presented simultaneously

masking, maximum in audiometry, the highest level of masking that can be used before overmasking occurs

masking, release from reduction in the effectiveness of masking as a result of a change in some aspect of the masking signal or the signal being masked; e.g., binaural release from masking, in which a change in phase of binaural tones causes them to be audible in noise

masking, remote the masking of a low-frequency sound by an intense level of high-frequency sound; SYN: downward spread of masking

masking, spread of masking of a sound of one frequency by sound of another frequency, including upward spread of masking and downward or remote masking

masking, temporal the interference of one sound with another that is not presented simultaneously, increasing systematically as the interval between the signal and masker decreases

masking, upward spread of the masking of high-frequency sound by low-frequency sound, e.g., weaker high-frequency consonant sounds being masked by stronger low-frequency vowel sounds

masking efficiency relationship of the intensity level of a masker and the magnitude of the threshold shift that it produces

masking level difference MLD; improvement in binaural masked thresholds of signals that differ in some parameter over signals that are identical in both ears; clinically, binaural thresholds are tracked in noise for tones that are in phase and 180° out of phase

mass quantity of matter in a body

master hearing aid electronic device that simulates a wide range of electroacoustic parameters of a hearing aid, used in the prefitting selection of hearing aid gain and frequency response

mastoid conical projection of the temporal bone, lying posterior and inferior to the external auditory meatus, that creates a bony protuberance behind and below the auricle

mastoid air cells air-filled spaces throughout the mastoid, which are highly variable in number and shape

mastoid antrum enlarged space in the mastoid portion of the temporal lobe extending posteriorly from the epitympanic recess and connected via the aditus

mastoid artery artery in the mastoid portion of the temporal bone, branching from the occipital artery and supplying the posterior part of the mastoid bone

mastoid bone mastoid

mastoid cavity, radical cavity that remains following radical mastoidectomy, which is prone to recurrent serous or purulent discharge

mastoid emissary vein vein through the mastoid that carries blood from the scalp, entering the lateral venous sinus in its sigmoid portion

mastoid notch deep incisure at the medial limit of the mastoid process

mastoid process mastoid

mastoid shunt a surgically placed tube used in to drain the endolymphatic sac to relieve hydrops in Ménière's disease

mastoid wall posterior surface of the tympanic cavity, containing the opening or aditus to the mastoid antrum

mastoidectomy excision of the bony partitions forming the mastoid air cells to establish drainage for acute infections of the middle ear and mastoid that are unresponsive to drug therapy

mastoidectomy, modified radical surgical procedure for chronic suppurative infection of the middle ear and mastoid, consisting of excision of the mastoid air cells, posterior wall of the ear canal, and lateral wall of the epitympanic space, preserving the middle ear structures

mastoidectomy, radical surgical procedure performed to establish drainage for nonresponsive otitis media and mastoiditis, consisting of removal of the mastoid air cells, posterior wall of the ear canal, lateral wall of the epitympanic space, malleus, incus, and eardrum

mastoidectomy, simple excision of the bony partitions forming the mastoid air cells to establish drainage for acute infections of the middle ear and mastoid that are unresponsive to drug therapy

mastoiditis inflammation of the mastoid process

matching, impedance the process of equalizing impedances of two devices or media

matrix in hearing aid amplification, a group of electroacoustic gain curves and specifications designed to assist in the preselection of a frequency response

matrix approximation estimate of hearing aid matrix characteristics by prescriptive specification of gain and conversion of the desired insertion gain to coupler gain values

maturation process that leads to full development

mature fully developed

maximum acoustic output maximum power output

maximum length sequence MLS; signal-processing technique of interleaving sampling in groups or patterns that permits the presentation of stimuli at very high rates and the subsequent deconvolution of the interleaved patterns into their component responses

maximum masking in audiometry, the highest level of masking that can be used before overmasking occurs

maximum power output MPO; highest intensity level that a hearing aid can produce, regardless of input level; SYN: saturation sound pressure level

maximum tolerable pressure loudness discomfort level

MBC methotrexate, bleomycin, cisplatin; potentially ototoxic chemotherapy regimen used in the treatment of cervical cancer

MBD minimal brain dysfunction; early term used to describe a constellation of idiopathic behavioral, language, and learning disorders

MCL most comfortable loudness; intensity level at which sound is perceived to be most comfortable, usually expressed in dB HL

MCOs managed care organizations; HMOs, PPOs, insurance companies, and other organizations that participate in managed care

MCR message-to-competition ratio; in speech audiometry, the ratio in dB of the presentation level of a speech target to that of background competition; SYN: signal-to-noise ratio

MCT earmold minimal contact technology earmold; earmold designed to reduce the occlusion effect by limiting contact with the cartilaginous portion of the external auditory meatus and instead sealing around its perimeter at the medial tip

ME middle ear

mean statistical measure of central tendency derived from adding a set of values and dividing by the number of values; SYN: average

Meaningful Auditory Integration Scale MAIS; assessment scale, completed by parents of children with hearing impairment, that assesses the effectiveness of hearing aids or cochlear implants

measles highly contagious viral infection, characterized by fever, cough, conjunctivitis, and cutaneous rash, which can cause purulent labyrinthitis and consequent bilateral severe to profound sensorineural hearing loss

measles, German mild viral infection, characterized by fever and a transient eruption or rash on the skin resembling measles; when occurring in pregnancy, may result in abnormalities in the fetus, including sensorineural hearing loss; SYN: rubella

meatal pertaining to a meatus

meatoplasty reparative or reconstructive surgery of the external auditory meatus

meatus any anatomical passageway or channel, especially the external opening of a canal

meatus acusticus externus external auditory meatus; canal extending from the auricle to the tympanic membrane

meatus acusticus internus internal auditory meatus; opening on the posterior surface of the petrous portion of the temporal bone through which the auditory and facial nerves pass

mechanical tuning in hearing, the amount of frequency resolution or tuning attributable to the cochlea from the displacement caused by Békésy's traveling wave

mechanoreceptor any receptor responding to mechanical force

medial anatomical direction, referring to structures that are located toward the median plane or midline; ANT: lateral

medial geniculate MG; auditory nucleus of the thalamus, divided into central and surrounding pericentral nuclei, that receives primary ascending fibers from the inferior colliculus and sends fibers, via the auditory radiations, to the auditory cortex

medial geniculate body MGB; medial geniculate

medial inferior pontine syndrome vascular lesion of the inferior pons, with symptoms that include contralateral hemiplegia and ipsilateral facial weakness

medial nucleus of the trapezoid body MNTB or MTB; a nucleus of the superior olivary complex that receives primary ascending projections from the contralateral anterior ventral cochlear nucleus and sends projections to the ipsilateral lateral superior olive and lateral lemniscus

medial olivocochlear bundle efferent pathway of nerve fibers emanating from the periolivary nuclei surrounding the MSO, coursing through the ipsilateral and contralateral internal auditory canals along the vestibular nerve, and terminating on the bases of outer hair cells

medial rectus muscle muscle, innervated by the oculomotor nerve, responsible for horizontal eye movement toward the midline

medial superior olive MSO; one of the primary nuclei of the superior olivary complex, located in the hindbrain, receiving primary ascending projections directly from both the ipsilateral and contralateral anterior ventral cochlear nuclei

median statistical measurement of central tendency describing the midpoint of a set of ranked values, with half of the values below and half above

median plane anatomical plane of reference denoting a section projecting through the middle of the head; SYN: midsagittal plane

median plane localization perception of a fused sound as being centered in the middle of the head

medicolegal pertaining to medical jurisprudence

medium in acoustics, the substance through which sound travels

MEDLARS medical literature analysis

and retrieval system; computer-based index system of the U.S. National Library of Medicine

MEDLINE MEDLARS on-line; computer network of U.S. medical libraries and MEDLARS for rapid literature searches

medulla oblongata hindbrain portion of the central nervous system between the pons and spinal cord

MEE middle ear effusion; exudation of fluid from the membranous walls of the middle ear cavity, secondary to inflammation

MEG magnoencephalography; noninvasive technique, using scalp recordings, designed to measure spontaneous or sensory-evoked changes in magnetic fields of the cortex

megacephaly; megalocephaly abnormal enlargement of the head; SYN: macrocephaly

megahertz 1 million hertz

megaloencephaly abnormal largeness of the brain

mel unit of pitch equal to 1/1000 the pitch of a 1000-Hz tone at a specified intensity, so that a 1000-Hz tone at 40 dB HL has a pitch of 1000 mels

Melnick-Fraser syndrome autosomal dominant brachial arch syndrome with auricular anomalies and conductive, mixed, or sensorineural hearing loss; SYN: branchio-oto-renal syndrome

melotia congenital displacement of the auricle

membrane thin layer of pliable tissue that connects structures, divides spaces or organs, and lines cavities

membrane, basement thin membranous portion of Reissner's membrane that separates the mesothelial cell layer in the scala vestibuli from the epithelial cell layer in the scala media

membrane, basilar base of the membranous labyrinth of the cochlea, dividing it into the scala vestibuli and scala tympani, that supports the scala media and organ of Corti

membrane, mucous any epithelial lining of an organ or structure, such as the tympanic cavity, that secretes mucus

membrane, otolithic structure in the maculae of the utricle and saccule containing otoconia into which the stereocilia of the hair cells are embedded

membrane, Reissner's membrane within the cochlear duct, attached to the osseous spiral lamina and projecting obliquely to the outer wall of the cochlea, that separates the scala vestibuli and scala media

membrane, round window thin membrane covering the round window, sometimes referred to as the secondary tympanic membrane

membrane, Scarpa's round window

membrane, Shrapnell pars flaccida portion of the tympanic membrane

membrane, tectorial gelatinous membrane within the scala media projecting radially from the spiral limbus and overlying the organ of Corti, in which the cilia of the outer hair cells are embedded

membrane, tympanic TM; thin, membranous vibrating tissue terminating the external auditory meatus and forming the major portion of the lateral wall of the middle ear cavity, onto which the malleus is attached; COL: eardrum

membrane, vestibular Reissner's membrane, separating the scala vestibuli and scala media

membranous pertaining to or in the form of a membrane

membranous atresia congenital absence of the external auditory meatus due to a dense soft tissue plug between the external auditory canal and middle ear space; COM: bony atresia

membranous labyrinth soft-tissue, fluid-filled channels within the osseous labyrinth that contain the end organ structures for hearing and vestibular function

membranous semicircular ducts portions of the membranous labyrinth that courses through the semicircular canals

membranous wall lateral surface of the tympanic cavity, formed largely by the tympanic membrane

memory information-processing function of the central nervous system that receives, modifies, stores, and retrieves information in short-term or long-term form

memory, auditory assimilation, storage, and retrieval of previously experienced sound

memory, long-term aspect of the information-processing function of the central nervous system that receives, modifies, and stores information on a permanent basis for later retrieval

memory, short-term aspect of the information-processing function of the central nervous system that receives, modifies, and stores information briefly

memory span, auditory number of items that can be recalled following presentation of speech or other sounds

Memphis State University prescriptive procedure MSU procedure; gain and frequency response selection algorithm based on the theory that a hearing aid should amplify the long-term speech spectrum to a point halfway between threshold and the upper limit of comfortable loudness

Ménière's disease idiopathic endolymphatic hydrops, characterized by fluctuating vertigo, hearing loss, tinnitus, and aural fullness

Ménière's disease, cochlear atypical form of Ménière's disease in which only the characteristic auditory symptoms are present without vertiginous episodes

Ménière's disease, vestibular atypical form of Ménière's disease in which only the characteristic vestibular symptoms are present without hearing loss

Ménière's syndrome constellation of symptoms of episodic vertigo, hearing loss, tinnitus, and aural fullness

meninges the three membranes—arachnoidea, dura mater, and pia mater—covering the brain and spinal cord

meningioma benign tumor arising from the arachnoid villi of the sigmoid and petrosal sinuses at the posterior aspect of the petrous pyramid, which may encroach on the cerebellopontine angle, resulting in retrocochlear disorder

meningitis bacterial or viral inflammation of the meninges, which can cause significant auditory disorder due to suppurative labyrinthitis or inflammation of the lining of Cranial Nerve VIII

meningitis, otitic infection of the meninges secondary to otitis media or mastoiditis

meningo-neuro-labyrinthitis inflammation of the membranous labyrinth and Cranial Nerve VIII meninges, occurring as a predominant lesion in early congenital syphilis or in acute attacks of secondary and tertiary syphilis

meninx one of the meninges

meniscus crescent-shaped structure or form, used to describe the fluid line visible upon otoscopic examination of the tympanic membrane when middle ear effusion is present

mental age MA; intellectual age, as measured on standardized tests

mental-alerting tasks tasks, such as arithmetic problem solving, designed to maintain a patient's alertness during vestibular or other assessment

mental retardation intellectual function below the normal range

MEP multimodality evoked potentials; collective term referring to the sensory evoked potentials, including auditory, visual, and somatosensory electrophysiologic measures

mesencephalic referring to the mesencephalon

mesencephalon midbrain of the central nervous system, the auditory portion of which includes the nuclei of the lateral lemniscus and the inferior colliculus

mesenchyme connective tissue of the embryo

mesoderm middle of three primary embryonic germ layers that become the connective tissues, muscles, blood vessels, and lymph vessels at maturation

mesotympanum middle ear; tympanic cavity

message-to-competition ratio MCR; in speech audiometry, the ratio in dB of the presentation level of a speech target to that of background competition; SYN: signal-to-noise ratio

metabolism sum of physical and chemical processes that maintain a living organism

metacognition the process of thinking about the process of thought

metalinguistic pertaining to the use of language to think and communicate about language

metastasis the shift or spread of disease from one part of the body to another

metastatic neoplasm abnormal tissue growth in parts of the body remote from the original, primary tumor

meter measuring device

meter, decibel sound level meter

meter, otoadmittance early immittance measurement instrument designed to assess susceptance and conductance components of middle ear function

meter, sound level an electronic instrument designed to measure sound intensity in dB in accordance with an accepted standard

meter, VU volume unit meter; visual indicator on an audiometer showing intensity of an input signal in dB, where 0 dB is equal to the attenuator output setting

method of adjustment psychophysical procedure for determining absolute or differential threshold in which the observer controls the changes in the stimulus necessary to measure a threshold

method of constant stimuli psychophysical procedure for determining thresholds in which the same stimuli that fall into a discrete range about the threshold of interest are presented repeatedly until a 50% threshold is determined on a psychometric function

method of limits psychophysical procedure for determining absolute or differential threshold in which the stimuli are presented at levels well above or below threshold and changed in small increments until the boundary of sensation is reached

Metz test indirect measure of recruitment by comparing the behavioral pure-tone threshold to the acoustic stapedial reflex threshold; as the former approaches the latter, the difference is reduced, indicating disordered loudness growth, or recruitment

mg milligram; one-thousandth of a gram

MG medial geniculate; auditory nucleus of the thalamus, divided into central and surrounding pericentral nuclei, that receives primary ascending fibers from the inferior colliculus and sends fibers, via the auditory radiations, to the auditory cortex

mg per kg milligrams per kilogram; method of expressing dosage of a drug in terms of quantity per measure of body weight

MGB medial geniculate body; medial geniculate

mho unit of electrical conductance, expressed as the reciprocal of ohm

MHz megahertz; 1 million cycles per second

micro prefix denoting one-millionth

microbar unit of pressure, representing one-millionth of a bar

microcephalic having an abnormally small head

microcephaly abnormal smallness of the head

micropascal unit of pressure, representing one-millionth of a pascal

microphone transducer that converts sound waves into an electric signal

microphone, air-dielectric type of condenser microphone that derives its electrical output from changes in distance between two polarized plates, with air serving as the dielectric between the two plates

microphone, boom microphone that is suspended above a speaker's head

microphone, capacitor condenser microphone

microphone, carbon early microphone that used carbon granules to convert sound pressure into electrical energy

microphone, ceramic type of piezoelectric microphone in which electric current is generated by applied mechanical stress

microphone, condenser microphone in which the variation of capacitance in response to sound level controls the electrical signal; includes air-dielectric and electret microphones; SYN: electrostatic microphone

microphone, crystal early piezoelectric microphone in which mechanical stress was applied to generate electric current in crystals such as quartz and lithium sulfate

microphone, directional microphone with a transducer that is more responsive to sound from a focused direction; in hearing aids, the microphone is designed to be more sensitive to sounds emanating from the front than from behind

microphone, dynamic microphone consisting of a thin diaphragm that, as it moves, induces voltage in a coil in a magnetic field

microphone, electret type of condenser microphone that uses a permanently charged material as the dielectric between the two polarized plates

microphone, electrostatic condenser microphone in which the variation of capacitance in response to sound level controls the electrical signal

microphone, electrostatic condenser microphone in which the variation of capacitance in response to sound level controls the electrical signal

microphone, environmental EM; the microphone on a hearing aid that transduces airborne sound

microphone, lavalier small microphone hung around the neck

microphone, nondirectional omnidirectional microphone

microphone, omnidirectional microphone with a sensitivity that is similar regardless of the direction of incoming sound

microphone, piezoelectric transducer in which acoustic energy is converted to electric current by applied mechanical stress on ceramic or crystal

microphone, probe microphone transducer with a small-diameter probe-tube extension for measuring sound near the tympanic membrane

microphone, probe-tube probe microphone

microphone, reference a second microphone used to measure the stimulus level during probe-microphone measurements or to control the stimulus level during the probe-microphone equalization process

microphone, unidirectional microphone that is responsive predominantly to sound incident from a single position; SYN: directional microphone

microphonic, cochlear cochlear microphonic; alternating current electrical potential of the cochlea that resembles the input signal

microprocessor audiometer automatic audiometer characterized by its ability to carry out pure-tone audiometry under microprocessor control

microsecond one-millionth of a second

microtia abnormal smallness of the auricle

microvilli extensions of the cell membranes of the hair cells, projecting from their apical end to form the stereocilia

μV microvolt; one-millionth of a volt

microvolt μV; 1 microvolt equals 0.000001 volts; one-millionth of a volt

mid frequency nonspecific term referring to frequencies around 1000 Hz to 2000 Hz

mid-frequency hearing loss nonspecific term referring to hearing sensitivity loss occurring at frequencies around 1000 Hz to 2000 Hz

midbrain mesencephalon of the central nervous system, the auditory portion of which includes the nuclei of the lateral lemniscus and the inferior colliculus

middle ear portion of the hearing mechanism extending from the medial membrane of the tympanic membrane to the oval window of the cochlea, including the ossicles and middle ear cavity; serves as an impedance matching device of the outer and inner ears

middle ear cavity space in the temporal bone, including the tympanic cavity, epitympanum, and eustachian tube; SYN: middle ear space

middle ear cleft middle ear cavity

middle ear effusion MEE; exudation of fluid from the membranous walls of the middle ear cavity, secondary to inflammation

middle ear implant, allogeneic tissue, such as tympanic membrane and ossicles, from another individual used in reconstructive middle ear surgery

middle ear implant, alloplastic ossicular prosthesis made of inert material, such as ceramic or plastic, used in reconstructive middle ear surgery

middle ear muscle reflex reflexive contraction of the stapedius and tensor tympani muscles in response to loud sound; stapedius muscle dominates the reflex in humans; SYN: acoustic reflex

middle ear pressure, negative air pressure in the middle ear cavity that is below atmospheric pressure, resulting from an inability to equalize pressure due to eustachian tube dysfunction

middle ear pressure, positive air pressure in the middle ear cavity that is greater than atmospheric pressure, resulting from air being forced into the middle ear through the eustachian tube

middle ear space middle ear cavity

middle fossa approach surgical strategy used to preserve hearing during removal of tumors confined to the internal auditory canal

middle-latency auditory evoked response MLAER; auditory evoked potential, originating from the region of the auditory radiations and cortex, having as a

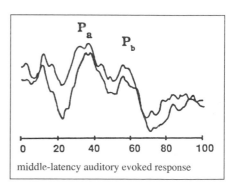

middle-latency auditory evoked response

primary component a vertex positive peak at 25 msec to 40 msec following signal presentation; SYN: auditory middle latency response

middle-latency response MLR; middle-latency auditory evoked response

middle-latency response, electrically evoked EMLR; auditory middle-latency response generated by electrical stimulation of the cochlea with either an extracochlear promontory electrode or a cochlear implant

midline at the middle

midsagittal plane anatomical plane of reference denoting a section projecting through the middle of the head; SYN: median plane

migration embryologic process during which young neurons move from their birth site to their adult location

mild hearing loss loss of hearing sensitivity of 25 dB HL to 40 dB HL

miliary tuberculosis infectious bacterial disease characterized by formation of tubercles of millet-seed size in the central nervous system; involvement of the auditory pathways can result in retrocochlear disorder

milli- prefix denoting one-thousandth

milligram mg; one-thousandth of a gram

millimeter of water mm H_2O; unit of air pressure used in tympanometry

millimho mmho; one-thousandth of a mho

millisecond msec; one-thousandth of a second

mini CROS CROS hearing aid with a short tube from the receiver on the good ear, designed to provide minimum gain to that ear

minimal auditory deficiency syndrome constellation of auditory deficits that may result from intermittent auditory stimulation during childhood as a result of conductive hearing loss secondary to recurrent otitis media

minimal brain dysfunction MBD; early term used to describe a constellation of idiopathic behavioral, language, and learning disorders

minimal contact technology earmold MCT earmold; earmold designed to reduce the occlusion effect by limiting contact with the cartilaginous portion of the external auditory meatus and instead sealing around its perimeter at the medial tip

minimal pairs test a two-alternative

closed-set word-recognition task for children that uses two pictures that vary by one segmental feature for both consonant and vowel contrast pairs

minimal response level lowest level to which a child will respond behaviorally to sound

minimum audible angle measure of the minimum detectable azimuth difference, an amount that varies as a function of azimuth and is best at 0°

minimum audible field MAF; binaural threshold of sensitivity to sound presented in a sound field via loudspeaker placed at 0° azimuth; COM: minimum audible pressure

minimum audible pressure MAP; monaural threshold of sensitivity to sound presented via earphones; COM: minimum audible field

minimum auditory capabilities battery MAC battery; group of tests designed to assess auditory perception of persons with profound hearing loss

minimum contralateral interference level on the Stenger test, the lowest intensity level of a signal presented to the allegedly poorer-hearing ear that causes the patient to stop responding, despite continued suprathreshold presentation to the better ear

mismatch, impedance condition in which two devices or media between which energy flows have different impedances

mismatched negativity MMN; auditory evoked potential recorded using an oddball paradigm, characterized by a negative peak at 100 msec to 200 msec, reflecting discrimination ability for different simple and complex sound features

mitochondrial disorders abnormalities of mitochondrial DNA that can result in isolated sensorineural hearing loss or hearing loss associated with other features of the disease, including encephalopathy, myopathy, seizure disorder, ataxia, and ophthalmoplegia

mixed hearing loss hearing loss with both a conductive and a sensorineural component

MLAER middle latency auditory evoked response; auditory evoked potential, originating from the region of the auditory radiations and cortex, having as a primary component a vertex positive peak at 25 msec to 40 msec following signal presentation; SYN: AMLR

MLB monaural loudness balance test; test of loudness recruitment that compares loudness growth at a frequency at which the patient has normal hearing to loudness growth at a frequency at which the patient has hearing loss in the same ear

MLD masking level difference; measure of binaural release from masking in which binaural thresholds are tracked in noise for tones that are in phase and 180 out of phase

MLR middle latency response; middle latency auditory evoked response

MLS maximum length sequence; signal processing technique of interleaved sampling in groups or patterns that permits the presentation of stimuli at very high rates

MLV monitored live voice; outdated speech audiometric technique in which speech signals were presented via a microphone with controlled vocal output; SYN: live-voice testing

mm H₂0 millimeter of water; unit of air pressure used in tympanometry

mmho millimho; one-thousandth of a mho

MMN mismatched negativity; auditory evoked potential recorded using an oddball paradigm, characterized by a negative peak at 100 msec to 200 msec, reflecting discrimination ability for different simple and complex sound features

MNTB medial nucleus of the trapezoid body; nucleus of the superior olivary complex that receives primary ascending projections from the contralateral AVCN and sends projections to the ipsilateral lateral superior olive and lateral lemniscus

mobile hearing conservation program hearing conservation service that uses a mobile test van to provide on-site industrial hearing screenings

mobile unit mobile van equipped to provide on-site industrial hearing screenings

mobilization of the stapes surgical procedure in cases of otosclerosis to free the footplate of the stapes from the oval window

Möbius syndrome severe congenital bilateral facial paralysis, associated with neurological, ocular, and musculoskeletal anomalies due to lesions of Cranial Nerves III, V, VI, VII, and XII, with associated middle ear anomalies and sensorineural hearing loss

modality any of the physical senses, including vision, hearing, smell, taste, and touch

mode statistical term describing the value that occurs most frequently in a set of values

moderate hearing loss loss of hearing sensitivity of 40 dB HL to 55 dB HL

moderately severe hearing loss loss of hearing sensitivity of 55 dB HL to 70 dB HL

modification change in structure or function

modification, earmold change in the structure of an earmold to alter the fit or the acoustic characteristics

modified peak clipping peak clipping in hearing aid amplification that removes the extremes of alternating current amplitude peaks at some predetermined level in a gradual manner that reduces distortion; SYN: soft peak clipping

modified pressure method in probe-microphone measurements, equalization method in which the field reference microphone is placed near the surface of the head, outside the acoustic influence of the external ear and the hearing aid

modified radical mastoidectomy surgical procedure for chronic suppurative infection of the middle ear and mastoid, consisting of excision of the mastoid air cells, posterior wall of the ear canal, and lateral wall of the epitympanic space, preserving the middle ear structures

modified Rainville test test of masked bone-conduction thresholds by establishing thresholds by air conduction with and without masking noise presented through a bone vibrator placed on the forehead; SYN: sensorineural acuity level (SAL) test

modified rhyme test closed-set word-recognition test in which the signal and foils rhyme

modified SISI test early test used in differential diagnosis in which short increments of 1 dB were superimposed on a carrier tone presented at a high intensity level; the ability to detect the increments is consistent with normal hearing or cochlear hearing loss

modified Stenger test Stenger test in which spondaic words are used in place of pure tones; SYN: speech Stenger

modiolus central bony pillar of the cochlea through which the blood vessels and nerve fibers of the labyrinth course

modulation periodic change in a particular stimulus dimension

modulation transfer function description of the ability of an acoustic or electronic transmission system to maintain the amplitude characteristics of a signal envelope

modulation, amplitude AM; the process of varying the magnitude of a radio wave or sound wave in relation to the strength of the carrier wave

modulation, frequency FM; the process of creating a complex signal by sinusoidally varying the frequency of a carrier wave

Mohr syndrome autosomal recessive craniofacial disorder, characterized by deformities of face, mouth, and fingers, associated with conductive hearing loss due to ossicular malformation

monaural pertaining to one ear

monaural hearing aid hearing aid worn on one ear only

monaural loudness balance test MLB; test of loudness recruitment that compares loudness growth at a frequency at which the patient has normal hearing to loudness growth at a frequency at which the patient has hearing loss in the same ear

Mondini dysplasia congenital anomaly of the osseous and membranous labyrinths, exhibiting a wide range of morphologic and functional abnormality, including severe loss of hearing and vestibular function

monesthetic pertaining to a single sense

mongolism Down syndrome

monitored live voice MLV; outdated speech audiometric technique in which speech signals are presented via a microphone with controlled vocal output; SYN: live-voice testing

monitoring continuous assessment of the integrity of function over time, such as intraoperative or ototoxicity monitoring

monitoring, intraoperative continuous assessment of integrity of cranial nerves during surgery; e.g., during acoustic tumor removal, Cranial Nerve VII is monitored because of proximity of the dissection, and Cranial Nerve VIII is monitored in an attempt to preserve hearing

monitoring, ototoxicity continuous assessment of hearing over the course of treatment with ototoxic drugs

monomeric tympanic membrane eardrum membrane that is missing a portion of the fibrous layer

monopolar electrode an electrode with one pole that is active for recording or de-

livering electrical signals; COM: bipolar electrode

monopolar stimulation 1. delivery of an electrical signal to one pole of an electrode array; 2. cochlear implant stimulation in which the active electrode is intracochlear and the indifferent electrode is extracochlear; COM: bipolar stimulation

monosyllabic word a word of one syllable

monosyllable-trochee-spondee test MTS test; speech-audiometric measure of word recognition and stress-pattern identification in children

monothermal caloric stimulation measure of vestibular function by irrigation of the external auditory meatus with warm, cool, or ice water only; COM: bithermal caloric stimulation

monotic presented to one ear

monotonic pertaining to a function that does not vary as the independent variable changes

montage in electrophysiology, the configuration of electrode positions used to record a given potential

Moro reflex normal reaction of infants to a variety of stimuli, characterized by a sudden extension and abduction of the arms, hands, and fingers

Moro reflex test test designed to assess the presence of a Moro reflex in response to the sudden presentation of sound

morpheme smallest unit of language that conveys meaning

morphology the qualitative description of an auditory evoked potential, related to the replicability of the response and the ease with which component peaks can be identified

Morquio syndrome rare autosomal recessive metabolic disorder, or mucopolysaccharidosis, characterized by dwarfism, major skeletal disorders, corneal clouding, and hearing loss

most comfortable loudness MCL; intensity level at which sound is perceived to be most comfortable, usually expressed in dB HL

motoneuron motor neuron

motoneurons, stapedial single-celled column of neurons, responsible for stapedius muscle contraction, located medially to the motor nucleus of Cranial Nerve VII and extended anteriorly to the area between the superior olivary complex and the motor nucleus

motor nerve efferent nerve carrying information from the central nervous system to a muscle or other effector

motor neuron efferent nerve fiber that conveys impulses from the central nervous system to peripheral muscles

motor nucleus of the facial nerve nucleus in the hindbrain sending projections to facial muscles, including the stapedius muscle

motorboating colloquial term to describe the sound that is sometimes generated by a hearing aid as the battery weakens

motoric compensation compensatory movement of the muscles in response to changes in gravitational pull

movement coordination test computerized dynamic posturography subtest in which forceplates, which measure leg movements, are subjected to a series of computer-driven movements during which motoric compensation is assessed

MPO maximum power output; highest intensity level that a hearing aid can produce, regardless of input level; SYN: saturation sound pressure level

MR mental retardation; intellectual function below the normal range

MRI magnetic resonance imaging; radiographic technique used to provide precise structural images

MS multiple sclerosis; demyelinating disease involving the white matter of the brainstem, resulting in diffuse neurologic symptoms, including hearing loss, speech-understanding deficits, and abnormalities of the acoustic reflexes and ABR

msec millisecond; one-thousandth of a second

MSO medial superior olive; one of the primary nuclei of the superior olivary complex, located in the hindbrain, receiving primary ascending projections directly from both the ipsilateral and contralateral anterior ventral cochlear nuclei

MSU prescriptive procedure Memphis State University procedure; gain and frequency response selection algorithm based on the theory that a hearing aid should amplify the long-term speech spectrum to a point halfway between threshold and ULCL

MTB medial nucleus of the trapezoid body; a nucleus of the superior olivary complex, receiving primary ascending projections from the contralateral anterior ventral cochlear nucleus and sending projections to the ipsilateral LSO and lateral lemniscus

MTS monosyllable-trochee-spondee test; speech-audiometric measure of word recognition and stress-pattern identification in children

μ mu; micro-; one-millionth

mu μ; micro-; one-millionth

Muckle-Wells syndrome autosomal dominant endocrine and metabolic disorder of teenage onset characterized by progressive nephropathy and renal failure, with coincident progressive sensorineural hearing loss

mucoid effusion thick, viscid, mucuslike fluid

mucoid otitis media inflammation of the middle ear, with mucoid effusion

mucopolysaccharides complex of protein and carbohydrates

mucopolysaccharidosis any of a group of rare diseases related to abnormal deposition of mucopolysaccharides in the central nervous system, including Hurler syndrome, Hunter syndrome, Sanfilippo syndrome, and Morquio syndrome

mucosa mucous membrane

mucosanguinous otitis media inflammation of the middle ear with effusion consisting of blood and mucus

mucous pertaining to mucus or a mucous membrane

mucous membrane any epithelial lining of an organ or structure, such as the tympanic cavity, that secretes mucus

mucous otitis mucoid otitis media

mucus clear, viscid fluid secreted by a mucous membrane

multichannel compression process in which a hearing aid separates the input signal into two or more frequency bands, each having independently controlled compression circuitry

multi-CROS a CROS hearing aid system that can be changed to a CROS, BICROS or conventional hearing aid configuration

multichannel processing signal processing in more than one channel, referring especially to cochlear implant configurations

multifrequency tympanometry tympanometric assessment of middle ear function with a conventional 220-Hz probe tone and with one or more additional probe-tone frequencies

multimodality evoked potentials MEP; collective term referring to the sensory evoked potentials, including auditory, visual, and somatosensory electrophysiologic measures

multiple lentigines syndrome autosomal dominant integumentary-pigmentary disorder, characterized by small brown spots on the neck and upper trunk and multiple anomalies, including sensorineural hearing loss

multiple-memory hearing aid hearing aid that can be programmed to contain more than one frequency response for use under different listening conditions

multiple sclerosis MS; demyelinating disease in which plaques form throughout the white matter of the brainstem, resulting in diffuse neurologic symptoms, including hearing loss, speech-understanding deficits, and abnormalities of the acoustic reflexes and ABR

multisensory approach aural habilitation approach using visual, auditory, and tactile stimulation to enhance communication learning

mumps contagious systemic viral disease, characterized by painful enlargement of parotid glands, fever, headache, and malaise; associated with sudden, permanent, profound unilateral sensorineural hearing loss; SYN: parotitis, epidemic parotitis

muscle fibrous contractile tissue, attached by a tendon to a bone or other structure, which produces motion upon stimulation

muscle, auricularis anterior muscle innervated by the facial nerve that inserts into the cartilage of the ear and may draw the auricle forward

muscle, auricularis posterior muscle innervated by the facial nerve that originates at the mastoid process and inserts into the cartilage of the ear and may draw the auricle backward

muscle, auricularis superior muscle innervated by the facial nerve that inserts into the cartilage of the ear and may raise the auricle

muscle, auricularis transverse muscle innervated by the facial nerve that inserts into the cartilage of the ear

muscle, lateral rectus muscle innervated by the abducens nerve responsible for

horizontal eye movement away from the midline

muscle, levator veli palatini along with the tensor veli palatini, one of two muscles of the nasophyarynx responsible for opening the end of the eustachian tube by medial displacement of the cartilage; innervated by the pharyngeal plexus

muscle, medial rectus muscle innervated by the oculomotor nerve responsible for horizontal eye movement toward the midline

muscle, oblique auricular one of four muscles attaching to the medial surface of the auricle

muscle, stapedius along with the tensor tympani, one of two striated muscles of the middle ear, classified as a pennate muscle, consisting of short fibers directed obliquely onto the stapedius tendon at the midline, innervated by the facial nerve, Cranial Nerve VII

muscle, tensor tympani along with the stapedius, one of two striated muscles of the middle ear, classified as a pennate muscle, consisting of short fibers directed obliquely onto the stapedius tendon at the midline, innervated by the trigeminal nerve, Cranial Nerve V

muscle, tensor veli palatini along with the levator veli palatini, one of two muscles of the nasophyarynx responsible for opening the end of the eustachian tube by medial displacement of the tube membrane, innervated by the trigeminal nerve, Cranial Nerve V

muscle artifact in the recording of auditory evoked potentials, the unwanted myogenic electrical activity generated from neck or other muscles

muscles, extraocular muscles located around the eye, including the lateral, medial, superior, and inferior rectus

muscles, intra-aural stapedius and tensor tympani muscles of the middle ear

muscles, tympanic stapedius and tensor tympanic muscles of the middle ear, which serve to suspend the ossicles of the middle ear, thereby reducing the effective mass of the ossicular chain

muscular dystrophy autosomal recessive disorder characterized by muscle wasting; severe infantile muscular dystrophy is associated with mild-to-moderate sensorineural hearing loss

musician's earplug hearing protection

device designed to attenuate sound equally across the frequency range to maintain the fidelity of sound, especially music

mutation alteration in a gene that produces a change in later generations of an organism

mute unable or unwilling to speak

mutism organic or functional absence of speech

MVAC methotrexate, vinblastine, adriamycin, cisplatin; potentially ototoxic chemotherapy regimen used in the treatment of bladder cancer

MX-41/AR cushion standard cushion mounted on a circumaural earphone used commonly in audiometry

mycomyringitis fungal inflammation of the tympanic membrane

myelin tissue enveloping the axon of myelinated nerve fibers, composed of alternating layers of lipids and protein

myelin sheath cover of myelin over nerve fibers

myelination formation of the myelin sheath around a nerve fiber

myeloarchitecture distribution of nerve fibers in an area

myoclonic pertaining to myoclonus

myoclonic epilepsy autosomal dominant nervous system disorder, characterized by myoclonic jerking and progressive ataxia; associated with late-onset progressive sensorineural hearing loss

myoclonus twitching of a muscle or group of muscles

myogenic originating in muscle; COM: neurogenic

myopia and congenital deafness autosomal recessive disorder, characterized by myopia and congenital moderate-to-severe sensorineural hearing loss

myositis ossificans dominant skeletal disorder, characterized by formation of osseous tissue in skeletal muscles, with associated conductive, mixed, or sensorineural hearing loss

myringectomy excision of the tympanic membrane; SYN: myringodectomy

myringitis inflammation of the tympanic membrane, usually associated with infection of the middle ear or external auditory meatus; SYN: tympanitis

myringitis, bullous acute painful viral inflammation of the tympanic membrane accompanied by bullae formation between layers of the tympanic membrane, commonly occurring in association with influenza

myringitis, granular focal or diffuse replacement of the dermis of the tympanic membrane with granulation tissue

myringodectomy myringectomy

myringomycosis fungal infection of the tympanic membrane and adjoining skin of the external auditory meatus

myringoplasty procedure in which a tissue graft, usually of fascia or vein, is used to close a perforation of the tympanic membrane

myringostapediopexy surgical technique in which the tympanic membrane or membrane graft is functionally connected to the head of the stapes

myringotomy passage of a needle through the tympanic membrane to remove effusion from the middle ear

myrinx tympanic membrane

N

N Newton; unit of physical force

N/m² Newton per square meter; unit of measure of pressure used as a reference for sound measurement

N₁ major negative peak of the late-latency auditory evoked potential, occurring at around 90 msec following stimulus onset

N₁-P₂ major peak complex of the late-latency auditory evoked potential, occurring at around 90 msec and 180 msec following stimulus onset

Nₐ major negative peak of the auditory middle latency response

Na+ chemical symbol for sodium, a substance found in high concentration in perilymph and low concentration in endolymph

NAD National Association of the Deaf

Nager syndrome branchial arch disorder characterized by mandibulofacial dysostosis with limb defects, particularly the absence of thumbs, with hearing loss secondary to outer ear and middle ear malformation; SYN: acrofacial dysostosis

NAL National Acoustic Laboratories in Australia; laboratory responsible for developing the widely used NAL prescriptive hearing aid fitting technique

NAL prescriptive procedure National Acoustic Laboratories procedure; gain and frequency response prescriptive strategy based on the theory that a hearing aid should amplify the long-term spectrum of speech so that it is equally and comfortably loud across frequency

NAL-R procedure revised NAL procedure

NAL-RM procedure modification of the revised NAL procedure for use in prescribing gain and frequency response in cases of severe and profound hearing loss

naproxen anti-inflammatory analgesic drug used to treat rheumatoid arthritis, which, although rarely ototoxic in usual doses, has been associated with sudden, severe, bilateral sensorineural hearing loss and nephrotoxicity

narrow-band filter an electronic filter that allows a specified band of frequencies to pass through while reducing or eliminating frequencies above and below the band; SYN: band-pass filter

narrow-band noise NBN; bandpass-filtered noise that is centered at one of the audiometric frequencies, used for masking in pure-tone audiometry

nasopharynx cavity of the nose and pharynx into which the eustachian tube opens

natal pertaining to birth

National Acoustic Laboratories prescriptive procedure NAL prescriptive procedure

National Association of the Deaf NAD; advocacy group of deaf persons

National Board for Certification in Hearing Instrument Sciences NBC-HIS; organization that sets standards for and awards certification in hearing instrument sciences

National Hearing Aid Society NHAS; former name of the International Hearing Society

National Hearing Conservation Association NHCA; professional association of specialists in hearing conservation

National Institute for Hearing Instrument Sciences NIHIS; educational wing of the International Hearing Society

National Institute for Occupational Safety and Health NIOSH; organization developed under the Occupational Safety and Health Act to fund and conduct research on occupational hazards and to develop criteria and recommend standards

natural auditory boundaries sound discrimination ability present at birth, attributable to the natural operation of the auditory perceptual mechanism

natural frequency frequency at which a secured mass will vibrate most readily when set into free vibration; SYN: resonant frequency

Nb secondary negative peak of the auditory middle latency response

NBC-HIS National Board for Certification in Hearing Instrument Sciences; organization that sets standards for and awards certification in hearing instrument sciences

NBN narrow-band noise; bandpass-filtered noise that is centered at one of the audiometric frequencies, used for masking in pure-tone audiometry

NDT noise-detection threshold; lowest intensity level at which a specified noise signal is audible

near ear   the aided ear in a test situation in which the signal is presented to the same side of the head; ANT: far ear

near field   1. area of a sound field, within about two wavelengths of a noise source, in which there is no simple relationship between distance and sound level; 2. in evoked potentials, condition in which the recording electrode is adjacent to the source

near-field recording   measurement of evoked potentials from electrodes adjacent to the source

neck of the malleus   portion of the malleus located between the head and the manubrium, from which the anterior process protrudes

neckloop   transducer worn as part of an FM amplification system, consisting of a cord from the receiver that is worn around the neck and that transmits signals via magnetic induction to the telecoil of a hearing aid

necrosis   localized pathologic death of body tissue

necrotizing otitis media   persistent inflammation of the middle ear that results in tissue necrosis

needle aspiration   removal by suction of fluid from the middle ear via a needle placed through the tympanic membrane; SYN: myringotomy

negative correlation   inverse relationship of the values of two sets of measures

negative middle ear pressure   air pressure in the middle ear cavity that is below atmospheric pressure, resulting from an inability to equalize pressure due to eustachian tube dysfunction

negative predictive value   probability that a disorder is not present when a diagnostic test is negative

neomycin   highly ototoxic aminoglycoside antibiotic used occasionally as a lifesaving measure in severe bacterial infections

neonatal   pertaining to the first 4 weeks after birth

neonatal intensive care unit   NICU; hospital unit designed to provide care for newborns needing greater than normal support and monitoring

neonate   infant during the first 4 weeks of life

neoplasm   abnormal new growth of tissue, resulting from an excessively rapid proliferation of cells that continue to grow even after cessation of the stimuli that initiated the new growth; SYN: tumor

neoplasm, metastatic   abnormal tissue growth in parts of the body remote from the original, primary tumor

neoplasm, secondary   metastatic neoplasm

neoplastic disease   pathologic process that results in the formation and growth of a neoplasm

nephritis   inflammation of the kidney

nephron   functional tissue of the kidney

nephrosis, urinary tract malformations   autosomal recessive renal disorder, characterized by kidney degeneration, digital anomalies, bifurcation of the uvula, and congenital conductive hearing loss

nephrotoxic   having a poisonous action on the nephrons of the kidney

nephrotoxicity   property of being toxic to kidney cells, a condition that can enhance the ototoxicity of a substance because of failure of the damaged kidneys to filter the noxious toxins

nerve   cordlike structure made of nerve fibers surrounded by connective tissue sheath through which nervous impulses are conducted to and from the central nervous system

nerve, abducens   Cranial Nerve VI; cranial nerve that provides efferent innervation to the lateral rectus muscles involved in eye movement

nerve, accessory   Cranial Nerve XI; cranial and spinal nerve that provides efferent innervation to muscles of the larynx and neck

nerve, acoustic   Cranial Nerve VIII; auditory nerve, consisting of a vestibular and cochlear branch

nerve, Arnold's   nerve formed by a portion of Cranial Nerve X, the inferior branch of which is joined by fibers from the facial nerve to provide cutaneous sensation to a region of the posterior surface of the external auditory canal

nerve, auditory   AN; Cranial Nerve VIII, consisting of a vestibular and cochlear branch; SYN: vestibulocochlear nerve

nerve, cochlear   auditory branch of Cranial Nerve VIII, arising from the spiral ganglion of the cochlea and terminating in the cochlear nuclei of the brainstem

nerve, cranial   any of 12 pairs of neuron bundles exiting the brainstem above the first cervical vertebra

nerve, eighth   Cranial Nerve VIII, consisting of the auditory and vestibular nerves

nerve, facial   Cranial Nerve VII; cranial

nerve that provides efferent innervation to the facial muscles and afferent innervation from the soft palate and tongue

nerve, glossopharyngeal   Cranial Nerve IX; cranial nerve that provides efferent innervation to pharyngeal muscles and the parotid gland and afferent innervation from the auricle, eustachian tube, and posterior one-third of the tongue

nerve, greater superficial pretrosal branch of Cranial Nerve VII from which the nerve to the stapedius muscle arises

nerve, horizontal ampullary   nerve fiber bundle from the hair cells of the crista ampullaris of the horizontal semicircular canal that joins with similar bundles from the other semicircular canals, the utricle, and the saccule to form the vestibular branch of Cranial Nerve VIII

nerve, hypoglossal   Cranial Nerve XII; cranial nerve that provides efferent innervation to the muscles of the tongue

nerve, inferior vestibular   division of the vestibular portion of Cranial Nerve VIII, consisting of neurons from the cristae of the posterior semicircular canal and the main portion of the macula of the saccule

nerve, Jacobson's   nerve arising from Cranial Nerve IX, providing the main sensory fibers to the mucosa of the mesotympanum and eustachian tube; SYN: tympanic nerve

nerve, lateral ampullary   horizontal ampullary nerve

nerve, lesser superficial petrosal   part of the sensory nerve system of the ear formed by the joining of the tympanic nerve and the caroticotympanic nerve

nerve, motor   efferent nerve carrying information from the central nervous system to a muscle or other effector

nerve, oculomotor   Cranial Nerve III; cranial nerve that primarily provides efferent innervation to the extraocular muscles involved in eye movement

nerve, olfactory   Cranial Nerve I; cranial nerve that provides afferent innervation from the nose

nerve, optic   Cranial Nerve II; cranial nerve that provides afferent innervation from the eyes

nerve, posterior ampullary   nerve fiber bundle from the hair cells of the crista ampullaris of the posterior semicircular canal that joins with similar bundles from the

other semicircular canals, the utricle, and the saccule to form the vestibular branch of Cranial Nerve VIII

nerve, saccular   nerve fiber bundle from the hair cells of the macula of the saccule that joins with similar bundles from the semicircular canals and the utricle to form the vestibular branch of Cranial Nerve VIII

nerve, sensory   afferent nerve carrying information from a sense organ to the central nervous system

nerve, statoacoustic   auditory and vestibular branches combined to form Cranial Nerve VIII

nerve, superior ampullary   nerve fiber bundle from the hair cells of the crista ampullaris of the superior semicircular canal that joins with similar bundles from the other semicircular canals, the utricle, and the saccule to form the vestibular branch of Cranial Nerve VIII

nerve, superior vestibular   division of the vestibular portion of Cranial Nerve VIII, consisting of neurons from the cristae of the superior and lateral semicircular canals, the macula of the utricle, and the anterosuperior part of the macula of the saccule

nerve, trigeminal   Cranial Nerve V; cranial nerve that provides efferent innervation to the mastication muscles, including the tensor tympani, and afferent innervation from the face

nerve, trochlear   Cranial Nerve IV; cranial nerve that provides efferent innervation to the superior oblique muscle involved in eye movement

nerve, tympanic   nerve branch arising from the inferior ganglion of Cranial Nerve IX, providing the main sensory fibers to the mucosa of the tympanum and eustachian tube; SYN: Jacobson's nerve

nerve, utricular   nerve fiber bundle from the hair cells of the utricular macula that joins with similar bundles from the semicircular canals and the saccule to form the vestibular branch of Cranial Nerve VIII

nerve, vagus   Cranial Nerve X; cranial nerve that provides efferent and afferent innervation to the thoracic and abdominal viscera, pharynx, and larynx

nerve, vestibular   portion of Cranial Nerve VIII consisting of nerve fibers from the maculae of the utricle and saccule and the cristae of the superior, lateral, and posterior semicircular canals

nerve, vestibulocochlear Cranial Nerve VIII, consisting of a vestibular and a cochlear branch

nerve, Voit's saccular branch of the vestibular nerve

nerve cell neuron

nerve deafness misnomer for sensorineural hearing loss

nerve fiber axon or dendrite of a neuron

nervous system the entirety of nerve cells and tissues in an organism

nervous system, autonomic ANS; that portion of the nervous system that regulates glandular and visceral responses

nervous system, central CNS; that portion of the nervous system to which sensory impulses and from which motor impulses are transmitted, including the cortex, brainstem, and spinal cord

nervous system, central auditory CANS; portion from Cranial Nerve VIII to the auditory cortex that involves hearing, including the cochlear nucleus, superior olivary complex, lateral lemniscus, inferior colliculus, medial geniculate, and auditory cortex

netilmicin aminoglycoside used for short-term treatment of serious bacterial infections; can be ototoxic in high doses

neural pertaining to a structure composed of nerve cells

neural plasticity the capacity of the nervous system to change over time in response to changes in sensory input

neural presbyacusis loss of cochlear and higher-order neurons associated with the aging process

neuralgia pain emanating along the course or distribution of a nerve

neurectomy surgical excision of a segment of a nerve

neurilemoma a benign encapsulated neoplasm of a nerve sheath; SYN: neurinoma; neurilemoma; Schwannoma

neurinoma neurilemoma

neuritis inflammation of a nerve with corresponding sensory or motor dysfunction

neuritis, acoustic inflammation of the auditory portion of Cranial Nerve VIII, often of a viral nature, resulting in acute retrocochlear disorder

neuritis, cochlear acoustic neuritis

neuritis, vestibular inflammation of the vestibular nerve, often of a viral nature, resulting in a single episode of severe vertigo

that is prolonged and gradually subsides over a period of days or weeks

neuritis vestibularis viral inflammation of Cranial Nerve VIII, resulting in acute rotary vertigo, vegetative symptoms, and auditory disorder

neuroaudiology branch of audiologic science specializing in the assessment and diagnosis of impairment of the peripheral and central auditory nervous systems

neurodevelopmental pertaining to development of the nervous system

neurofibroma benign nonencapsulated tumor resulting from proliferation of Schwann cells in a poorly defined pattern that may include nerve fibers

neurofibromatosis I NF1; autosomal dominant disorder, characterized by childhood-onset multiple neurofibromas, located on any nerve, with associated sequelae; SYN: von Recklinghausen's disease

neurofibromatosis II NF2; autosomal dominant disorder characterized by bilateral cochleovestibular Schwannomas, which are faster growing and more virulent than the unilateral type; associated with secondary hearing loss and other intracranial tumors

neurogenic originating in nervous tissue; COM: myogenic

neuroglia non-neuronal supporting tissues of the nervous system

neurolemma the sheath encasing a nerve fiber

neurologic pertaining to the nervous system

neuroma generic term used to describe any neoplasm derived from cells of the nervous system, including cochleovestibular Schwannoma

neuron basic unit of the nervous system, consisting of an axon, cell body, and dendrite

neuron, first-order nerve fiber carrying information from a sensory end organ to the point of its first synaptic connection; in the auditory system, first-order neurons emanate from the cochlear hair cells and terminate at the cochlear nucleus

neuron, second-order nerve-fiber carrying information beyond the point of the first synapse from a specialized nerve ending; in the auditory system, all second-order neurons emanate from the cochlear nucleus and terminate throughout the auditory nervous system

neuronitis inflammation of nervous tissue

neuronitis vestibularis neuritis vestibularis

neuro-otology neurotology

neuropathogenesis the origin of a neuropathy

neuropathy any disorder involving the cranial or spinal nerves

neurophysiology science concerned with the function of the nervous system

neurotology branch of medical science specializing in the study, diagnosis, and treatment of diseases of the peripheral and central auditory and vestibular nervous systems

neurotoxic poisonous to the nervous system

neurotransmitters chemical agents released by a presynaptic cell upon excitation that cross the synapse and excite or inhibit the postsynaptic cell

nevi benign proliferative lesions of the skin and mucosa

newborn neonatal

Newton N; unit of physical force

NF1 neurofibromatosis 1; autosomal dominant disorder, characterized by childhood-onset multiple neurofibromas, located on any nerve, with associated sequelae; SYN: von Recklinghausen's disease

NF2 neurofibromatosis II; autosomal dominant disorder characterized by bilateral cochleovestibular Schwannomas, which are faster growing and more virulent than the unilateral type; associated with secondary hearing loss and other intracranial tumors

NHAS National Hearing Aid Society; former name of the International Hearing Society

NHCA National Hearing Conservation Association; professional association of specialists in hearing conservation

NHHHI Nursing Home Hearing Handicap Index; self- and staff-assessment scale designed to evaluate the handicapping influence of hearing impairment on aging residents of nursing homes

nHL normalized hearing level; the decibel level of a sound that lacks a standardized reference, referred to behaviorally determined normative levels, expressed as dB nHL

niche small recess or indentation in the wall of a hollow organ

NICU neonatal intensive care nursery; hospital unit designed to provide care for newborns needing extensive support and monitoring

NIDCD National Institute on Deafness and other Communication Disorders

NIHIS National Institute for Hearing Instrument Sciences; educational wing of the International Hearing Society

NIHL noise-induced hearing loss; permanent sensorineural hearing loss caused by acoustic trauma from exposure to excessive sound levels

NIOSH National Institute for Occupational Safety and Health; organization developed under the Occupational Safety and Health Act to fund and conduct research on occupational hazards and to develop criteria and recommend standards

NIPTS noise-induced permanent threshold shift; permanent change in hearing sensitivity that occurs as a result of acoustic trauma from exposure to excessive levels of sound

nitrogen mustard chemotherapeutic anticancer agent that can be ototoxic if administered by total-body perfusion

NITTS noise-induced temporary threshold shift; transient change in hearing sensitivity that occurs as a result of exposure to excessive levels of sound; SYN: temporary threshold shift

NLL nuclei or nucleus of the lateral lemniscus

Noah registered name of a computer program for hearing aid fitting, developed to serve as an industry-standard software platform for programming hearing devices

noise 1. any unwanted sound; 2. highly complex sound, produced by random oscillation

noise, ambient surrounding sounds in an acoustic environment

noise, back-end source of noise located in the power amplifier or receiver segments of a hearing aid

noise, background extraneous surrounding sounds of the environment; SYN: ambient noise

noise, broad-band BBN; sound with a wide bandwidth, containing a continuous spectrum of frequencies, with equal energy per cycle throughout the band

noise, circuit unwanted signal in the output of a circuit created by the functioning of the circuit

noise, community environmental noise, such as aircraft and traffic noise, that affects residents of a community

noise, external noise source in a hearing aid resulting from anything before the microphone portion of the instrument; ANT: internal noise

noise, extraneous ambient or unwanted noise

noise, flat-spectrum noise with equal energy content across a continuous band of frequencies

noise, front-end source of noise located in the microphone, pre-amplifier, or volume control of a hearing aid

noise, gaussian noise with equal energy at all frequencies; SYN: white noise

noise, impact intermittent noise of short duration, usually produced by nonexplosive mechanical impact such as pile driving or riveting; distinguishable from impulse noise by longer rise times and longer duration

noise, impulse intermittent noise with an instantaneous rise time and short duration that creates a shock wave, usually produced by gunfire or explosion; distinguishable from impact noise by shorter rise time and duration

noise, industrial zone industrial noise emanating from within a circumscribed area surrounding the noise source

noise, input-referred specification of front-end noise of a hearing instrument

noise, internal in a hearing aid, any sound not related to the input signal; e.g., circuit noise; ANT: external noise

noise, narrow-band NBN; bandpass-filtered noise that is centered at one of the audiometric frequencies, used for masking in pure-tone audiometry

noise, nonstationary noise characterized by substantial variation in level over time

noise, notched broad band of noise with a discrete frequency region removed, used in auditory brainstem response testing in an attempt to derive frequency-specific estimates of hearing sensitivity

noise, pink broad-band noise with a spectrum that is inversely proportional to frequency

noise, pseudorandom complex sound wave in which a sequence of component amplitudes, frequencies, and phases vary periodically over time

noise, random complex sound wave in which component amplitudes, frequencies, and phases vary randomly over time

noise, saw-tooth noise, composed of a fundamental frequency of 60 Hz and its harmonics together in random phase, that has a saw-tooth waveform and a buzz-saw quality

noise, 60-cycle unwanted electrical activity emanating from the 60-Hz electric energy commonly available to power lights, appliances, etc.

noise, speech broad-band noise that is filtered to resemble the speech spectrum

noise, stationary noise with negligible fluctuation of level

noise, thermal broad-band noise having constant energy at all frequencies

noise, white broad-band noise having similar energy at all frequencies

noise, wide-band white noise

noise control use of administrative or engineering strategies to limit the duration and level of noise exposure

noise control, administrative reduction of noise exposure by limiting employee exposure time

noise control, engineering reduction of noise exposure by controlling workplace noise at the source by quieting the noise-generating machinery

noise-criterion curves values used in determining noise limits, plotted as a curve representing a fixed numerical criterion for noise as a function of frequency band and the sound pressure level to reach the criterion within each band

noise-detection threshold NDT; lowest intensity level at which a specified noise signal is audible

noise-emission level standard measure of intensity of environmental or industrial noise, expressed as the decibel level at a specified distance and direction from a noise source in an open environment

noise exposure level and duration of noise to which an individual is subjected

noise exposure, nonoccupational exposure to excessive levels of noise outside of the workplace

noise exposure, occupational exposure to excessive levels of sound while on the job in the workplace

noise floor in any amplification system, the continuous baseline-level of background activity or noise from which a signal or response emerges

noise generator noise-producing source

noise-induced hearing loss NIHL; permanent sensorineural hearing loss caused by acoustic trauma from exposure to excessive sound levels

noise-induced permanent threshold shift NIPTS; permanent change in hearing sensitivity that occurs as a result of acoustic trauma from exposure to excessive levels of sound; SYN: permanent threshold shift

noise-induced temporary threshold shift NITTS; transient change in hearing sensitivity that occurs as a result of exposure to excessive levels of sound; SYN: temporary threshold shift

noise interference level level at which noise masks the recognition of speech targets

noise level, perceived expression in dB of the annoyance or unacceptability of loud sound, based on subjective ratings of noisiness; used primarily to assess the perception related to single-event aircraft flyover noise

noise notch pattern of audiometric thresholds associated with noise-induced hearing loss, characterized by sensorineural hearing loss predominantly at 4000 Hz

noise pollution level community noise level, expressed as the sum of the equivalent continuous sound level and an estimate of the increase of annoyance attributable to fluctuations of the sound levels

noise rating any of various quantitative descriptors of the aversiveness or the specific effects of a given environmental noise

noise rating, composite CNR; a scale used to rate and predict the total noise environment in a specified geographic area, such as around an airport, for evaluating compatible land use

noise reduction 1. decrease in the sound pressure level; 2. the difference in sound pressure level of a noise at two different locations

noise-reduction coefficient number describing absorptive properties of materials, expressed as the arithmetic average of absorption coefficients at 250 Hz, 500 Hz, 1000 Hz, and 2000 Hz

noise-reduction rating NRR; standardized specifications of the attenuation properties of hearing-protection devices, expressed as the number of dB of attenuation at specified frequencies throughout the frequency range

noise spectrum spectral content of a noise

noise trauma 1. damage to hearing from a transient, high-intensity sound; 2. long-term insult to hearing from excessive noise exposure; SYN: acoustic trauma

nondirectional microphone omnidirectional microphone

noninvasive pertaining to a procedure that does not involve penetration of the skin, such as the use of surface electrodes in auditory evoked potential measurement

noninverting electrode electrode that is attached to the positive-voltage side of a differential amplifier that does not invert the input; the active or vertex electrode in conventional auditory brainstem response recordings; ANT: inverting electrode

nonlinear amplification amplification whose gain is not the same for all input levels

nonlinear distortion reduction in fidelity of an amplified signal as a result of an output level that varies with input level

nonlinear hearing aid hearing aid that incorporates compression circuitry producing nonlinear amplification

nonlinear hearing protection device amplitude-sensitive hearing protection device that provides little or no attenuation of low-intensity sound and increasing attenuation of increasing sound intensity

nonoccluding earmold open earmold with a small outside-diameter canal portion that allows unamplified low-frequency sound to pass around the mold and directs amplified sound through the canal portion tubing; used in high-frequency hearing loss and CROS fittings

nonoccupational noise exposure exposure to excessive levels of noise outside the workplace

nonorganic hearing loss apparent loss in hearing sensitivity in the absence of any organic pathologic change in structure; used to describe hearing loss that is feigned; SYN: functional hearing loss

nonpenetrance condition in which a genetic trait, although appropriately present genetically, does not manifest itself in the phenotype

nonsense syllable single-syllable speech utterance that has no meaning, used in speech audiometric measures

nonsense syllable test NST; speech-audiometric measure of nonsense-syllable recognition

nonstationary noise noise characterized by substantial variation in level over time

nonsuppurative not containing, forming, or discharging pus

nonsuppurative otitis media inflammation of the middle ear with effusion that is not infected, including serous and mucoid otitis media

nonsyndromic hearing loss autosomal recessive or dominant genetic condition in which there are no other significant features besides hearing loss; SYN: recessive nonsyndromic hearing loss; ANT: syndromic hearing loss

nontest ear in audiometry, the ear that is not intended to be the test ear, or the ear with masking

nonverbal pertaining to communication without oral language

norepinephrine chemical secreted by the adrenal gland that functions as a neurotransmitter

norm standard derived from a representative sampling of a population considered to be normal for the characteristic of interest

normal 1. not pathologic; 2. at or near average

normal hearing hearing ability, including threshold of sensitivity and suprathreshold perception, that falls within a specified range of normal capacity

normal hearing, range of dispersion of hearing threshold levels around audiometric zero for the population of those with normal hearing

normalized hearing level nHL; the decibel level of a sound that lacks a standardized reference, referred to behaviorally determined normative levels, expressed as dB nHL

Norrie syndrome X-linked recessive ocular disorder, characterized by progressive eye degeneration, mental retardation, and late-onset, progressive, bilateral, symmetric sensorineural hearing loss; SYN: oculoacousticocerebral degeneration

Northwestern University Auditory Test Number 6 NU-6; monosyllabic word-recognition measure, designed to be phonetically balanced within a word list

notch, Carhart's pattern of bone-conduction audiometric thresholds associated with otosclerosis, characterized by reduced bone-conduction sensitivity predominantly at 2000 Hz; after Raymond Carhart

notch, noise pattern of audiometric thresholds associated with noise-induced hearing loss, characterized by sensorineural hearing loss predominantly at 4000 Hz

notch filter filtering network that removes a discrete portion of the frequency range, used in evoked potential measurement to remove 60-Hz noise and in hearing aids to limit amplification in a discrete frequency region of better hearing

notched noise broad band of noise with a discrete frequency region removed, used in auditory brainstem response testing in an attempt to derive frequency-specific estimates of hearing sensitivity

noy basic unit of subjective noisiness, expressed in terms of perceived noise level

NPO non per os; nothing by mouth; referring to instructions given to patients or parents before certain procedures, such as those requiring sedation

NR no response

NRR noise-reduction rating; standardized specifications of the attenuation properties of hearing-protection devices, expressed as the number of dB of attenuation at specified frequencies throughout the frequency range

NST nonsense syllable test; speech-audiometric measure of nonsense-syllable recognition

NU-6 Northwestern University Auditory Test Number 6; monosyllabic word-recognition measure, designed to be phonetically balanced within a word list

nuclei, periolivary PON; group of nuclei of the superior olivary complex surrounding the lateral and medial superior olives that receive projections from the intermediate acoustic stria

nuclei, vestibular superior, lateral, medial, and inferior nuclei of the vestibular system, located in the upper medulla oblongata, and serving as the initial obligatory stop for vestibular nerve fibers

nucleus pl. nuclei 1. mass of specialized protoplasm, constituting the central core of a neuron; 2. a group of nerve cells in the brain

nucleus, abducens nucleus of Cranial Nerve VI, responsible for controlling the lateral rectus muscles for horizontal eye movement

nucleus, caudate elongated, arched mass of gray matter that is part of the basal ganglia or inner portion of the cerebrum

nucleus, central central core of the inferior colliculus

nucleus, cochlear CN; cluster of cell bodies of second-order neurons on the lateral edge of the hindbrain in the central auditory nervous system at which fibers from Cranial Nerve VIII have an obligatory synapse

nucleus, oculomotor brainstem motor nucleus of Cranial Nerve III, responsible for controlling the medial rectus muscle for horizontal eye movement

nucleus, pericentral area surrounding the central nucleus of the medial geniculate through which parallel, not primary, ascending auditory fibers course

null hypothesis H_o; in statistics, the working hypothesis of the null or no difference between sets of data

numbness, facial peculiar sensation of the face due to impaired cutaneous perception, associated with facial nerve disorder

nursery, intensive care ICN; hospital unit designed to provide care for newborns needing extensive support and monitoring

nursery, intermediate care ICN; hospital unit designed as a step-down facility for newborns leaving the intensive care unit prior to discharge

nursery, well-baby hospital unit designed to provide care for healthy newborns

Nursing Home Hearing Handicap Index NHHHI; self- and staff-assessment scale designed to evaluate the handicapping influence of hearing impairment on aging residents of nursing homes

Nyquist frequency frequency equal to one-half of the analog-to-digital sampling rate, determining the highest frequency that can be sampled without distortion from aliasing

Nyquist theorem rule for determining how fast to digitally sample a signal without missing relevant frequency information; states that the sampling rate must be at least twice the highest frequency of interest in the input signal

nystagmograph instrument for measuring electrical muscle potentials related to the amplitude and velocity of eye movements

nystagmography electrical recording of nystagmus

nystagmus pattern of eye movement, characterized by a slow component in one direction that is periodically interrupted by a saccade, or fast component in the other; results from the anatomical connection between the vestibular and ocular systems

nystagmus, ageotropic positional nystagmus that beats in a direction that is away from the ground

nystagmus, alcohol positional nystagmus that occurs regularly after moderate ingestion of alcohol

nystagmus, benign paroxysmal sudden, transient burst of nystagmus during the Dix-Hallpike maneuver, which disappears within 10 seconds once the head position is achieved

nystagmus, bilateral horizontal gaze nystagmus that beats to the right on right gaze and beats to the left on left gaze

nystagmus, bilateral unequal gaze nystagmus that is present in both gaze directions, but of different magnitude in one direction, consistent with central nervous system pathology

nystagmus, caloric characteristic nystagmus eye movement pattern induced by vestibular labyrinthine stimulation with warm or cold water in the external auditory meatus

nystagmus, down-beating 1. vertical nystagmus in which the fast phase is downward; 2. pathologic down-beating vertical nystagmus, characterized by increased nystagmus velocity on downward gaze, consistent with central vestibular pathology

nystagmus, gaze nystagmus that occurs during horizontal gaze to one or both sides of midline

nystagmus, geotropic positional nystagmus that changes direction in relation to gravity, right beating when the right ear is down and left beating when the left ear is down

nystagmus, idiopathic nonpathologic horizontal spontaneous nystagmus of unknown cause

nystagmus, induced nystagmus that occurs expectedly as a result of specific stimulation such as rotation and caloric stimulation; ANT: spontaneous nystagmus

nystagmus, jerk general term for reciprocating movement of the eyes with different velocities in the two directions, including horizontal, vertical, oblique, or rotatory nystagmus

nystagmus, left-beating horizontal nys-

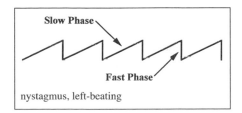
nystagmus, left-beating

tagmus in which the fast phase is toward the left

nystagmus, ocular nystagmus that occurs as a result of stimulation or pathology of the visual pathways, independent of vestibular input

nystagmus, optokinetic OKN; normally symmetric ocular nystagmus that occurs during optokinetic stimulation, reflecting the eye's attempt at smooth pursuit of alternating vertical stripes

nystagmus, paroxysmal abrupt-onset nystagmus that occurs following achievement of head position after the Dix-Hallpike maneuver

nystagmus, periodic alternating pathologic spontaneous horizontal nystagmus, occurring with eyes open or closed, characterized by cyclic beating in one direction and then the other; consistent with disorder of the cerebellomedullary region

nystagmus, positional usually abnormal presence of nystagmus that occurs with the head placed in a particular position; subtypes

are classified as geotropic or ageotropic and direction-changing or direction-fixed nystagmus; COM: positioning nystagmus

nystagmus, positional alcoholic positional nystagmus that occurs regularly after moderate ingestion of alcohol

nystagmus, positioning normal presence of nystagmus that occurs during head movement

nystagmus, right-beating horizontal nystagmus in which the fast phase is toward the right

nystagmus, rotary nystagmus characterized by rotation of the eyes in clockwise or counterclockwise direction

nystagmus, secondary phase caloric nystagmus that reverses its direction prior to 140 seconds following onset of irrigation, consistent with central vestibular pathology; SYN: premature caloric reversal

nystagmus, spontaneous ocular nystagmus that occurs in the absence of stimulation; ANT: induced nystagmus

nystagmus, up-beating vertical nystagmus in which the fast movement is upward, enhanced by upward or downward gaze, consistent with central vestibular pathology

nystagmus, vertical gaze nystagmus in upward or downward gaze directions, consistent with central nervous system pathology

nystagmus, vertical spontaneous normal nystagmus in the vertical direction with eyes closed

O

OAE otoacoustic emission; low-level sound emitted by the cochlea, either spontaneously or as an echo or other sound evoked by an auditory stimulus, related to the function of the outer hair cells of the cochlea

objective physically measurable; independent of subjective interpretation; COM: subjective

objective audiometry measurement of hearing sensitivity based on predictions made from physiologic responses to sound; COM: behavioral audiometry

objective tinnitus ringing or other head noises that can be heard and measured by an examiner

objective vertigo a sensation of external objects spinning or whirling; COM: subjective vertigo

oblique auricular muscle one of four muscles attaching to the medial surface of the auricle

OCB olivocochlear bundle; crossed and uncrossed bundles of efferent fibers from the medial and lateral superior olives directly to the outer hair cells or to nerve fiber dendrites leading to the inner hair cells

occlude to block or obstruct

occluded gain, real-ear REOG; probe-microphone measurement of the difference, in dB as a function of frequency, between the SPL in the ear canal and the SPL at a field reference point for a specified sound field with a hearing aid in place and turned off

occluded response, real-ear REOR; probe-microphone measurement of the sound pressure level, as a function of frequency, at a specified point near the tympanic membrane with a hearing aid in place and turned off; expressed in absolute SPL or as gain relative to stimulus level

occlusion a blockage or obstruction

occlusion effect low-frequency enhancement in the loudness level of bone-conducted signals due to occlusion of the ear canal

occupational hearing conservation program OHCP; industrial program designed to quantify the nature and extent of hazardous noise exposure, monitor the effects of exposure on hearing, provide abatement of sound, and provide hearing protection when necessary

occupational hearing conservationist OHC; person who is certified by CAOHC to provide a comprehensive array of services related to hearing conservation

occupational hearing loss noise-induced hearing loss due to exposure to excessive sound levels on the job

occupational noise exposure exposure to excessive levels of sound on the job

Occupational Noise Exposure Regulation regulation adopted in 1981 by OSHA to limit exposure to dangerous noise levels on the job; includes 1983 Hearing Conservation Amendment

Occupational Safety and Health Act 1970 U.S. federal legislation that created OSHA, NIOSH, and OSHRC in an effort to assure a healthy and safe working environment

Occupational Safety and Health Administration OSHA; U.S. federal agency responsible for regulating occupational health and safety hazards, including the setting of minimum standards for industrial hearing conservation programs, and for enforcing the regulations

Occupational Safety and Health Review Commission OSHRC; organization developed under the Occupational Safety and Health Act to adjudicate disputes that arise between OSHA and employers over the enforcement of regulations

octave frequency interval between two tones with a 2 to 1 ratio, so that one frequency is twice the frequency of the other

octave band division of the frequency range into octave intervals

octave filter filter in which the upper bandpass limit is twice the frequency of the lower limit

octopus cells specialized cells of the posterior ventral cochlear nucleus with tentaclelike dendrites that sample information from a number of fibers representing a broad range of frequencies

ocular dysmetria eye-movement disorder, associated with cerebellar pathology, in which the eyes consistently undershoot or overshoot a fixed target and require additional saccades to reach the target or bring the eyes back to the target

ocular flutter eye-movement disorder,

associated with brainstem pathology, characterized by one or more spiky overshoots of a fixed target

ocular nystagmus nystagmus that occurs as a result of stimulation or pathology of the visual pathways, independent of vestibular input

oculoacousticocerebral degeneration autosomal recessive ocular disorder, characterized by progressive eye degeneration, mental retardation, and late-onset, progressive, bilateral, symmetric sensorineural hearing loss; SYN: Norrie syndrome

oculoauricovertebral dysplasia congenital disorder characterized by musculoskeletal anomalies, including microtia and atresia of the external auditory meatus; SYN: Goldenhar syndrome

oculomotor pertaining to movements of the eyes

oculomotor nerve Cranial Nerve III; cranial nerve that primarily provides efferent innervation to the extraocular muscles involved in eye movement

oculomotor nucleus brainstem motor nucleus of Cranial Nerve III, responsible for controlling the medial rectus muscle for horizontal eye movement

oddball paradigm technique used to elicit event-related potentials in which a series of standard signals are interspersed with an occasional rare, or oddball, signal that differs in some aspect; waveforms are usually recorded independently for frequent and rare event

odynacusis auditory hypersensitivity, with reported pain in response to loud sounds

offset neurons neurons that fire only in response to the offset of a stimulus

OHC 1. occupational hearing conservationist; 2. outer hair cell

OHCP occupational hearing conservation program; industrial program designed to quantify the nature and extent of hazardous noise exposure, monitor the effects of exposure on hearing, provide abatement of sound, and provide hearing protection if necessary

ohm unit of resistance of a conductor to electrical or other forms of energy

Ohm's law law of electrical energy stating that current, or the rate at which charge flows, equals voltage divided by resistance, or the force that is dissipated by opposition to the flow of current

OKN optokinetic nystagmus; normally symmetric ocular nystagmus that occurs during optokinetic stimulation, reflecting the eye's attempt at smooth pursuit of alternating vertical stripes

olfactory nerve Cranial Nerve I; cranial nerve that provides afferent innervation from the nose

oligodendrocytes cells that form the myelin sheaths in the central auditory pathways, much as Schwann cells form the myelin sheath of Cranial Nerve VIII

olivocochlear bundle, crossed COCB; group of efferent nerve fibers of the medial olivocochlear bundle, coursing from the periolivary nuclei near the medial superior olive, across the brainstem and along the vestibular nerve, to the outer hair cells of the contralateral cochlea

olivocochlear bundle, lateral efferent pathway of nerve fibers emanating from the periolivary nuclei surrounding the LSO, coursing through the ipsilateral internal auditory meatus along the vestibular nerve, and terminating on afferent dendrites at the bases of inner hair cells

olivocochlear bundle, medial efferent pathway of nerve fibers emanating from the periolivary nuclei surrounding the MSO, coursing through the ipsilateral and contralateral internal auditory canals along the vestibular nerve, and terminating on the bases of outer hair cells

olivocochlear bundle OCB; crossed and uncrossed bundles of efferent fibers coursing from the periolivary nuclei surrounding the medial and lateral superior olives directly to the outer hair cells or to nerve fiber dendrites leading of the inner hair cells

olivocochlear efferents efferent fiber system of the olivocochlear bundles

OM otitis media; inflammation of the middle ear, resulting predominantly from eustachian tube dysfunction

OME otitis media with effusion; inflammation of the middle ear with an accumulation of any of several types of effusion in the middle ear cavity

omnidirectional microphone microphone with a sensitivity that is similar regardless of the direction of incoming sound

on time signal duration

onset neurons neurons that fire only in response to the onset of a stimulus

onset response synchronous firing of onset neurons in response to rapid-onset click stimuli used in auditory brainstem response measurement

ontogeny development of the individual

onychodystrophy autosomal recessive skin disorder, characterized by rudimentary fingernails and toenails, triphalangeal thumbs, and congenital, severe sensorineural hearing loss

open captioning printed text of the dialogue or narrative on television or video that is visible without the use of an adapter or special circuitry

open-ear response sound pressure at the eardrum of a person placed in a sound field; SYN: real-ear unaided response

open earmold nonoccluding earmold with a small outside-diameter canal portion that allows unamplified low-frequency sound to pass around the mold and directs amplified sound through the canal portion tubing; used in high-frequency hearing loss and CROS fittings

open-loop caloric irrigation method of warm or cool stimulation of the vestibular system in which water is delivered directly into the ear canal; ANT: closed-loop caloric irrigation

open-set test speech audiometric test in which the targeted syllable, word, or sentence is chosen from among all available targets in the language; ANT: closed-set test

ophthalmoplegia, internuclear eye movement disorder resulting from lesions of the medial longitudinal fasciculus

OPK optokinetic; pertaining to ocular tracking of repetitive moving targets

optic atrophy and diabetes mellitus autosomal recessive disorder, characterized by childhood-onset visual impairment and diabetes mellitus, with associated progressive sensorineural hearing loss

optic atrophy and polyneuropathy autosomal recessive disorder, characterized by progressive bilateral optic atrophy, childhood polyneuropathy, and progressive sensorineural hearing loss

optic nerve Cranial Nerve II; cranial nerve that provides afferent innervation from the eyes

opticocochleodentate degeneration rare autosomal recessive nervous system disorder, characterized by progressive visual loss, progressive spastic quadriplegia, and progressive sensorineural hearing loss

optokinetic OPK; pertaining to ocular tracking of repetitive moving targets

optokinetic asymmetry poorly formed nystagmus with optokinetic stimulation in one direction, but not in the other, consistent with cortical pathology

optokinetic drum rotating cylinder with alternating black and white stripes used to measure optokinetic nystagmus during electronystagmography testing

optokinetic nystagmus OKN; normally symmetric ocular nystagmus that occurs during optokinetic stimulation, reflecting the eye's attempt at smooth pursuit of alternating vertical stripes

optokinetic testing component of electronystagmography in which the patient focuses on a pattern of black vertical stripes alternating with white stripes moving horizontally, designed to assess the smooth- or slow-pursuit eye movement system

OR 1. operating room; 2. orienting reflex

oral-aural communication method of communicating that involves hearing, speaking, and speechreading

oralism method of deaf education that emphasizes the use of verbal communication to the exclusion of manual communication

ordinate vertical or Y access on a graph

organ of Corti hearing organ, composed of sensory and supporting cells, located on the basilar membrane in the cochlear duct

organ, spiral hearing organ, composed of sensory and supporting cells, located on the basilar membrane in the cochlear duct; SYN: organ of Corti

organic hearing loss hearing loss due to a pathologic process in the auditory system; ANT: functional hearing loss, nonorganic hearing loss

orientation, hearing aid process of teaching a new hearing aid wearer proper use and application of amplification

orienting reflex OR; reflexive head turn toward the source of a sound

ORL otorhinolaryngology; branch of medicine specializing in the diagnosis and treatment of diseases of the ear, nose, and throat

ORL—HNS otorhinolaryngology—head and neck surgery; branch of medicine specializing in the diagnosis and treatment of diseases of the ear, nose, and throat, including diseases of related structures of the head and neck

oscillation 1. periodic vibration back and forth between two points; 2. a state of acoustic feedback

oscillator electronic instrument designed to produce pure-tone oscillation

oscillator, bone-conduction electromechanical vibrator designed to stimulate the cochlea via transmission of vibrations through the bones of the skull

oscillopsia oculomotor disorder, characterized by blurring of vision during movement, that occurs due to uncoupling of the vestibulo-ocular reflex caused by bilateral vestibular disorder

oscilloscope electronic instrument that displays voltage of acoustic or other signals as a function of time

OSHA Occupational Safety and Health Administration; agency responsible for regulating occupational health and safety hazards, including the setting of minimum standards for industrial hearing conservation programs, and for enforcing the regulations

OSHRC Occupational Safety and Health Review Commission; organization developed under the Occupational Safety and Health Act to adjudicate disputes that arise between OSHA and employers over the enforcement of regulations

OSPL90 output sound pressure level for 90-dB input; ANSI standard term for saturation sound pressure level

osseotympanic bone conduction minor contribution to bone-conducted hearing from the cochlear reception of sound energy radiated into the osseous external auditory meatus

osseous labyrinth intricate maze of connecting channels in the petrous portion of each temporal bone that contains the membranous labyrinth; SYN: bony labyrinth

osseous spiral lamina bony shelf in the cochlea projecting out from the modiolus onto which the inner margin of the membranous labyrinth attaches and through which the nerve fibers of the hair cells course

ossicles the three small bones of the middle ear—the malleus, incus, and stapes—extending from the tympanic membrane through the tympanic cavity to the oval window

ossicular chain the ossicles considered collectively

ossicular chain disruption disarticulation of the ossicular chain

ossicular disarticulation detachment or break in the bones of the ossicular chain

ossicular discontinuity ossicular disarticulation

ossiculectomy removal of one or more of the ossicles of the middle ear

ossiculoplasty surgical repair of the ossicles of the middle ear

ossiculotomy division of the ossicles of the middle ear or mobilization of an ankylosis between any ossicles

ossification a change into bone

osteitis inflammation of bone

osteogenesis formation of bone

osteogenesis imperfecta autosomal dominant disorder, characterized by symptoms related to having brittle bones; symptoms include multiple fractures at birth, weak joints, bone deformities, nerve-root compression, and temporal bone malformation; SYN: Van Der Hoeve syndrome

osteoma benign, slowly growing mass of bony tissue, sometime occurring at the junction of bone and cartilage in the external auditory meatus

osteopetrosis autosomal recessive craniofacial and skeletal disorder characterized by brittle bones; may include disarticulated ossicular chain and progressive sensorineural hearing loss; SYN: Albers-Schönberg disease

otalgia ear pain

OTE hearing aid over-the-ear; seldom used term for behind-the-ear hearing aid

otic pertaining to the ear

otic capsule osseous portion of the cochlea containing the membranous labyrinth

otic placode thickened plate of cells on the lateral aspect of the neural fold, which forms about the 20th day of embryonic development

otic vesicle otocyst developed from the otic placode during the fourth week of gestation that eventually forms into the inner ear

otitic pertaining to otitis

otitic barotrauma traumatic inflammation of the middle ear caused by a rapid marked change in atmospheric pressure, during descent from altitude or ascent from diving; results in sudden severe negative air pressure in the middle ear cavity; SYN: aerotitis media

otitic meningitis infection of the meninges secondary to otitis media or mastoiditis

otitis inflammation of the ear

otitis externa   inflammation of the outer ear, usually the external auditory meatus

otitis media   OM; inflammation of the middle ear, resulting predominantly from eustachian tube dysfunction

otitis media, acute   AOM; inflammation of the middle ear having a duration of fewer than 21 days

otitis media, acute serous   acute inflammation of middle ear mucosa, with serous effusion

otitis media, acute suppurative   acute inflammation of the middle ear with infected effusion containing pus

otitis media, adhesive   inflammation of the middle ear caused by prolonged eustachian tube dysfunction resulting in severe retraction of the tympanic membrane and obliteration of the middle ear space

otitis media, catarrhal   middle ear inflammation resulting from catarrh of the nasopharynx with congestion of the eustachian tube

otitis media, chronic   COM; persistent inflammation of the middle ear having a duration of greater than 8 weeks

otitis media, chronic adhesive   long-standing inflammation of the middle ear caused by prolonged eustachian tube dysfunction resulting in severe retraction of the tympanic membrane and obliteration of the middle ear space

otitis media, chronic atticoantral suppurative   persistent purulent inflammation of the attic and mastoid antrum of the middle ear

otitis media, chronic suppurative   CSOM; persistent inflammation of the middle ear with infected effusion containing pus

otitis media, mucoid   inflammation of the middle ear, with mucoid effusion

otitis media, mucosanguinous   inflammation of the middle ear with effusion consisting of blood and mucus

otitis media, necrotizing   persistent inflammation of the middle ear that results in tissue necrosis

otitis media, nonsuppurative   inflammation of the middle ear with effusion that is not infected, including serous and mucoid otitis media

otitis media, persistent   middle-ear inflammation with effusion for 6 weeks or longer following initiation of antibiotic therapy

otitis media, purulent   inflammation of the middle ear with infected effusion containing pus; SYN: suppurative otitis media

otitis media, recurrent   middle ear inflammation that occurs 3 or more times in a 6-month period

otitis media, reflux   inflammation of the middle ear mucosa resulting from the passage of nasopharyngeal secretions through the eustachian tube

otitis media, sanguineous   inflammation of the middle ear, accompanied by bloody effusion

otitis media, secretory   otitis media with effusion, usually referring to serous or mucoid effusion

otitis media, seromucinous   inflammation of the middle ear with an accumulation of fluid of varying viscosity in the middle ear cavity and other pneumatized spaces of the temporal bone; SYN: otitis media with effusion

otitis media, serous   SOM; inflammation of middle ear mucosa, with serous effusion

otitis media, subacute   inflammation of the middle ear ranging in duration from 22 days to 8 weeks

otitis media, suppurative   inflammation of the middle ear with infected effusion containing pus

otitis media, tuberculous   chronic inflammation of the middle ear and mastoid secondary to tuberculosis, resulting in early perforation and suppurative otorrhea

otitis media, unresponsive   middle ear inflammation that persists after 48 hours of initial antibiotic therapy, occurring more frequently in children with recurrent otitis media

otitis media with effusion   OME; inflammation of the middle ear with an accumulation of fluid of varying viscosity in the middle ear cavity and other pneumatized spaces of the temporal bone; SYN: seromucinous otitis media

otitis media with perforation   inflammation of the middle ear, with secondary perforation of the tympanic membrane

otitis media without effusion   inflammation of the middle ear

otitis prone   being inclined to develop otitis media

OTO   otolaryngology

oto block   a small piece of plastic foam or other material that is inserted in the external auditory meatus before an earmold impression is made to prevent impression material from reaching the tympanic membrane

oto-spondylo-megaepiphyseal dysplasia autosomal recessive disorder characterized by severe to profound sensorineural hearing loss, short extremities, and abnormally thick joints

otoacoustic emission OAE; low-level sound emitted by the cochlea, either spontaneously or as an echo or other sound evoked by an auditory stimulus, related to the function of the outer hair cells of the cochlea

otoacoustic emission, click-evoked transient otoacoustic emission elicited by click stimuli

otoacoustic emission, distortion-product DPOAE; otoacoustic emission, measured as the cubic distortion product that occurs at the frequency represented by $2f_1-f_2$, resulting from the simultaneous presentation of two pure tones (f_1 and f_2)

otoacoustic emission, distortion-product evoked distortion-product otoacoustic emission

otoacoustic emission, evoked EOAE; otoacoustic emission that occurs in response to acoustic stimulation

otoacoustic emission, spontaneous SOAE; measurable low-level sound that is emitted by the cochlea in the absence of stimulation; related to the function of the outer hair cells

otoacoustic emission, transient TOAE; transient evoked otoacoustic emission

otoacoustic emission, transient evoked TEOAE; low-level acoustic echo emitted by the cochlea in response to a click or transient auditory stimulus; related to the integrity and function of the outer hair cells of the cochlea

otoadmittance meter early immittance measurement instrument designed to assess susceptance and conductance components of middle ear function

otocleisis closure of the external auditory meatus by a new growth or impacted cerumen

otoconia structures in the maculae of the utricle and saccule, located on the gelatinous material in which the stereocilia of the hair cells are embedded, which increase the sensitivity of the underlying hair cells to linear acceleration; SYN: statoconia

otocup earphone enclosure, containing a standard earphone and cushion, that fits completely over the auricle; designed to attenuate ambient noise

otocyst auditory vesicle formed from the otic placode during the fourth week of embryonic development that eventually forms into the inner ear

otodynia earache

otogenic originating from within the ear or secondary to an inflammation of the ear

otogenic suppurative labyrinthitis inflammation of the labyrinth caused by bacterial invasion from the middle ear into the vestibule, resulting in severe vertigo and hearing loss

otolaryngologist physician specializing in the diagnosis and treatment of diseases of the ear, nose, and throat, including diseases of related structures of the head and neck

otolaryngology branch of medicine specializing in the diagnosis and treatment of diseases of the ear, nose, and throat; SYN: otorhinolaryngology

otolaryngology—head and neck surgery branch of medicine specializing in the diagnosis and treatment of diseases of the ear, nose, and throat, including diseases of related structures of the head and neck

otolithic catastrophe atypical form of Ménière's disease in which patients experience abrupt falling attacks of brief duration

otolithic membrane structure in the maculae of the utricle and saccule containing otoconia into which the stereocilia of the hair cells are embedded

otologic pertaining to otology

otologist physician specializing in the diagnosis and treatment of ear disease

otology otolaryngology subspecialty devoted to the study, diagnosis, and treatment of diseases of the ear and related structures

otomycosis fungal infection of the external auditory meatus

otoneurology science involving the study, diagnosis, and treatment of nervous system diseases of the auditory and vestibular systems

otopalatodigital syndrome X-linked recessive disorder characterized by generalized bone dysplasia, resulting in conductive hearing loss, cleft palate, wide spacing of toes, broad thumbs, and other signs of dysplasia

otopathy any disease of the ear

otoplasty surgical repair or restoration of the auricle

otorhinolaryngology ORL; branch of medicine specializing in the diagnosis and treatment of diseases of the ear, nose, and throat; SYN: otolaryngology

otorhinolaryngology—head and neck surgery ORL—HNS; branch of medicine specializing in the diagnosis and treatment of diseases of the ear, nose, and throat, including diseases of related structures of the head and neck

otorrhagia bleeding from the external auditory meatus

otorrhea discharge from the ear

otosclerosis remodeling of bone, by resorption and new spongy formation around the stapes and oval window, resulting in stapes fixation and related conductive hearing loss

otosclerosis, cochlear disease process involving new formation of spongy bone near the oval window resulting in sensorineural or mixed hearing loss

otosclerosis, malignant severe active otosclerosis involving the oval window, round window, and most of the bony labyrinth, resulting in a mixed hearing loss that eventually progresses to severe or profound levels

otoscope a speculumlike instrument for visual examination of the external auditory meatus and tympanic membrane

otoscopy inspection of the external auditory meatus and tympanic membrane with an otoscope

otoscopy, pneumatic inspection of the motility of the tympanic membrane with an otoscope capable of varying air pressure in the external auditory meatus

otoscopy, video endoscopic examination of the external auditory meatus and tympanic membrane displayed on a video monitor

otosteal pertaining to the ossicles of the ear

otosteon one of the ossicles of the ear

otosyphilis membranous labyrinthitis secondary to syphilis infection, resulting in sensorineural hearing loss

ototoxic having a poisonous action on the ear, particularly the hair cells of the cochlear and vestibular end organs; COM: cochleotoxic, vestibulotoxic

ototoxic drug any of a variety of antibiotics and other chemotherapeutic agents that are toxic to the ear, usually affecting the cochlear and/or vestibular hair cells

ototoxicity property of being ototoxic; COM: cochleotoxicity, vestibulotoxicity

ototoxicity monitoring continuous assessment of hearing over the course of treatment with ototoxic drugs

ototoxicity, aspirin temporary threshold shift and tinnitus caused by excessive doses of aspirin

outer ear peripheral most portion of the auditory mechanism, consisting of the auricle, external auditory meatus, and lateral surface of the tympanic membrane; SYN: external ear

outer hair cells OHC; motile cells within the organ of Corti with rich efferent innervation, which appear to be responsible for fine-tuning frequency resolution and potentiating the sensitivity of the inner hair cells

outer hair cell electromotility the capacity of the outer hair cells to change shape in response to electrical stimulation

outer pillars supporting pillars that stabilize the hair cells, extending from the basilar membrane to the top of the organ of Corti, forming the lateral wall of the tunnel of Corti; ANT: inner pillars

output energy or information released from or directed out of a system

output compression process in which a hearing aid compresses a signal after the volume control, resulting in an expanded dynamic range for low gain settings and a lower kneepoint for high gain settings; COM: input compression

output limiting restriction of the maximum output of a hearing aid by peak clipping or amplitude compression

output-limiting compression method of limiting maximum output of a hearing aid with compression circuitry

output, acoustic sound waves emanating from an amplification system

oval window opening in the labyrinthine wall of the middle ear space, leading into the scala vestibuli of the cochlea, into which the footplate of the stapes fits; SYN: vestibular window; fenestra vestibuli

over-the-ear hearing aid OTE hearing aid; seldom-used term for a hearing aid that fits over the ear and is coupled to the ear canal via an earmold; SYN: BTE hearing aid, postauricular hearing aid

overall sound pressure level total sound energy throughout the frequency range, measured without any frequency weighting

overamplification 1. the provision of excessive gain by a hearing aid; 2. hearing aid amplification of sufficient magnitude to cause additional, noise-induced, hearing loss

overlay, functional 1. exaggeration of an organic disorder; 2. non-organic consequence of an organic disorder

overload distortion of a system by excessive input

overmasking condition in which the intensity level of masking in the nontest car is sufficient to contralateralize to the test ear, thereby elevating the test-ear threshold

overrecruitment excessive growth in loudness perception with increasing intensity, so that loudness of a high-intensity tone in an impaired ear exceeds that in a normal ear; SYN: hyper-recruitment

overt reaction behavior that is readily observable

overtone multiple of the fundamental frequency of a sound

oxyacoia hypersensitivity to sound related to stapedius muscle paralysis

P

P₂ major positive peak of the late-latency auditory evoked potential, occurring around 180 msec following stimulus onset

P₃ major peak of the endogenous event-related potential, occurring around 300 msec following acoustic stimulus onset; SYN: P300

P300 P₃

Pₐ major positive peak of the auditory middle latency response occurring 25 msec to 40 msec following stimulus onset

Pa Pascal; unit of measure of pressure; reference sound pressure for 0 dB SPL is 0.00002 Pa or 20 μPa

PAC platinol (cisplatin), adriamicin, cyclophosphamide; potentially ototoxic chemotherapy regimen used in the treatment of ovarian cancer

pachyotia abnormally thick and coarse auricles

pad attenuator circuit on an audiometer or other instrument whose removal results in a specified amount of additional intensity

paed. pediatrics

Paget disease autosomal recessive skeletal disorder in which bones progressively soften, thicken, and deform; involves the auditory system when the temporal bone is affected

paired comparison psychophysical technique in which two hearing aid circuits or devices are compared on the basis of a specified parameter, such as sound quality or speech intelligibility, usually in a two-alternative forced-choice format

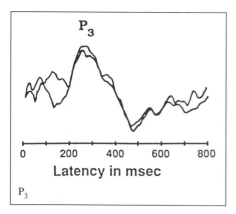

P₃

PAL PB-50 Psycho-Acoustic Laboratory (Harvard University) phonetically balanced 50 (word list); one of the earliest word-recognition measures, designed to be phonetically balanced within a word list

palsy paralysis, often referring to paresis

palsy, facial impairment or loss of voluntary movement of the face due to facial nerve disorder

palsy, saccadic eye-movement disorder in which saccadic movements are normal in one direction but impaired in the opposite direction, consistent with unilateral cortical lesion

PAM postauricular muscle or myogenic (potential); electrical potential generated from muscles of the neck that occurs around 20 msec and can be of sufficient magnitude to obscure the neurogenic auditory middle latency response

panesthesia sum of sensations experienced at one time

panotitis general inflammation of the structures of the ear

paracentesis passage of a needle into a cavity, such as the middle ear, to remove fluid

paracousis paracusis

paracusis hearing impairment

paracusis, false apparent hearing improvement in noisy surroundings due to others speaking louder; SYN: paracusis willisiana

paracusis duplicata auditory condition in which one sound is heard as two; SYN: diplacusis

paracusis loci loss or diminution of ability to localize sound

paracusis willisiana paradoxical phenomenon in which a person with conductive hearing loss hears better in a noisy environment, related to the elevated level at which others speak in noise

paradigm an example or model

paradox seemingly contradictory occurrence

paraganglionic tissue cells derived from the ganglionic neural crest that may form into neoplasms, including glomus tumors

parallel vent vent that runs parallel to the bore for the entire length of an earmold

paralysis functional loss of muscle movement due to injury or disease of the nerve supply; SYN: palsy

parameter a measurable characteristics of an object, subject, or population

paramyxovirus genus of viruses that includes those causing measles and mumps

paraneoplastic pertaining to neurologic or other disorders that are secondary to malignant neoplasms but not related directly to their invasion

paresis partial or incomplete paralysis

paresthesia abnormal sensation, such as burning or tingling, in an extremity

parietal pertaining to the wall of a cavity

parotic near the ear

parotid gland salivary gland near the ear

parotiditis contagious systemic viral disease, characterized by inflammation and enlargement of parotid, associated with sudden, permanent, profound unilateral sensorineural hearing loss; SYN: mumps; parotitis

parotitis parotiditis

paroxysm abrupt, recurrent onset of a symptom

paroxysmal occurring in paroxysms

paroxysmal nystagmus abrupt-onset nystagmus that occurs following achievement of head position after the Dix-Hallpike maneuver

paroxysmal positioning vertigo a recurrent, acute form of vertigo due to semicircular canal dysfunction, occurring in clusters in response to positional changes; SYN: benign paroxysmal positioning vertigo

paroxysmal vertigo sudden, brief episodes of dizziness and nystagmus, often accompanied by nausea and vomiting

pars part or portion of a structure or area

pars flaccida smaller and more compliant or flaccid portion of the tympanic membrane, containing two layers of tissue, located superiorly; COM: pars tensa

pars tensa larger and stiffer portion of the tympanic membrane, containing four layers of tissue; COM: pars flaccida

pars tympanica curved plate of bone, located anterior to the mastoid process, constituting the tympanic portion of the temporal bone and forming much of the wall of the external auditory meatus

partial in acoustics, any single frequency component of a complex tone

partial recruitment condition in which the loudness of a high-intensity tone in an ear with hearing loss approaches, but remains less than, the loudness of a tone of the same

intensity in an ear with normal hearing; COM: complete recruitment, decruitment

Pascal Pa; unit of pressure, expressed in Newtons per square meter

Pascoe prescriptive procedure hearing aid selection algorithm designed to prescribe a gain and frequency response that amplifies the long-term speech spectrum to a point that represents a specified percentage of the difference between threshold and MCL

pass-fail criterion specified outcome used as the determination point for whether a screening or test result was positive or negative for a disorder

passband filter an electronic filter that allows a specified band of frequencies to pass, while reducing or eliminating frequencies above and below the band; SYN: band-pass filter

passive filter filter circuit in which the response is constant, regardless of amplifier gain

Patau syndrome chromosomal disorder, trisomy 13, characterized by numerous anomalies, including microcephaly, severe mental retardation, low-set ears, auricular malformation, atresia, and middle ear and inner ear malformation

patent open; unobstructed; SYN: patulous

patent PE tube unobstructed, functional pressure-equalization tube

pathogen any agent or microorganism causing disease

pathogenic causing disease

pathognomonic distinctive or characteristic of a particular disease

pathologic pertaining to or caused by disease

pathology scientific study of disease

pathophysiology study of the functional consequences of disease

pathway functionally and anatomically circumscribed collection of axons carrying nerve impulses from one group of nerve cells to another

patulous eustachian tube abnormally patent eustachian tube, resulting in sensation of stuffiness, autophony, tinnitus, and audible respiratory noises

P_b secondary positive peak of the auditory middle latency response occurring 50 msec to 75 msec following stimulus onset

PB phonetically balanced; descriptive of a list of words containing speech sounds that occur with the same frequency as in conversational speech

PB max highest percentage-correct score obtained on monosyllabic word-recognition measures (PB word lists) presented at several intensity levels

PB min the lowest percentage-correct score obtained on monosyllabic word-recognition measures (PB word lists) at an intensity level above that at which PB max occurs

PB word list phonetically balanced word list; list of words used in word-recognition testing that contain speech sounds that occur with the same frequency as those of conversational speech

PB words phonetically balanced words; misnomer for PB word list

PBK word lists phonetically balanced kindergarten word lists; lists of words used in word-recognition testing, designed both to be phonetically balanced and to contain words that are at a vocabulary level appropriate for use with young school children

PE platinol (cisplatin), etoposide; potentially ototoxic chemotherapy regimen used in the treatment of testicular cancer

pe SPL peak equivalent sound pressure level: decibel level of a 1000-Hz tone at an amplitude equivalent to the peak of a transient signal; used to express the intensity level of click stimuli used in auditory evoked potential testing

PE tube pressure-equalization tube; small tube or grommet inserted in the tympanic membrane following myringotomy to provide equalization of air pressure within the middle ear space as a substitute for a nonfunctional eustachian tube

PE tube, patent unobstructed, functional pressure-equalization tube

peak acoustic gain amount of gain at a point along the frequency response of a hearing aid at which gain is maximal

peak amplitude maximum instantaneous displacement of a waveform in a specified time interval

peak clipping 1. process of limiting maximum output intensity of a hearing aid or amplifier by removing alternating current amplitude peaks at a fixed level; 2. distortion of an acoustic waveform resulting from hearing aid amplifier saturation

peak clipping, hard output-limiting technique in hearing aid amplification that removes the extremes of alternating current amplitude peaks at some predetermined level; COM: soft peak clipping

peak clipping, modified soft peak clipping

peak clipping, soft peak clipping in hearing aid amplification that removes the extremes of alternating current amplitude peaks at some predetermined level in a gradual manner that reduces distortion

peak equivalent SPL pe SPL: decibel level of a 1000-Hz tone at an amplitude equivalent to the peak of a transient signal; used to express the intensity level of click stimuli used in auditory evoked potential testing

peak-to-peak amplitude difference in amplitude between the positive and negative extremes of a waveform

peaks, spectral narrow ranges of high energy in the amplitude spectrum of a sound

pediacoumeter early visual-reinforcement device used in pure-tone audiometry with small children, in which the appearance of a puppet served to reinforce a correct response

pediatric audiologist audiologist with a subspecialty interest in the evaluation and treatment of hearing disorders in children

pediatric audiology audiology subspecialty devoted to the study, evaluation, and treatment of hearing disorders in children

pediatric intensive care unit PICU; hospital unit designed to provide care for young children needing extensive support and monitoring

pediatric speech intelligibility test PSI test; closed-set test of word and sentence recognition, in quiet and in a background of speech competition, designed to assess speech perception ability of children ages 2.5 to 6 years

pediatrician physician specializing in the development and care of children and in the diagnosis and treatment of their diseases

pediatrics branch of medicine concerned with the development and care of children and in the diagnosis and treatment of their diseases

peep show audiometer pediacoumeter

Pelizaeus-Merzbacher disease X-linked demyelinating disorder, characterized by childhood onset of nystagmus, ataxia, dysarthria, and psychomotor dysfunction, with associated sensorineural hearing loss due to both cochlear and auditory brainstem pathway disorder

Pendred syndrome autosomal recessive

endocrine metabolism disorder resulting in goiter and congenital, symmetric, moderate-to-profound sensorineural hearing loss

pendular tracking component of the electronystagmography test battery in which an object or spot of light moving sinusoidally is tracked horizontally and vertically to assess the smooth- or slow-pursuit eye movement system

penetrance the frequency with which a genetic trait expresses its characteristics in the population of those possessing it

penetrating trauma damage to the ear as a result of any sharp object traversing the external auditory meatus, with auditory disorder ranging from minor perforation of the tympanic membrane to ossicular destruction and oval window fistula

perceived noise level expression in dB of the annoyance or unacceptability of loud sound, based on subjective ratings of noisiness; used primarily to assess the perception related to single-event aircraft flyover noise

perception awareness, recognition, and interpretation of sensory stimuli received in the brain

perception, speech awareness, recognition, and interpretation of speech signals received in the brain

perceptive hearing loss early term for sensorineural hearing loss

perceptual analysis the subjective assessment of sound in terms of pitch, loudness, and quality

percutaneous through unbroken skin

perfect pitch rare capability of identifying the pitch of a note; SYN: absolute pitch

perforation abnormal opening in a tissue or structure

perforation, attic perforation of the pars flaccida portion of the tympanic membrane

perforation, marginal hole at the edge or margin of the tympanic membrane

perforation, tympanic membrane abnormal opening in the tympanic membrane

performance, real-world the effectiveness of hearing aids or hearing protection devices as measured under normal conditions of use

performance-intensity function PI function; graph of percentage-correct speech-recognition scores as a function of presentation level of the target signals

pericentral nucleus area surrounding the central nucleus of the medial geniculate

through which parallel, not primary, ascending auditory fibers course

perichondritis, auricular inflammation of the connective tissue membrane around the cartilage of the auricle

perichondrium nutritive connective tissue covering, such as that of the auricle

perilabyrinthitis diffuse inflammation of tissue around the labyrinth

perilymph cochlear fluid, found in the scala vestibuli, scala tympani, and spaces within the organ of Corti, which is high in sodium and calcium and has an ionic composition that resembles cerebrospinal fluid

perilymphatic fistula abnormal passageway between the perilymphatic space and the middle ear, resulting in the leak of perilymph at the oval or round window, caused by congenital defects or trauma

perilymphatic gusher abnormal spontaneous or surgically induced, profuse, jet-like outflow of perilymphatic fluid from the oval window

perinatal pertaining to the period around the time of birth, from the 28th week of gestation through the 7th day following delivery

perineurium sheath of connective tissue surrounding the fibers of a peripheral nerve

period length of time for a sine wave to complete one cycle

periodic recurring at regular time intervals

periodic alternating nystagmus pathologic spontaneous horizontal nystagmus, occurring with eyes open or closed, characterized by cyclic beating in one direction and then the other; consistent with disorder of the cerebellomedullary region

periodic sound wave sound wave in which the pattern of vibration, however complex, repeats itself regularly as a function of time

periodicity pitch the perception of a pitch, in the absence of physical energy at the frequency corresponding to the perceived pitch, that occurs when a tone is amplitude modulated or a sound is turned on and off rapidly

periolivary nuclei PON; group of nuclei of the superior olivary complex surrounding the lateral and medial superior olives that receive projections from the intermediate acoustic stria

peripheral 1. toward the outer surface or part; 2. located outside the central nervous system

peripheral auditory system hearing mechanism, including the external ear, middle ear, cochlea, and Cranial Nerve VIII; COM: central auditory system

peripheral lesion in the auditory system, a lesion occurring at a site ranging from the auricle to and including Cranial Nerve VIII

peripheral vestibular neurons neurons of the superior and inferior division of the vestibular portion of Cranial Nerve VIII, located in the internal auditory meatus

permanent threshold shift PTS; irreversible hearing sensitivity loss following exposure to excessive noise levels; COM: temporary threshold shift

permanent threshold shift, noise-induced NIPTS; SYN: permanent threshold shift

permissible exposure limits the highest intensity level in dB to which an employee can be exposed for a specified duration of time and still meet occupational safety guidelines

persistent otitis media middle ear inflammation with effusion for 6 weeks or longer following initiation of antibiotic therapy

personal FM system a wearable assistive listening device consisting of a remote microphone/transmitter worn by a speaker that sends signals via FM to a receiver worn by a listener; designed to enhance the signal-to-noise ratio

perstimulatory occurring during stimulation

perstimulatory fatigue auditory adaptation, or the reduction in loudness or audibility of sound, during prolonged stimulation; COM: poststimulatory fatigue

petromastoid canal channel in the temporal bone through which the subarcuate artery runs, supplying blood to the otic capsule and anteromedial portion of the mastoid

petrosa the petrous portion of the temporal bone

petrosal pertaining to the petrous portion of the temporal bone

petrositis inflammation in the pneumatized perilabyrinthine areas and apical region of the temporal bone

petrous resembling the hardness of stone

petrous bone section of the temporal bone of the skull that houses the sensory organ of the peripheral auditory system

PFL platinol (cisplatin), fluorouracil, leucovorin calcium; potentially ototoxic chemotherapy regimen used in the treatment of head and neck cancer

PGR psychogalvanic response; psychogalvanic skin response

PGSR psychogalvanic skin response; change in skin resistance resulting from an emotional response to a stimulus; SYN: galvanic skin response

PGSR audiometry method of determining hearing sensitivity in suspected functional hearing loss by measuring psychogalvanic skin response to sound, following conditioning of the patient to the sound paired with a mild shock; SYN: electrodermal audiometry

PHAB Profile of Hearing Aid Benefit; self-assessment inventory designed to evaluate perceived benefit from the use of hearing aids

PHAP Profile of Hearing Aid Performance; self-assessment inventory designed to assess the perceived performance received from the use of hearing aid amplification

phase 1. any stage in a cycle; 2. relative position in time of a point along a periodic waveform, expressed in degrees of a circle

phase, fast component of nystagmus that represents the saccadic system of eye movement control required to reposition a visual target on the retinal fovea

phase, in condition in which the pressure waves of two signals crest and trough at the same time; SYN: homophasic

phase, slow component of nystagmus that represents the smooth continuous eye movement required to maintain a visual target on the retinal fovea

phase locking tendency of nerve fibers to fire at a particular phase of the stimulating waveform

phenotype 1. the observable expression of the genetic constitution (genotype) of an individual; 2. group to which an individual may be assigned based on observable genetic characteristics

phon unit of measure of the subjective loudness of a tone, referenced to that of a 1000-Hz pure tone at a specified intensity level; e.g., a 500-Hz signal of 30 dB that is judged equal in loudness to a 1000-Hz tone of 20 dB has a loudness level of 20 phon

phonal pertaining to sound or voice

phone an individual speech sound

phoneme smallest distinctive class of phones in a language that represents the set of variations of a speech sound that are considered the same sound and represented by the same symbol

phonemic pertaining to a phoneme

phonemic regression age-related reduction in word-recognition ability beyond that which would be predicted from the degree of hearing sensitivity loss

phonetic pertaining to phones

phonetic alphabet alphabet containing symbols that represent speech sounds

phonetically balanced descriptive of a list of words containing speech sounds that occur with the same frequency as in conversational speech phonetically balanced kindergarten word lists

PBK word lists; lists of words used in word-recognition testing, designed to be phonetically balanced and to contain words that are at a vocabulary level appropriate for use with young school children

phonetically balanced word lists PB word list; list of words used in word-recognition testing that contain speech sounds that occur with the same frequency as those of conversational speech

phonetics, acoustic branch of phonetics devoted to the study of sound and auditory perception of speech sounds

photoplastic pertaining to a plastic material used in some hearing aid shells that cures when exposed to ultraviolet light

phylogenetic; phylogenic pertaining to the evolutionary development of a group of organisms

physical volume test PVT; subtest of immittance audiometry in which the volume of the ear canal is estimated; e.g., a large volume is found in the case of a tympanic membrane perforation or a patent PE tube and a small volume in the case of impacted cerumen

physiogenic resulting from physiologic activity

physiologic pertaining to physiology

physiology science of the function of living organisms and their components

PI function performance-intensity function; graph of percentage-correct speech-recognition scores as a function of presentation level of the target signals

PI-PB performance intensity (PI) function for phonetically balanced (PB) word lists

PI-SSI performance intensity (PI) function for the synthetic sentence identification (SSI) test

PICU pediatric intensive care unit; hospital unit designed to provide care for young children needing extensive support and monitoring

pidgin jargon using words and grammar from different languages

piebaldness recessive, X-linked, or dominant forms of skin-pigmentary syndromes, characterized by patchy absence of pigment of scalp hair; may include profound congenital sensorineural hearing loss

Pierre Robin syndrome autosomal dominant craniofacial-skeletal disorder, characterized by micrognathia and abnormal smallness of the tongue, often with cleft palate, severe myopia, congenital glaucoma, retinal detachment, and conductive or sensorineural hearing loss

piezoelectric microphone transducer in which acoustic energy is converted to electric current by applied mechanical stress on ceramic or crystal

pigment any coloring tissue in the body

pili torti [L. twisted hair] recessive skin disorder, characterized by dry, brittle twisted hair of the scalp, eyebrows, and eyelashes; often with bilateral sensorineural hearing loss

PILL programmable increases at low levels; type of automatic signal processing in a hearing aid that uses level-dependent control of frequency response, reducing either low-frequency or high-frequency gain as input level increases

pillar cells two groups of supporting cells in the organ of Corti, the inner and outer pillars, that have their bases on the basilar membrane and that lean toward each other and articulate at their tops, forming the tunnel of Corti

pillars of Corti inner and outer pillar cells

pillars, inner supporting pillars that stabilize the hair cells, extending from the basilar membrane to the top of the organ of Corti, forming the medial wall of the tunnel of Corti

pillars, outer supporting pillars that stabilize the hair cells, extending from the basilar membrane to the top of the organ of Corti, forming the lateral wall of the tunnel of Corti

pineal tumor neoplasm derived from the pineal gland; SYN: pinealoma

pinealoma pineal tumor

pink noise broad-band noise with a spectrum that is inversely proportional to frequency

pinna; pl. pinnae external cartilaginous portion of the ear; SYN: auricle

pinna, cleft congenital fissure of the pinna

pinna malformation structural defect of the auricle due to failure of normal development

pinna reflex reflexive orienting of the pinnae in many animals in response to altering sounds

pit, auditory depression for the formation of an ear on the side of the head of an embryo; SYN: otic pit

pit, preauricular craniofacial anomaly characterized by a small hole of variable depth lying anterior to the auricle

pitch perception or psychological impression of the frequency of sound

pitch, absolute perfect pitch

pitch, perfect rare capability of identifying the pitch of a note

pitch, periodicity the perception of a pitch, in the absence of physical energy at the frequency corresponding to the perceived pitch, that occurs when a tone is amplitude modulated or a sound is turned on and off rapidly

PL 101-336 United States public law (PL) 101–336; Americans with Disabilities Act of 1990

PL 101-431 United States public law (PL) 101–336; Television Decoder Circuitry Act of 1990

PL 94-142 United States public law (PL) 94–142, known as the Education for All Handicapped Children Act of 1975 and renamed the Individuals with Disabilities Education Act, mandating free and appropriate public education for all children who are handicapped

PL 99-457 United States public law (PL) 99–457, passed in 1986; bill that reauthorized PL 94–142, extended it to include children aged 3 to 5 years, and encouraged the provision of services to infants and toddlers from birth to 3 years

place theory well-documented theory that frequency perception is based on the location of maximum traveling-wave displacement along the basilar membrane

placode local thickening in an embryonic epithelial layer from which organs and structures develop

placode, auditory otic placode

placode, otic thickened plate of cells on the lateral aspect of the neural fold in the human embryo that develops into the otic capsule and inner ear

plaque 1. a small, defined deposit of material, as on the tympanic membrane; 2. focused area of demyelination in multiple sclerosis

plasticity the capacity to be formed or molded

plasticity, neural the capacity of the nervous system to change over time in response to changes in sensory input

plateau in audiometry, the level between undermasking and overmasking at which a patient's threshold in the test ear does not vary as masking in the nontest ear is increased or decreased over a 10 dB to 20 dB range

plateau method method of masking the nontest ear in which masking is introduced progressively over a range of intensity levels until a plateau is reached, indicating the level of masked threshold of the test ear

plateau time time that a signal is on at its maximum intensity

play audiometry behavioral method of hearing assessment of young children in which the correct identification of a signal presentation is rewarded with the opportunity to engage in any of several play-oriented activities

plexus tympanicus network of interjoining nerves and blood vessels on the promontory formed by the tympanic nerve, a branch of the facial nerve, and branches of the internal carotid artery

PLL preferred loudness level; signal level at which speech is rated as most comfortable

plosive stop-consonant speech sound produced by releasing impounded air pressure in the airway, such as [p], [t], and [g] sounds in the initial consonant position

pneumatic otoscopy inspection of the motility of the tympanic membrane with an otoscope capable of varying air pressure in the external auditory meatus

pneumatization development of air cells

pneumolabyrinth abnormal entrance of air into the labyrinth by traumatic or surgical fistulization, resulting in acute vertigo and hearing loss

POGO II prescriptive procedure prescription of gain and output II; modification of the POGO gain rule in which the gain is increased at each frequency by one-half the decibel amount that the hearing loss exceeds 65 dB HL

POGO prescriptive procedure prescription of gain and output; hearing aid selection algorithm designed to prescribe a gain and frequency response that is based on a half-gain rule at frequencies above 500 Hz and reductions from half gain of -5 dB and -10 dB at 500 Hz and 250 Hz

polar directivity pattern expression of the directional characteristics of a hearing aid microphone, usually displayed in a polar plot that depicts the relative amplitude output of a hearing aid as a function of angle of sound incidence

polarity 1. the property of having two opposite magnetic poles or having opposite characteristics; 2. the direction or orientation of an opposing characteristic

polarity, alternating characteristic of auditory evoked potential stimuli in which the rarefaction and condensation polarity of a click or tone burst are alternated successively

Politzer bag early instrument used to force air through the eustachian tube to aerate the middle ear

politzerization early technique in which air is forced through the eustachian tube to aerate the middle ear

polychondritis connective tissue disorder, characterized by inflammation and loss of multiple cartilage, including that of the auricle and eustachian tube; SYN: relapsing polychondritis

polyethylene hard earmold material that can be used in cases of allergic reaction to conventional materials

polyotia presence of an additional auricle on one or both sides of the head

polyp mass of tissue that grows outward from a surface

polyp, aural benign lesion in the external auditory meatus, protruding from a perforation of the tympanic membrane

PON periolivary nuclei; group of nuclei of the superior olivary complex surrounding the lateral and medial superior olives that receive projections from the intermediate acoustic stria

pons portion of the hindbrain between the medulla oblongata and the midbrain, containing the cochlear nuclei, superior olivary complex, and nuclei of the lateral lemniscus

pontine pertaining to the pons

pontine paramedian reticular formation PPRF; nucleus in the pons that carries afferent information from the contralateral semicircular canal and vestibular nucleus to the motor nucleus of Cranial Nerve VI

positional alcoholic nystagmus positional nystagmus that occurs regularly after moderate ingestion of alcohol

positional nystagmus usually abnormal presence of nystagmus that occurs with the head placed in a particular position; subtypes are classified as geotropic or ageotropic and direction-changing or direction-fixed nystagmus; COM: positioning nystagmus

positional nystagmus, central direction-changing abnormal positional nystagmus in which nystagmus changes direction when the head is kept in the same position, characteristic of central pathology

positional nystagmus, direction-fixed abnormal positional nystagmus that beats in the same direction regardless of head position, characteristic of peripheral vestibular pathology

positional nystagmus, peripheral direction-changing abnormal positional nystagmus in which nystagmus changes directions with changes in head position, characteristic of nonlocalized vestibular pathology

positional testing component of electronystagmography test battery in which eye movements are recorded as the patient is moved slowly into several test positions; used to identify the presence of nystagmus elicited by head positions that do not involve head movement

positional vertigo dizziness that occurs when the head is placed in a certain position and that does not involve head movement

positioning nystagmus normal presence of nystagmus that occurs during head movement; COM: positional nystagmus

positive correlation direct relationship of the values of two sets of measures

positive middle ear pressure air pressure in the middle ear cavity that is greater than atmospheric pressure, resulting from air being forced into the middle ear through the eustachian tube

positive predictive value probability that a disorder is present when a diagnostic test is positive

positive venting valve PVV; series of small inserts, with holes of graduated diameter, that fit in the lateral end of an earmold vent to permit alteration of vent size

postauricular located posterior to the auricle

postauricular hearing aid a hearing aid that fits over the ear and is coupled to the ear canal via an earmold; SYN: behind-the ear hearing aid, over-the-ear hearing aid

postauricular muscle or myogenic potential PAM potential; electrical potential generated from muscles of the neck that occurs around 20 msec and can be of sufficient magnitude to obscure the neurogenic auditory middle latency response

posterior anatomical direction, referring to structures that are located toward the back or behind; SYN: dorsal; ANT: anterior

posterior ampulla bulging portion of the posterior semicircular canal that contains the crista ampullaris

posterior ampullary nerve nerve fiber bundle from the hair cells of the crista ampullaris of the posterior semicircular canal that joins with similar bundles from the other semicircular canals, the utricle, and the saccule to form the vestibular branch of Cranial Nerve VIII

posterior auricular muscle one of four muscles attaching to the medial surface of the auricle

posterior canal posterior semicircular canal

posterior incudal ligament one of several ligaments responsible for maintaining the position of the ossicles, extending from the short process of the incus to the posterior wall of the middle ear cavity

posterior malleolar fold one of two ligamentous bands on the tympanic membrane, coursing superiorly and posteriorly from the lateral process of the malleus to the tympanic sulcus

posterior semicircular canal one of three bony canals of the vestibular apparatus containing sensory epithelia that respond to angular motion

posterior semicircular duct one of three membranous canals of the vestibular apparatus containing sensory epithelia that respond to angular motion

posterior ventral cochlear nucleus PVCN; portion of the cochlear nucleus that receives nerve fibers from the posterior branch of Cranial Nerve VIII and sends fibers, via the intermediate acoustic stria, to the periolivary nuclei and contralateral nuclei of the lateral lemniscus

posterior vestibular artery branch of the vestibulocochlear artery that supplies the macula of the saccule, the crista and membranous canal of the posterior semicircular canal, and the inferior surface of the utricle and saccule

postlingual postlinguistic

postlinguistic occurring after the time of speech and language development

postlinguistic deafness deafness occurring after speech and language have developed

postnatal after birth

poststimulatory fatigue temporary change in hearing sensitivity following exposure to sound; SYN: temporary threshold shift; COM: perstimulatory fatigue

postural control maintenance of body posture by the interaction of sensory perception, central nervous system integration, and motor function

posturography, computerized dynamic dynamic platform posturography

posturography, dynamic platform quantitative assessment of the integrated function of the balance system for postural stability during quiet and perturbed stance; performed by a computer-based moving platform and motion transducers

pot potentiometer

potassium K+; chemical found in low concentration in perilymph and in high concentration in endolymph

potassium bromate colorless, odorless, tasteless neutralizer used in hairstyling solutions, food preservatives, and other commercial applications, associated with nephrotoxicity and ototoxicity

potential 1. electric tension; 2. consequence of a temporary change in membrane potential of nerve or muscle tissue upon excitation

potential, action AP; 1. synchronous change in electrical potential of nerve or muscle tissue; 2. in auditory evoked potential measures, whole-nerve or compound action potential of Cranial Nerve VIII, the main component of ECochG and Wave I of the ABR

potential, corneoretinal CRP; electrical potential generated by the voltage difference between the relatively positive cornea and the relatively negative retina

potential, electrical amount of available electromotive force

potential, endocochlear EP; electrical potential or voltage of endolymph in the scala media

potential, endolymphatic electrical potential within the endolymphatic space and cells of approximately 70 millivolts to 90 millivolts positive relative to the perilymph

potential, event-related ERP; evoked potential elicited by an endogenous response to an external event, such as the P3 or CNV

potential, evoked EP; electrical activity of the brain responding to sensory stimulation

potential, intracellular ionic potential within a cell

potential, postauricular muscle PAM potential; electrical potential generated from muscles of the neck that occurs around 20 msec and can be of sufficient magnitude to obscure the neurogenic auditory middle latency response

potential, receptor in the auditory system, either of the cochlear microphonic or summating potentials generated by the cochlea in response to sound

potential, resting membrane voltage developed across a membrane at rest

potential, summating SP; a direct-current electrical potential of cochlear origin that follows the envelope of acoustic stimulation and is measured with electrocochleography

potential, vertex any evoked potential that is most prominent when recorded at the vertex

potentiation synergistic enhancement of one structure or function by another

potentiometer a resistor connected across a voltage that permits variable change of a current or circuit

power CROS monaural power hearing aid fitting that uses a contralateral routing of signals (CROS) strategy by placing the microphone on the opposite ear to reduce the potential for feedback

PPO preferred provider organization; managed care organization in which providers and employers or third-party administrators

contract to provide services to a defined population at agreed-upon, usually discounted, fees

PPRF pontine paramedian reticular formation; nucleus in the pons that carries afferent information from the contralateral semicircular canal and vestibular nucleus to the motor nucleus of Cranial Nerve VI

practolol beta blocker used to inhibit stimulation of the heart for management of cardiac arhythmia and angina pectoris; associated with sensorineural hearing loss due to ototoxicity

preauricular located anterior to the auricle

preauricular abnormalities autosomal dominant craniofacial disorders, characterized by preauricular pits or tags, branchial fistulas, mandibular anomalies, facial paralysis, external auditory meatal atresia, and conductive, mixed, or sensorineural hearing loss

preauricular pits craniofacial anomaly characterized by a small hole of variable depth lying anterior to the auricle

preauricular tag craniofacial anomaly characterized by a small appendage, often containing cartilage, lying anterior to the auricle

precedence effect perception of a fused image originating from one of a pair of loudspeakers placed on opposite sides of the head out of which the earlier of two identical signals is presented; interspeaker delay causing the effect is normally on the order of 0.5 msec

precipitous steep

precipitous hearing loss sensorineural hearing loss characterized by a steeply sloping audiometric configuration

predictive value, negative probability that a disorder is not present when a diagnostic test is negative

predictive value, positive probability that a disorder is present when a diagnostic test is positive

preferred loudness level signal level at which speech is rated as most comfortable

preferred provider organization PPO; managed care organization in which providers and organizations such as employers or third-party administrators contract to provide services to a defined population at agreed-upon, usually discounted, fees

prefitting, gain the use of probe-microphone measurement prior to ordering a custom hearing device to provide individual corrections to the desired coupler values for gain and output

prelim preliminary; used colloquially to refer to an initial draft of a patient report

prelingual prelinguistic

prelinguistic occurring prior to the time of speech and language development

prelinguistic deafness deafness occurring prior to speech and language development

premature caloric reversal caloric nystagmus that reverses its direction prior to 140 seconds following onset of irrigation, consistent with central vestibular pathology; SYN: secondary phase nystagmus

prenatal before birth

preponderance, directional DP; superiority in one direction or the other of the slow-phase velocity of nystagmus; e.g., for caloric labyrinthine stimulation, right-beating nystagmus (RW+LC) is compared to left-beating nystagmus (RC+LW), where R = right, L = left, W = warm, and C = cool

presbyacusis; presbycusis age-related hearing impairment

presbyacusis, neural loss of cochlear and higher-order neurons associated with the aging process

presbyacusis, sensory age-related hearing loss caused by hair cell loss at the basal end of the cochlea

presbyacusis, strial age-related hearing loss due to patchy atrophy of the stria vascularis in the middle and apical turns of the cochlea

prescribed gain gain and frequency response of a hearing aid that is determined by any of several prescriptive formulae

prescription of gain and output POGO; hearing aid selection algorithm designed to prescribe a gain and frequency response that is based on a half-gain rule at frequencies above 500 Hz and reductions from half gain of -5 dB and -10 dB at 500 Hz and 250 Hz

prescription of gain and output II POGO II; modification of the POGO gain rule in which the gain is increased at each frequency by one-half the decibel amount that the hearing loss exceeds 65 dB HL

prescriptive fitting strategy for fitting hearing aids by the calculation of a desired gain and frequency response, based on any

of a number of formulas that incorporate pure-tone audiometric thresholds and may incorporate uncomfortable loudness information

prescriptive gain target the desired gain and frequency response of a hearing aid, generated by a formula, against which the actual output of a hearing aid is compared

prescriptive procedure, Berger first comprehensive hearing aid selection algorithm designed to prescribe gain and frequency response based on the pure-tone audiogram, with different weighting factors at each of six frequencies from 500 Hz to 6000 Hz

prescriptive procedure, DSL method of choosing gain and frequency response of a hearing aid so that the long-term spectrum of speech is amplified to the desired sensation levels, estimated across the frequency range from audiometric thresholds

prescriptive procedure, MSU Memphis State University procedure; gain and frequency response selection algorithm based on the theory that a hearing aid should amplify the long-term speech spectrum to a point halfway between threshold and the upper limit of comfortable loudness

prescriptive procedure, NAL National Acoustic Laboratories procedure; gain and frequency response prescriptive strategy based on the theory that a hearing aid should amplify the long-term spectrum of speech so that it is equally and comfortably loud across frequency

prescriptive procedure, Pascoe hearing aid selection algorithm designed to prescribe a gain and frequency response that amplifies the long-term speech spectrum to a point that represents a specified percentage of the difference between threshold and MCL

prescriptive procedure, POGO prescription of gain and output; hearing aid selection algorithm designed to prescribe a gain and frequency response that is based on a half-gain rule at frequencies above 500 Hz and reductions from half gain of -5 dB and -10 dB at 500 Hz and 250 Hz

prescriptive procedure, POGO II prescription of gain and output II; modification of the POGO gain rule in which the gain is increased at each frequency by one-half the decibel amount that the hearing loss exceeds 65 dB HL

preset gain control secondary gain control in a hearing aid, which is inaccessible to the wearer, that can be manipulated by the fitter to limit the range of amplification available to the wearer

pressure force exerted per unit area, expressed in dynes per square centimeter, Newtons per square meter, or Pascals

pressure, reference pressure against which a measured pressure is compared in the decibel notation

pressure-equalization tube PE tube; small tube or grommet inserted in the tympanic membrane following myringotomy to provide equalization of air pressure within the middle ear space as a substitute for a nonfunctional eustachian tube; SYN: tympanostomy tube

pressure vent small vent in an earmold or hearing aid to provide pressure equalization in the external auditory meatus

prevalence number of existing cases of a specific disease or condition in a given population at a given time

preverbal prelinguistic

primary auditory neurons first-order neurons of the cochlear branch of Cranial Nerve VIII, with dendrites from the inner hair cells to cell bodies of the spiral ganglion to axons synapsing on the cochlear nucleus

primary auditory pathway neural pathway in the central nervous system that carries the primary afferent input from the cochlea to the cortex

probe microphone microphone transducer with a small-diameter probe-tube extension for measuring sound near the tympanic membrane

probe-microphone measurements electroacoustic assessment of the characteristics of hearing aid amplification near the tympanic membrane using a probe microphone

probe tone in immittance measurement, the pure tone that is held at a constant intensity level in the external auditory meatus; used to indirectly measure changes in energy flow through the middle ear mechanism

probe-tube microphone probe microphone

process in anatomy, a projection or outgrowth

processing, auditory peripheral and central auditory system manipulation of acoustic signals

processing, CA compressed analog processing

processing, central auditory CAP; function of the central auditory nervous system, including sound localization, lateralization, binaural processes, speech perception, etc.

processing, CIS continuous interleaved sampling processing

processing, compressed analog CA processing; cochlear implant processing strategy in which speech signals are divided into frequency bands and delivered to corresponding implant electrodes

processing, continuous interleaved sampling CIS processing; cochlear implant processing strategy designed to deliver nonsimultaneous pulses at a high rate of stimulation to multiple implant electrodes

processing, digital signal DSP; manipulation by mathematical algorithms of a signal that has been converted from analog to digital form

processing, $f_0/f_1/f_2$ cochlear implant processing strategy designed to extract frequency and amplitude estimates of f_1 and f_2 from a speech signal and deliver them to an electrode corresponding to each frequency band at a pulse rate equal to f_0

processing, interleaved pulses early cochlear implant processing strategy in which trains of pulses, representing both speech features and waveform representation, were delivered to electrodes with temporal offsets to eliminate overlap across channels

processing, multichannel signal processing in more than one channel, referring especially to cochlear implant configurations

processing, real-time instantaneous manipulation of signals or information by a computer at a rate fast enough to be imperceptible

processing, signal manipulation of specified characteristics of a signal

processing, single-channel hearing aid signal processing in one frequency band only, typically the entire frequency band

processing, spectral maxima sound SMSP; cochlear implant signal-processing strategy in which the highest six amplitudes of 16 processed bands are delivered in a nonoverlapping sequence to electrode locations mapped to the identified channels

processing disorder, auditory APD;

reduction in the ability to manipulate acoustic signals, despite normal hearing sensitivity and regardless of language, attention, and cognition ability

processing disorder, central auditory CAPD; disorder in function of central auditory structures, characterized by impaired ability of the central auditory nervous system to manipulate and use acoustic signals, including difficulty understanding speech in noise and localizing sounds

Profile of Hearing Aid Benefit PHAB; self-assessment inventory designed to evaluate perceived benefit from the use of hearing aids

Profile of Hearing Aid Performance PHAP; self-assessment inventory designed to assess the perceived performance received from the use of hearing aid amplification

profound hearing loss loss of hearing sensitivity of greater than 90 dB HL

prognosis prediction of the course or outcome of a disease or proposed treatment

programmable hearing aid digitally controlled analog or digital signal processing hearing aid in which the parameters of the instrument are under computer control

programmable increases at low levels PILL; type of automatic signal processing in a hearing aid that uses level-dependent control of frequency response, reducing either low-frequency or high-frequency gain as input level increases

progressive advancing, as in a disease

progressive adult-onset hearing loss autosomal dominant nonsyndromic hearing loss with onset in adulthood, characterized by progressive, symmetric sensorineural hearing loss

prolapsed canal external auditory meatus that is occluded by cartilaginous tissue that has lost rigidity; SYN: collapsed canal

proliferation second in a series of embryologic processes, which in the auditory system includes transformation of the otic placode into the otic pit and subsequent development of the cochlear duct epithelium and auditory neurons

promontory bony prominence in the labyrinthine wall of the middle ear cavity, separating the oval and round windows and serving as the wall of the basal turn of the cochlea

promontory stimulation delivery of electrical stimulation to the promontory via a transtympanic electrode to elicit an electrically evoked action potential

promontory testing pre-operative promontory stimulation of the cochlear implant candidate to assess the status of Cranial Nerve VIII

prone, otitis being inclined to develop otitis media

prophylaxis prevention of disease or disorder, such as by the use of ear protection to prevent noise-induced hearing loss or the use of antibiotics to prevent the occurrence of otitis media

prosody modulations of characteristics of the voice such as pitch, quality, and intensity that are perceived as stress and intonation

prospective capitated payment model in healthcare reimbursement, a model in which the provider receives payment on a monthly capitated basis before rendering services

prosthesis; pl. prostheses device replacing or augmenting a missing or dysfunctional part

protection, hearing broad category of devices and techniques designed to attenuate hazardous levels of noise

protection device, hearing HPD; any of a number of devices used to attenuate excessive environmental noise to protect hearing, including those that block the ear canal or cover the external ear

protocol precise, detailed plan for the administration of a test or for a regimen of treatment

proximal toward the center or point of origin; ANT: distal

pseudobinaural hearing aid early, single body-worn hearing aid with Y-cord transmission to earmolds in both ears

pseudohypoacusis; pseudohypacusis hearing sensitivity loss that is exaggerated or feigned; SYN: functional hearing loss

pseudorandom noise complex sound wave in which a sequence of component amplitudes, frequencies, and phases vary periodically over time

PSI pediatric speech intelligibility test; closed-set test of word and sentence recognition, in quiet and in a background of speech competition, designed to assess speech perception ability of children ages 2.5 to 6 years

psychoacoustics branch of psychophysics concerned with the quantification of auditory sensation and the measurement of the psychological correlates of the physical characteristics of sound

psychogalvanic skin response   PGSR; change in skin resistance as a result of an emotional response to a stimulus; SYN: galvanic skin response

psychogalvanic skin response audiometry   PGSR audiometry; method of determining hearing sensitivity in cases of suspected functional hearing loss by measuring psychogalvanic skin response to sound, following conditioning to the sound paired with a mild shock; SYN: electrodermal audiometry

psychogenic deafness   rare disorder characterized by apparent, but nonorganic, hearing loss resulting from psychological trauma

psychophysical procedures   behavioral procedures designed to assess the relationship between the subjective sensation to and physical magnitude of sensory stimuli

psychophysical scales   scales of measurement describing the relationship between the magnitude of subjective sensations to and the magnitude of physical attributes of sensory stimuli

psychophysical tuning curve   psychophysically determined plot of the level of a variable-frequency masking tone that just masks a fixed-frequency probe tone as a function of the frequency of the masker

psychophysics   science of the relationship between sensory perception and the physical attributes of stimuli

PT   platinol (cisplatin), taxol; potentially ototoxic chemotherapy regimen used in the treatment of ovarian cancer

PTA   pure-tone average; average of hearing sensitivity thresholds to pure-tone signals at 500 Hz, 1000 Hz, and 2000 Hz

PTA0   pure-tone average 0; low-frequency average of hearing sensitivity thresholds to pure-tone signals at 250 Hz, 500 Hz, and 1000 Hz

PTA2   pure-tone average 2; high-frequency average of hearing sensitivity thresholds to pure-tone signals at 1000 Hz, 2000 Hz, and 4000 Hz

PTS   permanent threshold shift; irreversible hearing sensitivity loss following exposure to excessive noise levels; COM: temporary threshold shift

Public Law 101-336   United States public law (PL) 101–336; Americans with Disabilities Act of 1990

Public Law 101-431   United States public law (PL) 101–336; Television Decoder Circuitry Act of 1990

Public Law 94-142   United States public law (PL) 94–142, known as the Education for All Handicapped Children Act of 1975 and renamed the Individuals with Disabilities Education Act, mandating free and appropriate public education for all children who are handicapped

Public Law 99-457   United States public law (PL) 99–457, passed in 1986; bill that reauthorized PL 94–142, extended it to include children aged 3 to 5 years, and encouraged the provision of services to infants and toddlers from birth to 3 years

pulsatile tinnitus   objective tinnitus, characterized by pulsing sound, that results from vascular abnormalities such as glomus tumor, arterial anomaly, and heart murmurs

pumping and breathing   audible fluctuations in the output of a hearing aid that occur when a compression circuit with a short release time is activated by a rapidly fluctuating input signal

pure tone   sound wave having only one frequency of vibration

pure-tone air-conduction threshold   lowest level at which a pure-tone stimulus, presented through earphones, is audible

pure-tone audiogram   graph of the threshold of hearing sensitivity, expressed in dB HL, as determined by pure-tone air-conduction and bone-conduction audiometry at octave and half-octave frequencies ranging from 250 Hz to 8000 Hz

pure-tone audiometer   instrument for presenting pure-tone stimuli of selected frequencies at calibrated output levels for the determination of an audiogram

pure-tone audiometry   measurement of hearing sensitivity thresholds to pure-tone stimuli by air and bone conduction

pure-tone average   PTA; average of hearing sensitivity thresholds to pure-tone signals at 500 Hz, 1000 Hz, and 2000 Hz

pure-tone bone-conduction threshold   lowest level at which a pure-tone stimulus, presented via a vibrating oscillator placed on the forehead or mastoid, is audible

pure-tone threshold   lowest level at which a pure-tone stimulus is audible

pursuit, saccadic   abnormal presence of saccades during smooth pursuit due to failure of the eyes to maintain fixation on the moving target, requiring saccadic movements to refixate; consistent with cortical, brainstem, or cerebellar disorder

pursuit, slow SYN: smooth pursuit

pursuit, smooth eye movement used to track slowly and smoothly moving objects; SYN: slow pursuit

purulent pertaining to the formation of pus; SYN: suppurative

purulent effusion fluid containing pus

purulent otitis media inflammation of the middle ear with infected effusion containing pus; SYN: suppurative otitis media

pus fluid containing debris of dead cells and tissue, resulting from inflammation

PVCN posterior ventral cochlear nucleus; portion of the cochlear nucleus that receives nerve fibers from the posterior branch of Cranial Nerve VIII and sends fibers, via the intermediate acoustic stria, to the PON and contralateral lateral lemniscus

PVT physical volume test; subtest of immittance audiometry in which the volume of the ear canal is estimated; e.g., a large volume is found in the case of a tympanic membrane perforation and a small volume in the case of impacted cerumen

PVV positive venting valve; series of small inserts, with holes of graduated diameter, that fit in the lateral end of an earmold vent to permit alteration of vent size

Pyle disease autosomal recessive craniofacial-skeletal disorder, which may include nystagmus and progressive mixed or sensorineural hearing loss

pyramidal eminence pyramid-shaped prominence, near the middle of the mastoid wall of the middle ear cavity, that contains the body of the stapedius muscle

Q

quality in psychoacoustics, the perception or psychological impression of the spectrum of sound

quarter-wave resonator air-filled tube, open at one end and closed at the other, the fundamental resonance of which is four times the length of the tube

quasi-digital hearing aid early term for digitally controlled analog hearing aid

quinine antimalarial drug, which, taken during pregnancy, can affect the auditory system of the fetus, or, taken in large doses, can cause temporary or permanent hearing loss in the person taking the drug

R

R   resistance; opposition to energy flow due to dissipation

radial fibers   tissue fibers, constituting one of two middle layers of the tympanic membrane, that radiate from the center toward the periphery and are unevenly spaced to resemble the spokes in a wheel

radiating arterioles   two sets of blood vessels, branching from the main cochlear artery, that supply the internal and external walls of the cochlea

radiation   x-rays or any other rays used in diagnosis and treatment of disease

radical mastoid cavity   cavity that remains following radical mastoidectomy, which is prone to recurrent serous or purulent discharge

radical mastoidectomy   surgical procedure performed to establish drainage for nonresponsive otitis media and mastoiditis, consisting of removal of the mastoid air cells, posterior wall of the ear canal, lateral wall of the epitympanic space, malleus, incus, and eardrum

radiography   diagnostic examination of structures of the body by means of x-rays

radiologic   pertaining to radiology

radiology   branch of medical science devoted to diagnostic examination and treatment of structures of the body by means of x-rays

radionecrosis   death of tissue due to excessive exposure to radiation, which in the auditory system may occur immediately or have later onset and is characterized by atrophy of the spiral and annular ligaments resulting in degeneration of the organ of Corti

radiotherapy   treatment of disease by use of radiation

Rainville technique   test of masked bone conduction in which thresholds are established by air conduction with and without masking noise presented through a bone vibrator placed on the mastoid; precursor to the sensorineural acuity level (SAL) test

raised threshold   elevated or abnormal threshold of hearing sensitivity

Ramsay Hunt syndrome   herpes zoster infection that lingers in the ganglia and can be activated by systemic disease, resulting in vesicular eruptions of the auricle, facial nerve palsy, and sensorineural hearing loss; SYN: herpes zoster oticus

randfasernetz   lateral process of the tectorial membrane

random noise   complex sound wave in which component amplitudes, frequencies, and phases vary randomly over time

range   statistical measurement of dispersion, expressed as the magnitude of the difference between data extremes

range, dynamic   1. amplitude range over which an electronic instrument operates; 2. the difference in dB between a person's threshold of sensitivity and threshold of discomfort

range, fitting   range of hearing loss for which a specific hearing aid circuit, configuration, earmold, etc. is appropriate

range of comfortable loudness   difference, in dB, between threshold of audibility and loudness discomfort level for a specified acoustic signal

range of normal hearing   dispersion of hearing threshold levels around audiometric zero for the population of those with normal hearing

rapid speech-transmission index   RASTI; assessment of the integrity of signal transmission in a room, expressed as the reduction in signal modulation of amplitude-modulated broad-band noise centered at 500 Hz and 2000 Hz

rapidly alternating speech perception   RASP; test of sentence recognition in which the signal is alternated between ears at rates ranging from 200 msec to 400 msec, designed to assess auditory brainstem integrity

rare event   in event-related potential measurement, the target stimulus that occurs less often; ANT: frequent event

rarefaction   in the propagation of sound waves, the time during which the density of air molecules is decreased below its static value; ANT: condensation

rarefaction click   rapid-onset, short-duration, broad-band sound produced by delivering a negative-polarity electric pulse to an earphone; ANT: condensation click

RASP   rapidly alternating speech perception; test of sentence recognition in which the signal is alternated between ears at rates ranging from 200 msec to 400 msec, designed to assess auditory brainstem integrity

RASTI rapid speech transmission index; assessment of the integrity of signal transmission in a room, expressed as the reduction in signal modulation of amplitude-modulated broad-band noise centered at 500 Hz and 2000 Hz

ratio, compression the decibel ratio of acoustic input to amplifier output in a hearing aid; e.g., a hearing aid with a compression ratio of 2:1 will increase output by 1 dB for every 2 dB increase in input

ratio, consonant-vowel relationship between the intensity of a consonant and its neighboring vowel

ratio, critical a measure of the limited effective bandwidth of a noise masker, taken as the difference in dB between a masked threshold and the level per cycle of the masker

ratio, message-to-competition MCR; in speech audiometry, the ratio in dB of the presentation level of a speech target to that of background competition; SYN: signal-to-noise ratio

ratio, signal-to-noise S/N; relative difference in dB between a sound of interest and a background of noise

RCT rotary chair testing; test of vestibular function, in which a computer-driven chair rotates in regulated variable-velocity clockwise and counterclockwise motion, with simultaneous electronystagmographic recording

reactance X; opposition to energy flow due to storage

reactance, elastic reduction of low-frequency vibrations due to stiffness of the vibrating object

reaction time time elapsed between a stimulus presentation and a response

REAG real-ear aided gain; measurement of the difference, in dB as a function of frequency, between the SPL in the ear canal and the SPL at a field reference point for a specified sound field with the hearing aid in place and turned on

real-ear aided gain REAG; measurement of the difference, in dB as a function of frequency, between the SPL in the ear canal and the SPL at a field reference point for a specified sound field with the hearing aid in place and turned on

real-ear aided response REAR; probe-microphone measurement of the sound pressure level, as a function of frequency, at

a specified point near the tympanic membrane with a hearing aid in place and turned on; expressed in absolute SPL or as gain relative to stimulus level

real-ear attenuation probe-microphone measurement of the attenuation characteristic of hearing protection devices, expressed as the difference between the real-ear unaided response and the real-ear occluded response

real-ear coupler difference RECD; measurement of the difference, in dB as a function of frequency, between the output of a hearing aid measured by a probe microphone in the ear canal and the output measured in a 2-cc coupler

real-ear dial difference REDD; measurement of the difference, in dB, between a signal measured by a probe microphone in the ear canal and the dial reading of that signal on the audiometer

real-ear gain nonspecific term referring generally to the gain of a hearing aid at the tympanic membrane, measured as the difference between the SPL in the ear canal and the SPL at the field reference point for a specified sound field

real-ear insertion gain REIG; probe-microphone measurement of the difference, in dB as a function of frequency, between the real-ear unaided gain and the real-ear aided gain at the same point near the tympanic membrane

real-ear insertion response REIR; probe-microphone measurement of the difference, in dB as a function of frequency, between the real-ear unaided response and the real-ear aided response at the same point near the tympanic membrane

real-ear masker response REMR; probe-microphone measurement of tinnitus masker output

real-ear occluded gain REOG; probe-microphone measurement of the difference, in dB as a function of frequency, between the SPL in the ear canal and the SPL at a field reference point for a specified sound field with a hearing aid in place and turned off

real-ear occluded response REOR; probe-microphone measurement of the sound pressure level, as a function of frequency, at a specified point near the tympanic membrane with a hearing aid in place and turned off; expressed in absolute SPL or as gain relative to stimulus level

real-ear saturation response RESR; probe-microphone measurement of the SPL, as a function of frequency, at a specified point near the tympanic membrane with a hearing aid in place and turned on, with sufficient stimulus level to drive the hearing aid at its maximum output

real-ear unaided gain REUG; probe-microphone measurement of the difference, in dB as a function of frequency, between the SPL in an unoccluded ear canal and the SPL at the field reference point for a specified sound field

real-ear unaided response REUR; probe-microphone measurement of the sound pressure level, as a function of frequency, at a specified point near the tympanic membrane in an unoccluded ear canal

real-time captioning computerized captioning of a person's speech with little or no time delay

real-time processing instantaneous manipulation of signals or information by a computer at a rate fast enough to be imperceptible

real-world performance the effectiveness of hearing aids or hearing protection devices as measured under normal conditions of use

REAR real-ear aided response; probe-microphone measurement of the sound pressure level, as a function of frequency, at a specified point near the tympanic membrane with a hearing aid in place and turned on

recall memory

RECD real-ear coupler difference; measurement of the difference, in dB as a function of frequency, between the output of a hearing aid measured by a probe microphone in the ear canal and the output measured in a 2-cc coupler

receiver 1. device that converts electrical energy into acoustic energy, such as an earphone or a loudspeaker in a hearing aid; 2. portion of an FM system worn by the listener that receives signals from the FM transmitter

receiver operator characteristic curve ROC curve; graph used in signal detection theory in which the hit rate, or probability of a positive response to a signal, is plotted as a function of the false-alarm rate, or probability of a positive response in the absence of a signal

receptor sensory nerve terminal

receptor, distance sensory organ that can perceive stimuli at some distance from the body

receptor potential in the auditory system, either of the cochlear microphonic or summating potentials generated by the cochlea in response to sound

receptors, sensory in the ear, the sensory epithelia, including the inner hair cells, the cristae ampullares, and the utricular and sacular maculae

recess a small indentation

recessive hereditary sensorineural hearing loss most common inherited hearing loss, in which both parents are carriers of the gene but only 25% of offspring are affected; occurring in either nonsyndromic or syndromic form

recognition, speech the ability to perceive and identify speech targets; SYN: speech intelligibility, speech discrimination

recognition, word the ability to perceive and identify a word; SYN: word discrimination, word intelligibility

recording, far-field measurement of evoked potentials from electrodes on the scalp at a distance from the source

recording, near-field measurement of evoked potentials from electrodes adjacent to the source

recovery time release time

recreational audiology audiology subspecialty devoted to the conservation of hearing during recreational activities, such as shooting, listening to music, boating, etc.

recruitment exaggeration of nonlinearity of loudness growth in an ear with sensorineural hearing loss, wherein loudness grows rapidly at intensity levels just above threshold but may grow normally at high intensity levels; SYN: loudness recruitment

recruitment, complete condition in which the loudness of a tone in an ear with hearing loss is equal to the loudness of a tone of the same intensity in an ear with normal hearing, at high intensity levels

recruitment, loudness SYN: recruitment

recruitment, partial condition in which the loudness of a high-intensity tone in an ear with hearing loss approaches, but remains less than, the loudness of a tone of the same intensity in an ear with normal hearing

recurrence return of the symptoms of a disease

recurrent otitis media middle ear inflammation that occurs 3 or more times in a 6-month period

REDD real-ear dial difference; measurement of the difference, in dB, between a signal measured by a probe microphone in the ear canal and the dial reading of that signal on the audiometer

redundancy in speech audiometry, the abundance of information available to the listener due to the substantial informational content of a speech signal and to the capacity inherent in the richly innervated pathways of the central auditory nervous system

redundancy, extrinsic the abundance of information present in the speech signal

redundancy, intrinsic the abundance of information present in the central auditory system due to the capacity inherent in its richly innervated pathways

reference electrode inverting electrode attached to that side of a differential amplifier that inverts the input by 180; earlobe electrode in conventional auditory brainstem response recordings; COM: active electrode

reference equivalent threshold sound pressure level RETSPL; ANSI standard specification of the sound-pressure levels that correspond to audiometric zero for a specific earphone

reference microphone a second microphone used to measure the stimulus level during probe-microphone measurements or to control the stimulus level during the probe-microphone equalization process

reference pressure pressure against which a measured pressure is compared in the decibel notation

reference test frequencies frequencies of 1000 Hz, 1600 Hz, and 2500 Hz at which reference test gain is established

reference test gain ANSI standard gain level with a 60-dB-SPL input and the volume control of the hearing aid adjusted so that the gain at the reference test frequencies is 17 dB less than that at SSPL-90

refixations rapid eye movements that occur to maintain the image of fast-moving objects on the fovea; SYN: saccades

reflex involuntary response to a stimulus

reflex, acoustic reflexive contraction of the intra-aural muscles in response to loud sound, dominated by the stapedius muscle in humans; SYN: acoustic stapedial reflex

reflex, acousticopalpebral auropalpebral reflex

reflex, audito-oculogyric AOR; rapid turning of the eyes toward the source of a sudden sound

reflex, auropalpebral APR; eyeblink or twitch at the canthus caused by a sudden loud sound

reflex, Babinski normal extension and fanning of the toes on stimulation of the sole of the foot, a lack of which is consistent with neurologic disorder

reflex, cochlear acoustic reflex

reflex, cochleo-orbicular auropalpebral reflex

reflex, cochleopalpebral auropalpebral reflex

reflex, cochleostapedial acoustic reflex

reflex, Gault's eyeblink or twitch at the canthus caused by a sudden loud sound; SYN: auropalpebral reflex

reflex, intra-aural reflexive contraction of the intra-aural muscles in response to loud sound; stapedius muscle dominates the reflex in humans; SYN: acoustic reflex

reflex, light bright triangular reflection on the surface of the tympanic membrane of the illumination used during otoscopic examination; SYN: cone of light

reflex, middle ear muscle reflexive contraction of the stapedius and tensor tympani muscles in response to loud sound; stapedius muscle dominates the reflex in humans; SYN: acoustic reflex

reflex, Moro normal reaction of infants to a variety of stimuli, characterized by a sudden extension and abduction of the arms, hands, and fingers

reflex, orienting OR; reflexive head turn toward the source of a sound

reflex, pinna reflexive orienting of the pinna in many animals in response to altering sounds

reflex, stapedial reflexive contraction of the stapedius muscle in response to loud sound; SYN: acoustic reflex

reflex, startle normal reflexive extension and abduction of the limb and neck muscles in an infant when surprised by a sudden sound; SYN: Moro reflex

reflex, vestibulo-ocular VOR; reflex arc between the vestibular system and extraocular muscles, activated by asymmetric neural firing rate of the vestibular nerve, serving to maintain gaze stability by generating compensatory eye movements in response to head rotation

reflex arc functional pathway of the nervous system from a sensory receptor to a motor responder

reflex decay perstimulatory reduction in the amplitude of an acoustic reflex in response to continuous stimulus presentation

reflex decay test measure of auditory adaptation in which a signal is presented at 10 dB above an acoustic reflex threshold and the amplitude is monitored for a clinically significant reduction of over 50% of initial amplitude within 10 seconds of stimulus onset

reflexogenic vertigo nystagmus and vertigo resulting from stimulation of the utricular macula when positive pressure is placed on the stapes footplate, via pneumatic otoscopy, tympanometry, stapedius muscle contraction, etc.,

reflux otitis media inflammation of the middle ear mucosa resulting from the passage of nasopharyngeal secretions through the eustachian tube

refraction change in direction or deflection of a sound wave as it moves from one medium into another

refractory period time following the major phase of an action potential during which a nerve cannot discharge again regardless of the magnitude of stimulation

Refsum syndrome autosomal recessive eye disorder, characterized by retinitis pigmentosa, peripheral neuropathy, and cerebellar ataxia, with associated progressive, asymmetric sensorineural hearing loss

register, high-risk 1. record of names of infants who are at risk for hearing loss; 2. list of factors that put a child at risk for having or developing hearing loss

rehabilitation partial or total restoration of function following disease or injury

rehabilitation, aural treatment of persons with adventitious hearing impairment to improve the efficacy of overall communication ability, including the use of hearing aids, auditory training, speech reading, counseling, and guidance

REIG real-ear insertion gain; probe-microphone measurement of the difference, in dB as a function of frequency, between the real-ear unaided gain and the real-ear aided gain at the same point near the tympanic membrane

reimbursement payment for services rendered by a third party

REIR real-ear insertion response; probe-microphone measurement of the difference, in dB as a function of frequency, between the real-ear unaided response and the real-ear aided response at the same point near the tympanic membrane

Reissner's membrane membrane within the cochlear duct, attached to the osseous spiral lamina and projecting obliquely to the outer wall of the cochlea, that separates the scala vestibuli and scala media

relapse recurrence or exacerbation of a disease or its symptoms

relapsing polychondritis connective tissue disorder, characterized by inflammation and loss of cartilage, usually involving the auricles first; associated with conductive hearing loss secondary to eustachian tube collapse and sensorineural hearing loss

relationship, direct the condition in which the values of two sets of measures are positively correlated, so that the greater the magnitude of one, the greater the magnitude of the other

relationship, inverse the condition in which the values of two sets of measures are negatively correlated so that the greater the magnitude of one, the smaller the magnitude of the other

relative bone conduction early term used to describe bone-conduction thresholds established with the ears unoccluded; COM: absolute bone conduction

release from masking reduction in the effectiveness of masking as a result of a change in some aspect of the masking signal or the signal being masked; e.g., binaural release from masking, in which a change in phase of binaural tones causes them to be audible in noise

release time in compression circuitry, the time it takes for an amplifier to return to its steady state following cessation of a compression-eliciting signal; SYN: recovery time

release time, variable a characteristic of some compression circuits in which the compression release time changes in direct relation to duration of the input, e.g., the shorter the compression-activating input, the shorter the release time

reliability extent to which a test yields consistent scores on repeated measures

reliability coefficient coefficient of cor-

relation between successive administrations of a test or two forms of a test

remodeling, synapse changes in innervation pattern that occur during embryologic development; e.g., early in development, both afferent and efferent fibers contact the inner hair cells, but with development, efferent fibers relocate onto the afferent terminals

remote control hand-held unit that permits volume and/or program changes in a programmable hearing aid

remote masking the masking of a low-frequency sound by an intense level of high-frequency sound; SYN: downward spread of masking

REMR real-ear masker response; probe-microphone measurement of tinnitus masker output

renal pertaining to the kidney

renal-genital syndrome autosomal recessive disorder, characterized by renal anomalies and internal genital malformation, with low-set auricles, stenotic ear canals, and malformed middle ears with associated conductive hearing loss

REOG real-ear occluded gain; probe-microphone measurement of the difference in dB between the SPL in the ear canal and the SPL at a field reference point for a specified sound field with a hearing aid in place and turned off

REOR real-ear occluded response; probe-microphone measurement of the sound pressure level, as a function of frequency, at a specified point near the tympanic membrane with a hearing aid in place and turned off

repair strategies compensatory strategies used by individuals with hearing impairment to clarify missed or misunderstood utterances

repetition rate number of times a stimulus is presented or an event occurs in a specified period of time

replicate to repeat an experiment or condition exactly

resection surgical excision of a segment or part

reserve gain the remaining gain in a hearing aid; the difference between use gain and the gain at which feedback occurs

residual hearing the remaining hearing ability in a person with hearing loss

residual inhibition temporary cessation of tinnitus following masking

resistance R; opposition to energy flow due to dissipation

resistor device that controls the flow of electricity

resolution, frequency the ability to distinguish among sounds of different frequencies presented simultaneously

resolution, temporal ability to perceive or discriminate as separate events sound segments spaced closely in time

resonance condition of peak vibratory response obtained on excitation of a system that can vibrate freely

resonance theory of hearing early assumption that transverse fibers in the basilar membrane act as resonators, each of which is tuned to a different frequency

resonant frequency frequency at which a secured mass will vibrate most readily when set into free vibration; SYN: natural frequency

resonator system that is set into forced vibration by another vibration

resonator, Helmholtz early device for studying acoustics that had variously sized cavities with a protruding tube for insertion in the ear, designed for observation and measurement of the resonant effects of the shape and size of the cavities

resonator, quarter-wave air-filled tube, open at one end and closed at the other, the fundamental resonance of which is four times the length of the tube

resonator earmold earmold in which the sound channel has been altered to enhance resonance in the high frequencies

resorption loss of substance by pathologic absorption

resorptive pertaining to resorption

response 1. in behavioral audiometry, the observable reaction to signal presentation; 2. in hearing aid amplification, the magnitude of the output of a device as a function of frequency

response level, minimal lowest level to which a child will respond behaviorally to sound

response time interval between stimulus delivery and occurrence of a measurable event

RESR real-ear saturation response; probe-microphone measurement of the SPL at a specified point near the tympanic membrane, with a hearing aid in place and turned on and with sufficient stimulus level to drive the hearing aid at its maximum output

resting membrane potential voltage developed across a membrane at rest

retardation delay or limitation in any process

retardation, mental intellectual function below the normal range

reticular lamina delicate netlike structure forming the continuous surface of the organ of Corti, comprising the phalangeal processes, tops of the pillars, and cuticular plates of the inner and outer hair cells

retraction of the tympanic membrane a drawing back of the eardrum into the middle ear space due to negative pressure formed in the cavity secondary to eustachian tube dysfunction

retraction pocket invagination into the middle ear space of a weakened portion of the tympanic membrane

retrocochlear pertaining to the neural structures of the auditory system beyond the cochlea, especially Cranial Nerve VIII and the auditory portions of the brainstem

retrocochlear disorder hearing disorder resulting from a neoplasm or other lesion located on Cranial Nerve VIII or beyond in the auditory brainstem or cortex

retrograde degeneration neural degeneration backward along pathways

retrolabyrinthine retrocochlear

retrospective fee for service reimbursement traditional healthcare reimbursement system in which the provider receives payment only for services rendered, after those services are rendered

RETSPL reference equivalent threshold sound pressure level; ANSI standard specification of the sound-pressure levels that correspond to audiometric zero for a specific earphone

REUG real-ear unaided gain; probe-microphone measurement of the difference, in dB as a function of frequency, between the SPL in an unoccluded ear canal and the SPL at the field reference point for a specified sound field

REUR real-ear unaided response; probe-microphone measurement of the sound pressure level, as a function of frequency, at a specified point near the tympanic membrane in an unoccluded ear canal

reverberation prolongation of sound by multiple reflections

reverberation room specialized testing room designed for minimal sound absorption

reverberation time rate of sound decay, defined as the time required for a sound to decay to a specified level following cessation of the sound source

reversal in adaptive psychophysical procedures, a point of change in the direction of a stimulus parameter

reverse curve fitting hearing aid gain and frequency response shaped to fit a rising hearing loss configuration in which low-frequency hearing sensitivity is poorer than high-frequency sensitivity

reverse horn bore tapered bore in an earmold that is wider in diameter at its lateral aspect, designed to reduce high-frequency amplification

rheobase minimum strength of an electrical signal required to cause excitation of a nerve or muscle

rhinitis inflammation of the mucous membrane of the nasal cavity

Richards-Rundle syndrome autosomal recessive nervous system disorder, characterized by ataxia, muscle wasting, and severe mental retardation, with early-onset, progressive sensorineural hearing loss; SYN: ataxia-hypogonadism syndrome

right-beating nystagmus horizontal nystagmus in which the fast phase is toward the right

right-ear advantage tendency in most individuals for right-ear performance on speech-perception measures to be better than left-ear performance

Rinne test tuning-fork test in which the fork is alternately held to the mastoid for bone-conducted stimulation and near the auricle for air-conducted stimulation in an effort to detect the presence of a conductive hearing loss

rise time time required for a gated signal to reach a specified percentage of its maximum amplitude; ANT: fall time

risk factors health, environmental, and lifestyle factors that enhance the likelihood of having or developing a specified disease or disorder

RMS root mean square; overall effective level of a signal, expressed as the square root of the mean of the squared values of a signal integrated over a time period sufficient to characterize the signal

ROC curve receiver-operating characteristic curve; graph used in signal detection theory in which the hit rate, or probability of

---

Risk factors for hearing loss
— family history of childhood hearing loss
— congenital TORCH infections
— craniofacial anomalies
— birth weight < 1500 grams
— hyperbilirubinemia requiring exchange
— bacterial meningitis
— asphyxia
— ototoxic medication
— mechanical ventilation > 10 days
— syndromes that include hearing loss

risk factors

---

a positive response to a signal, is plotted as a function of the false-alarm rate, or probability of a positive response to noise

rods of Corti   two groups of supporting cells in the organ of Corti, the inner and outer pillars, that form the tunnel of Corti; SYN: pillars of Corti

roentgenography   radiography

rolloff   filter skirt or rate of attenuation of a filter, expressed in dB per octave

rollover   paradoxical decrease in speech-recognition ability with increasing level at high-intensity levels, consistent with retrocochlear disorder

roof of the tympanic cavity   thin plate of bone separating the tympanic cavity from the cranium and meningeal covering of the brain; SYN: tegmen tympani

root mean square, sound pressure level   RMS; overall effective level of a signal, expressed as the square root of the mean of the squared values of a signal integrated over a time period sufficient to characterize the signal

rostral   anatomical direction, referring to structures that are located toward the head, or, more accurately, toward the beak or nose; ANT: caudal; SYN: cranial, cephalad

rotary chair testing   RCT; test of vestibular function, in which a computer-driven chair rotates in regulated variable-velocity clockwise and counterclockwise motion, with simultaneous electronystagmographic recording

rotary stimulation   vestibular system stimulation created by rotating a chair sinusoidally about its vertical axis, first in one direction and then the other, with variable velocity

rotatory nystagmus   nystagmus characterized by rotation of the eyes in clockwise or counterclockwise direction

round-robin tournament   paired comparison technique for hearing aid circuit selection in which each condition is compared to all other conditions to establish ranking

round window   membrane-covered opening in the labyrinthine wall of the middle ear space, leading into the scala tympani of the cochlea; SYN: cochlear window; fenestra rotunda

round window fistula   passageway between the perilymphatic space and the middle ear occurring at the round window, caused by congenital defects or trauma, resulting in the leak of perilymph

round window membrane   thin membrane covering the round window, sometimes referred to as the secondary tympanic membrane

round window niche   small recess or indentation in the labyrinthine wall of the middle ear cavity containing the round window

rubella   mild viral infection, characterized by fever and a transient eruption or rash on the skin resembling measles; when occurring in pregnancy, may result in abnormalities in the fetus, including sensorineural hearing loss; SYN: German measles

rubella, congenital   teratogenic disorder caused by maternal rubella, characterized by cataract or glaucoma, cardiovascular defects, mental retardation, psychomotor retardation, and severe to profound sensorineural hearing loss

rubeola   1. SYN: rubella; 2. SYN: measles

Rudmose audiometer   early automatic audiometer in which the patient controlled the intensity level of the signal

Runge test   early variation of the Weber test in which the ear canal was filled with water and lateralization of bone-conducted signals was assessed

Rush Hughes test   early word-recognition measure using a distorted recording of the W-22 word lists that proved to be useful as a diagnostic speech audiometric test

Rx   prescription

S

S/N   signal-to-noise ratio; relative difference in dB between a sound of interest and a background of noise

S/N ratio   redundant term for S/N

sac   a pouch

SAC   Self Assessment of Communication; a self-assessment questionnaire designed to assess perceived communication ability of adults with hearing impairment

saccades   1. rapid voluntary eye movement from target to target; 2. rapid eye movements that maintain the image of fast-moving objects on the fovea, constituting the quick component of nystagmus

saccades, hypermetric   in ENG testing, condition in which the eyes overshoot the target during calibration, requiring additional saccades to bring them back to the target

saccades, hypometric   in ENG testing, condition in which the eyes undershoot the target during calibration

saccadic palsy   eye-movement disorder in which saccadic movements are normal in one direction but impaired in the opposite direction, consistent with unilateral cortical lesion

saccadic pursuit   abnormal presence of saccades during smooth pursuit due to failure of the eyes to maintain fixation on the moving target, requiring saccadic movements to refixate; consistent with cortical, brainstem, or cerebellar disorder

saccadic slowing   abnormally slow velocity during saccadic eye movement, consistent with internuclear ophthalmoplegia

saccular macula   sensory epithelium of the saccule that is responsive to linear acceleration

saccular nerve   nerve fiber bundle from the hair cells of the macula of the saccule that joins with similar bundles from the semicircular canals and the utricle to form the vestibular branch of Cranial Nerve VIII

saccular sensory epithelium   macula, consisting of Type I and Type II hair cells embedded in a gelatinous otolithic membrane

sacculotomy   surgical procedure used to fistulize the membranous labyrinth by introducing a needle through the stapes footplate to puncture the dilated saccule in Ménière's disease; SYN: cochleosacculotomy

sacculus   saccule

saddle nose and myopia   autosomal dominant disorder, characterized by severe myopia, cataracts, and a malformed nose, with congenital progressive sensorineural hearing loss; SYN: Marshall syndrome

sagittal plane   anatomical plane of reference, denoting a section dividing the head into left and right portions

SAL   sensorineural acuity level; method for quantifying the size of an air-bone gap by establishing air-conduction thresholds under earphones in quiet and in the presence of bone-conducted noise and comparing the shift in threshold to normative values

salicylic acid   a component of aspirin that causes temporary paralysis of cochlear outer hair cells by weakening their hydraulic system, resulting in a mild to moderate, reversible sensorineural hearing loss

salpingemphraxis   obstruction of the eustachian tube

salpingitis   inflammation of the eustachian tube

Sanfilippo syndrome   a type of mucopolysaccharidosis, characterized by severe mental retardation, minimal skeletal and visceral abnormalities, and hearing loss

sanguineous otitis media   inflammation of the middle ear, accompanied by bloody effusion

sarcoma   highly malignant connective tissue neoplasm

SAT   speech-awareness threshold; lowest level at which a speech signal is audible; SYN: speech-detection threshold

saturation   level in an amplifier circuit at which an increase in input signal no longer produces additional output

saturation response, real-ear   RESR; probe-microphone measurement of the SPL, as a function of frequency, at a specified point near the tympanic membrane with a hearing aid in place and turned on, with sufficient stimulus level to drive the hearing aid at its maximum output

saturation sound pressure level   maximum output generated by the receiver of a hearing aid, expressed as the root mean square sound pressure level

saturation sound pressure level 90   SSPL90; electroacoustic assessment of a hearing aid's maximum output, expressed as a frequency response curve to a 90-dB input with the hearing aid gain control set to full on; SYN: maximum power output

saw-tooth noise noise, composed of a fundamental frequency of 60 Hz and its harmonics together in random phase, that has a saw-tooth waveform and a buzz-saw quality

SBMPL simultaneous binaural median plane localization; early test of lateralization in which the intensity level of identical tones delivered simultaneously to the two ears was adjusted until a fused tone at the midline of the head was perceived

scala one of the three cavities of the cochlea spiraling around the modiolus

scala communis cochleae inner ear anomaly, characterized by a fissure in the bony partition separating the middle and apical turns of the cochlea, common in Mondini dysplasia

scala media middle of three channels of the cochlear duct, bordered by the basilar membrane, Reissner's membrane, and the spiral ligament, that is filled with endolymph and contains the organ of Corti; SYN: endolymphatic space

scala tympani lowermost of two perilymph-filled channels of the cochlear duct, separated by the scala media, terminating apically at the helicotrema and basally at the round window

scala vestibuli uppermost of two perilymph-filled channels of the cochlear duct, separated by the scala media, terminating apically at the helicotrema and basally in the vestibule at the oval window

scale, A-weighted sound level meter filtering network weighted to approximate an equal loudness contour at 40 phons; decibel level measured with this scale is usually designated dBA or dB(A)

scale, B-weighted sound level meter filtering network weighted to approximate an equal loudness contour at 70 phons; frequencies below 300 Hz are reduced by approximately 4 dB per octave

scale, C-weighted sound level meter filtering network designed to provide a uniform frequency response over the frequency range from 20 Hz to 10,000 Hz

scale, linear measurement scale in which each increment is equal to the next

scale, logarithmic measurement scale, such as the decibel scale, that is based on exponents of a base number

scalp electrode noninvasive surface electrode attached to the scalp by conductive paste or gel

SCAN test screening test of auditory processing abilities in children, including filtered-speech recognition, auditory figure-ground, auditory fusion, and competing-message subtests

scaphoid fossa normal boat-shaped depression of the auricle between the helix and antihelix

Scarpa's ganglia two adjacent cell-body masses of the peripheral vestibular neurons, located in the internal auditory canal, associated with the superior and inferior divisions of the vestibular nerve portion of Cranial Nerve VIII; SYN: vestibular ganglia

Scarpa's membrane round window

Scheibe dysplasia developmental abnormality of the phylogenetically newer parts of the inner ear, specifically the cochlea and saccule, and sparing of the utricle and semicircular canals, with associated sensorineural hearing loss

Schwabach test bone-conduction tuning-fork test in which the patient's ability to hear the vibrating fork applied to the mastoid is compared to the examiner's

Schwann cells cells that produce and maintain the myelin sheath of the axons of most cranial nerves

Schwannoma benign encapsulated neoplasm composed of Schwann cells

Schwannoma, cochleovestibular benign encapsulated neoplasm composed of Schwann cells arising from the intracranial segment, commonly the vestibular portion, of Cranial Nerve VIII; SYN: acoustic neuroma; acoustic neurilemoma

Schwartze sign reddish glow visualized through the tympanic membrane upon otoscopic examination, produced by increased vascularity of the promontory in some cases of otosclerosis

sclerectomy excision of fibrous adhesions formed in chronic otitis media

sclerosis a hardening of tissue, especially from inflammation

sclerosis, multiple MS; demyelinating disease in which plaques form throughout the white matter of the brainstem, resulting in diffuse neurologic symptoms, including hearing loss, speech-understanding deficits, and abnormalities of the acoustic reflexes and ABR

sclerosteosis subgroup of congenital disorders involving skeletal sclerosis, the autosomal dominant or malignant form of which often results in otic dysplasia and associated hearing loss

screening the application of rapid and simple tests, to a large population consisting of individuals who are undiagnosed and typically asymptomatic, to identify those who require additional diagnostic procedures

screening, immittance rapid assessment of middle ear function by tympanometry

screening audiometry rapid assessment of the ability of individuals to hear acoustic signals across a frequency range at a fixed criterion intensity level; designed to identify those who require additional audiometric procedures; SYN: identification audiometry

Screening Instrument For Targeting Educational Risk SIFTER; formalized teacher checklist designed to assess communication performance in the classroom of a child with hearing impairment

scroll ear auricular deformity in which the rim is rolled forward and inward

SD speech discrimination; old term for word recognition

SDS speech-discrimination score; old term for word-recognition score, expressed as the percentage of words presented in a list that are correctly identified

SDT speech-detection threshold; lowest level at which a speech signal is just audible; SYN: speech-awareness threshold

seal, hermetic airtight seal

second-order neuron nerve fiber carrying information beyond the point of the first synapse from a specialized nerve ending; in the auditory system, all second-order neurons emanate from the cochlear nucleus and terminate throughout the auditory nervous system

secondary acquired syphilis secondary stage of a syphilis infection, which can result in membranous labyrinthitis associated with acute meningitis

secondary neoplasm metastasis, or abnormal tissue growth in a part of the body remote from the original primary tumor

secondary phase nystagmus caloric nystagmus that reverses its direction prior to 140 seconds following onset of irrigation, consistent with central vestibular pathology; SYN: premature caloric reversal

secondary tympanic membrane round window membrane

secretion any substance produced by cellular or glandular activity

secretory pertaining to secretion

secretory otitis media otitis media with effusion, usually referring to serous or mucoid effusion

sedation, conscious sedated state wherein the patient retains protective reflexes and breathes independently, commonly attained with chloral hydrate

sedation, deep level of sedation in which patients are not easily aroused and may be unable to breathe independently

SEE1 Seeing Essential English

SEE2 Signing Exact English

Seeing Essential English contrived manual communication dialect based on American Sign Language that has been modified so that its syntax more closely resembles that of English

seizure sudden onset of a disease or symptoms, often referring to epilepsy

seizure, audiogenic seizure that is caused by sound

Select-a-vents proprietary name for inserts that can be used to modify the diameter of earmold vents

selective amplification hearing aid response with gain limited over a restricted frequency range, selected to match the audiometric configuration

selective listening focused attention on a particular sound source

Self Assessment of Communication SAC; a self-assessment questionnaire designed to assess perceived communication ability of adults with hearing impairment

Self Help for Hard of Hearing People SHHH; organization for persons with hearing impairment

semantic pertaining to meaning, or the relationship between symbols and their referents in language

semicanal of the tensor tympani canal in the temporal bone that opens into the carotid wall of the middle ear through which the tensor tympani muscle courses

semicircular canal, horizontal one of three bony canals of the vestibular apparatus containing sensory epithelia that respond to angular motion; SYN: lateral semicircular canal

semicircular canal, lateral horizontal semicircular canal

semicircular canal, posterior one of

three bony canals of the vestibular apparatus containing sensory epithelia that respond to angular motion

semicircular canal, superior one of three bony canals of the vestibular apparatus containing sensory epithelia that respond to angular motion

semicircular canals three canals in the osseous labyrinth of the vestibular apparatus containing sensory epithelia that respond to angular motion; the superior canal is oriented at a right angle to the posterior canal, and both are perpendicular to the lateral canal

semicircular duct, horizontal one of three membranous canals of the vestibular apparatus containing sensory epithelia that respond to angular motion; SYN: lateral semicircular duct

semicircular duct, lateral horizontal semicircular duct

semicircular duct, posterior one of three membranous canals of the vestibular apparatus containing sensory epithelia that respond to angular motion

semicircular duct, superior one of three membranous canals of the vestibular apparatus containing sensory epithelia that respond to angular motion

semicircular ducts three membranous canals of the vestibular apparatus, located within the superior, posterior, and lateral semicircular canals, containing the sensory epithelia, or cristae ampullares, that respond to angular motion

senescence the process of growing old

senescent pertaining to aging, growing old

senile pertaining to the characteristics of old age

senile dementia primary degenerative dementia occurring in old age, characterized by progressive cognitive deterioration, loss of memory, and emotional lability

senility sum of the cognitive and physiological expression of old age

sensation change in the state of awareness resulting from stimulation of an afferent nerve

sensation level SL; the intensity level of a sound in dB above an individual's threshold; usually used to refer to the intensity level of a signal presentation or a response above a specified threshold, such as pure-tone threshold or acoustic reflex threshold

sensation level, desired DSL; number of

dB above behavioral threshold required to amplify the long-term speech spectrum to a prescribed level across the frequency range

sensitive keenly susceptible to stimuli

sensitivity 1. capacity of a sense organ to detect a stimulus; 2. the ability of a test to detect the disorder that it was designed to detect, expressed as the percentage of positive results in patients with the disorder; COM: specificity

sensitivity, absolute the capacity of the auditory system to detect faint sound; SYN: auditory threshold

sensitivity, differential the capacity of the auditory system to detect differences between auditory signals that differ in intensity, frequency, time; SYN: auditory acuity

sensitivity, hearing capacity of the auditory system to detect a stimulus, most often described by audiometric pure-tone thresholds

sensitivity prediction from the acoustic reflex SPAR; test designed to predict the presence or absence of cochlear hearing loss by determining the difference between acoustic reflex thresholds elicited by pure tones and by broad-band noise, a difference that is smaller in ears with hearing loss

sensitivity threshold lowest level at which a signal is detectable

sensitization enhancement in sensitivity to one sound caused by the occurrence of a preceding sound

sensitized speech measures speech audiometric measures in which speech targets are altered in various ways to reduce their informational content in an effort to more effectively challenge the auditory system, including low-pass filtering and time compression

sensorimotor both sensory and motor

sensorineural pertaining to the sensory end organs and their nerve fibers

sensorineural acuity level test SAL test; method for quantifying the size of an air-bone gap by establishing air-conduction thresholds under earphones in quiet and in the presence of bone-conducted noise and comparing the shift in threshold to normative values

sensorineural hearing loss SNHL; cochlear or retrocochlear loss in hearing sensitivity due to disorders involving the cochlea and/or the auditory nerves fibers of Cranial Nerve VIII; COM: conductive hearing loss

sensory cells in the auditory system, hair cells in the cochlea

sensory epithelia in the ear, groups of sensory and supporting cells of the organ of Corti in the cochlea, the cristae ampullares in the semicircular canals, and the maculae in the utricle and saccule

sensory epithelium, saccular macula, consisting of Type I and Type II hair cells embedded in a gelatinous otolithic membrane

sensory epithelium, utricular macula, consisting of Type I and Type II hair cells embedded in a gelatinous otolithic membrane

sensory impairment abnormal functioning of one of the senses

sensory nerve afferent nerve carrying information from a sense organ to the central nervous system

sensory-neural sensorineural

sensory organization test SOT; component of computerized dynamic posturography designed to assess equilibrium with six different combinations of sensory input

sensory presbyacusis age-related hearing loss caused by hair cell loss at the basal end of the cochlea

sensory radicular neuropathy autosomal dominant nervous system disorder, characterized by young-adult-onset lightning pains in the distal extremities and painless ulcerations of the feet, with progressive sensorineural hearing loss

sensory receptors in the ear, the sensory epithelia, including the inner hair cells, the cristae ampullares, and the utricular and sacular maculae

sentential approximations contrived nonsense sentences, such as those used in the SSI test, designed to be syntactically appropriate but meaningless

SEP somatosensory evoked potential; evoked electrical activity of the brain created by stimulation of the somatosensory system, usually by electrical stimulation over a peripheral nerve or the spinal cord

sepsis presence of bacteria or other pathogens in blood or tissue

sequela; pl. sequelae a condition or disease following or occurring as a consequence of another condition or disease

sequencing, auditory perceptual process by which sounds and words are properly ordered

serial audiogram one of a series of audiograms obtained at regular intervals, usually on an annual basis as part of a hearing conservation program

seroma mass caused by a collection of serosanguineous fluid within tissue that can occur on the auricle following trauma

seromucinous otitis media inflammation of the middle ear with an accumulation of fluid of varying viscosity in the middle ear cavity and other pneumatized spaces of the temporal bone; SYN: otitis media with effusion

serosanguineous containing serum and blood

serous pertaining to serum

serous effusion thin, watery, sterile fluid secreted by a mucous membrane

serous labyrinthitis inflammation of the labyrinth caused by otogenic or meningogenic bacterial toxins or contamination during surgery; SYN: toxic labyrinthitis

serous otitis media SOM; inflammation of middle ear mucosa, with serous effusion

serum clear, thin fluid that moistens the surface of serous membranes

severe hearing loss loss of hearing sensitivity of 70 dB HL to 90 dB HL

sex-linked inheritance inheritance in which the disordered gene is on the X chromosome; SYN: X-linked inheritance

shadow audiogram an audiogram reflecting cross hearing from an unmasked nontest ear with normal or nearly normal hearing, obtained while testing an ear with a severe or profound hearing loss; indicative of the organicity of the loss in the test ear

shadow curve shadow audiogram

sheath tubular envelope of connective tissue covering nerves

sheath, myelin cover of myelin over nerve fibers

sheath of Schwann Schwann cells that envelop peripheral nerves, including Cranial Nerve VIII

shell earmold debulked, but otherwise full-sized earmold used for high-gain hearing aids when an acoustic seal is essential

short crus of the incus short leg of the incus that fits into the fossa incudis and serves as a pivotal point for the rocking motion of the ossicular chain

short-increment sensitivity index SISI; early test used in differential diagnosis based on differential sensitivity to 1-dB increments superimposed on a pure tone; the ability to perceive the increments is related to a cochlear site of disorder

short-term memory that aspect of the information-processing function of the central nervous system that receives, modifies, and stores information briefly

Shrapnell membrane pars flaccida portion of the tympanic membrane

Shrapnell membrane perforation attic perforation of the pars flaccida

shunt 1. to divert fluid; 2. fistulation or mechanical device used to divert fluid to prevent accumulation

shunt, endolymphatic surgical technique designed to create a hole in the membranous labyrinth in order to relieve endolymphatic hydrops

sibilant speech sound characterized by a hissing sound, such as [s] and [z]

Sickness Impact Profile SIP; standardized questionnaire designed to assess the physical and psychosocial impact of impairment on an individual

side band a group of frequencies on either side of a carrier frequency

SIFTER Screening Instrument For Targeting Educational Risk; formalized teacher checklist designed to assess communication performance in the classroom of a child with hearing impairment

sigmoid sinus portion of the lateral venous sinus, bulging prominently into the mastoid cavity, that serves as a principal conduit by which blood leaves the cranium

sign 1. any observable or measurable symptom of a disease; COM: symptom; 2. hand form and motion used in manual communication to symbolize a word or concept

sign language form of manual communication in which words and concepts are represented by hand positions and movements

signal a sound that conveys information or initiates action

signal averaging in auditory evoked potential measurement, the averaging of successive samples of EEG activity time-locked to an acoustic stimulus, designed to enhance the response (signal) evoked by the stimulus by reducing the unrelated EEG noise

signal-detection theory psychophysical model suggesting that detection of a signal involves establishing a decision criterion, the nature of which varies as a function of the probability of a signal being present and the costs and values related to being right or wrong

signal generator instrument that produces an electronic signal of known amplitude, frequency, and waveform

signal processing manipulation of specified characteristics of a signal

signal processing, automatic ASP; process in which hearing aid circuitry adjusts some parameter of the amplified output automatically or adaptively as the input signal reaches a certain criterion

signal-to-noise ratio S/N; relative difference in dB between a sound of interest and a background of noise

Signing Exact English SEE2; manual communication dialect based on a simplification of Seeing Essential English

SII speech intelligibility index; ANSI standard identifier of the articulation or audibility index; a measure of the proportion of speech cues that are audible

SIL speech-interference level; masking or interference effect of noise on the intelligibility of speech communication, originally expressed as the articulation index and later as sound pressure levels in various octave bands

silica gel moisture-absorbing agent often used in the storage of hearing aids

simple harmonic motion continuous, symmetric, periodic back and forth movement of an object that has been set into motion

simple mastoidectomy excision of the bony partitions forming the mastoid air cells to establish drainage for acute infections of the middle ear and mastoid that are unresponsive to drug therapy; COM: radical mastoidectomy

simplex procedure adaptive psychophysical procedure designed to compare electroacoustic characteristics of a hearing aid along a continuum on more than one dimension of the circuitry

simulator, audiometric computer-based instrument designed to simulate responses of patients with various audiometric configurations for training in audiometric skills

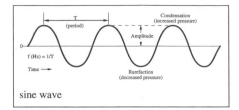

sine wave

simultaneous binaural bithermal calorics test modification of the open-loop calorics test of vestibular function in which both ears are irrigated simultaneously with cool water and then irrigated simultaneously with warm water

simultaneous binaural median plane localization SBMPL; early test of lateralization in which the intensity level of identical tones delivered simultaneously to the two ears was adjusted until a fused tone at the midline of the head was perceived

simultaneous method early term describing the communication habilitation method now referred to as total communication

sine trigonometric function, the shape of which is that of simple harmonic motion over time

sine wave graphic representation of simple harmonic motion as a function of time that is described by the trigonometric sine function

single-channel processing hearing aid signal processing in one frequency band only, typically the entire frequency band

single-gene disorder developmental defect resulting from the action of a single gene; may be either autosomal or X-linked and either dominant or recessive

sinistral pertaining to the left side

sintered filter small container of partially fused metal particles that can be controlled to provide attenuation of specific frequency ranges

sinus 1. a cavity or hollow in bone or other tissue; 2. a channel for the passage of blood or lymph

sinus, lateral largest of the venous sinuses, responsible for collecting blood from most of the head and neck

sinus, sigmoid portion of the lateral venous sinus, bulging prominently into the mastoid cavity, that serves as a principal conduit by which blood leaves the cranium

sinuses, venous collecting veins from the brain, temporal bone, and orbit located in the dura mater

sinusoid sine wave

sinusoidal pertaining to a sinusoid

sinusoidal wave sine wave

SIP Sickness Impact Profile; standardized questionnaire designed to assess the physical and psychosocial impact of impairment on an individual

SISI short increment sensitivity index; early test used in differential diagnosis based on differential sensitivity to 1-dB increments superimposed on a pure tone; the ability to perceive the increments is related to a cochlear site of disorder

SISI, high-level early diagnostic test for retrocochlear disorder; modification of the SISI procedure administered at a high-intensity level at which those with normal hearing or cochlear hearing loss should perceive the small increments in intensity

SISI, modified high-level SISI

sisomicin an antibiotic with a spectrum and application similar to gentamicin; potentially ototoxic in large doses

situ, in in position; e.g., in the case of hearing aids, on the patient in position for use

6-cc coupler metal cylinder with a 6-cc air space, designed to represent the average amount of air enclosed under an earphone placed on an ear; used in the output calibration of an audiometer with circumaural earphones

60-cycle noise unwanted electrical activity emanating from the 60-Hz electric energy commonly available to power lights, appliances, etc.

skeleton earmold earmold in which the bowl has been cut out, leaving an outer concha rim, but retaining the portion that seals the external auditory meatus

ski-slope hearing loss colloquial term referring to a hearing loss configuration characterized by normal hearing in the low frequencies and a precipitous loss in the high frequencies

skirt, filter rate of attenuation of a filter, expressed in dB per octave

SL sensation level; the intensity level of a sound in dB above an individual's threshold; usually used to refer to the intensity level of a signal presentation above a specified threshold, such as pure-tone threshold or acoustic reflex threshold

slit leak   leak of acoustic energy around the perimeter of an earmold or custom hearing aid

slow negative auditory evoked response SN10; averaged auditory electrical potential evoked by tone bursts, characterized as a broad vertex negative peak occurring around 10 msec following signal onset

slow phase   component of nystagmus that represents the smooth continuous eye movement required to maintain a visual target on the retinal fovea; ANT: fast phase

slow-phase velocity   SPV; commonly used measure of nystagmus strength, described as the size of the arc in degrees that the eyeball covers during the slow phase of nystagmus; SYN: vestibular eye speed

slow pursuit   eye movement used to track slowly and smoothly moving objects; SYN: smooth pursuit

slow-vertex response   auditory evoked potential, having two main waveform peaks—a vertex negative peak at approximately 90 msec following signal presentation and a vertex positive peak at approximately 180 msec following signal presentation; SYN: long-latency auditory evoked potential

SLP   speech-language pathologist; healthcare professional who is credentialed in the practice of speech-language pathology to provide a comprehensive array of services related to prevention, evaluation, and rehabilitation of speech and language disorders

smooth pursuit   eye movement used to track slowly and smoothly moving objects; SYN: slow pursuit

smoothing   the process of reducing irregularities in curves

SMSP   spectral maxima sound processor; cochlear implant signal-processing strategy in which the highest six amplitudes of 16 processed bands are delivered in a nonoverlapping sequence to electrode locations mapped to the identified channels

SN10   slow negative (auditory evoked response occurring at) 10 msec; averaged auditory electrical potential evoked by tone bursts, characterized as a broad vertex negative peak occurring around 10 msec following signal onset

SNHL   sensorineural hearing loss; cochlear or retrocochlear loss in hearing sensitivity due to disorders involving the cochlea and/or the auditory nerves fibers of Cranial Nerve VIII; COM: conductive hearing loss

SOAE   spontaneous otoacoustic emission; measurable low-level sound that is emitted by the cochlea in the absence of stimulation; related to the function of the outer hair cells; COM: evoked otoacoustic emissions

SOC   superior olivary complex; auditory nuclei in the hindbrain that relay information from the cochlear nucleus to the midbrain, including the lateral superior olive, medial superior olive, medial nucleus of the trapezoid body, and periolivary nuclei

social adequacy index   early measure designed to quantify hearing disability based on the relation of speech threshold and word-recognition ability

sociocusis   loss of hearing sensitivity due to the combined influences of aging, noise exposure, and environmental exposure

sodium   Na+; chemical found in high concentration in perilymph and low concentration in endolymph

soft peak clipping   peak clipping in hearing aid amplification that removes the extremes of alternating current amplitude peaks at some predetermined level in a gradual manner that reduces distortion; SYN: modified peak clipping

SOM   serous otitis media; inflammation of middle ear mucosa, with serous effusion

soma   neuronal cell body

somatosensory evoked potential   SEP; evoked electrical activity of the brain created by stimulation of the somatosensory system, usually by electrical stimulation over a peripheral nerve or the spinal cord

sone   unit of measure of the subjective loudness of a tone, referenced so that 1 sone is equal in loudness to a 1000-Hz pure tone at 40 dB SL and 2 sones is of a loudness of twice that magnitude

sonic   pertaining to sound

SOT   sensory organization test; component of computerized dynamic posturography designed to assess equilibrium with six different combinations of sensory input

sound   vibratory energy transmitted by pressure waves in air or other media that is the objective cause of the sensation of hearing

sound absorption   attenuation of sound energy by materials that prevent reflection

sound bore   hole in an earmold through which amplified sound is directed into the ear canal; SYN: earmold bore

sound field   circumscribed area or room

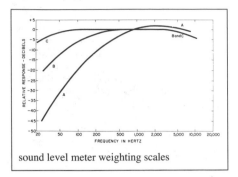

sound level meter weighting scales

into which sound is introduced via loudspeaker

sound field amplification   amplification of a classroom or other open area with a public address system or other small-room system to enhance the signal-to-noise ratio for all listeners

sound field testing   in pediatric audiometry or hearing aid fitting, the determination of hearing sensitivity or speech-recognition ability made with signals presented in a sound field through loudspeakers

sound intensity   1. sound power transmitted through a given area, expressed in watts/m2; 2. generic term for any quantity relating to the amount or magnitude of sound

sound level, equivalent   Leq; measurement of a time-varying sound, expressed as a time-weighted energy average, representing the total sound energy over a given time period as if the sound were unvarying; SYN: equivalent level

sound level meter   an electronic instrument designed to measure sound intensity in dB in accordance with an accepted standard

sound pressure level   SPL; magnitude or quantity of sound energy relative to a reference pressure, 0.0002 dynes/cm^2 or 20 μPa

sound pressure level, effective   intensity level of sufficient magnitude to produce a specified response

sound pressure level, overall   total sound energy throughout the frequency range, measured without any frequency weighting

sound pressure level, peak equivalent   pe SPL: decibel level of a 1000-Hz tone at an amplitude equivalent to the peak of a transient signal; used to express the intensity level of click stimuli used in auditory evoked potential testing

sound pressure level, reference equivalent threshold   RETSPL; ANSI standard specification of the sound pressure levels that correspond to audiometric zero for a specific earphone

sound pressure level, saturation   maximum output generated by the receiver of a hearing aid, expressed as the root mean square sound pressure level

sound-proof   impenetrable by sound energy

sound quality   perception or psychological impression of the spectrum of a sound

sound spectrum   entire extent of a specified sound, expressed as the magnitude of its frequency components

sound wave   energy generated by a vibrating body that transmits a series of alternating compressions and rarefactions of an elastic medium

sound wave, aperiodic   waveform that does not regularly repeat itself in a given period of time and that is not restricted to components at multiples of the fundamental frequency

sound wave, periodic   sound wave in which the pattern of vibration, however complex, repeats itself regularly as a function of time

SP   summating potential; a direct-current electrical potential of cochlear origin that follows the envelope of acoustic stimulation and is measured with electrocochleography

space of Nuel   space between the outer pillars and the first row of outer hair cells in the organ of Corti

space-occupying lesion   neoplasm that exerts its influence by growing and impinging on neural tissues, as opposed to a lesion caused by trauma, ischemia, or inflammation

SPAR   sensitivity prediction from the acoustic reflex; test designed to predict the presence or absence of cochlear hearing loss by determining the difference between acoustic reflex thresholds elicited by pure tones and by broad-band noise

specificity   the ability of a test to differen-

$$dB\ SPL = 20\ \log\ \frac{pressure}{pressure_r}$$

sound pressure level

tiate a normal condition from the disorder that the test was designed to detect, expressed as the percentage of negative results in patients without the disorder; COM: sensitivity

spectral contrast difference between the peaks and troughs of the formants of a speech signal, expressed in dB

spectral maxima sound processing SMSP; cochlear implant signal-processing strategy in which the highest six amplitudes of 16 processed bands are delivered in a nonoverlapping sequence to electrode locations mapped to the identified channels

spectral peaks narrow ranges of high energy in the amplitude spectrum of a sound

spectrogram short-term spectra, usually of a speech signal, displayed as a function of time

spectrograph electronic instrument that generates a three-dimensional graph of speech, plotting frequency on the ordinate, time on the abscissa, and intensity by the density of the tracing

spectrum; pl. spectra distribution of magnitudes of the frequency components of a sound

spectrum, amplified speech electroacoustic output of a hearing aid in response to speech-weighted noise or other signals representative of the speech spectrum

spectrum, band graphic representation of sound, displayed as sound pressure levels of specified frequency bands

spectrum, line graphic representation of the frequency content of a signal in which vertical lines are plotted for frequency bands as a function of magnitude of energy in each band

spectrum, long-term speech LTSS; overall level and frequency composition of speech energy that represents everyday speech

spectrum, noise spectral content of a noise

spectrum, sound entire extent of a specified sound, expressed as the magnitude of its frequency components

spectrum analyzer a sound level meter with bandpass filters used to determine the level of each frequency band of a complex sound

speculum instrument for enlarging the orifice of any cavity or canal to examine its interior

speculum, aural funnel-shaped instrument for enlarging the opening of the external auditory meatus to facilitate inspection of the ear canal and tympanic membrane

speech act of respiration, phonation, articulation, and resonation that serves as a medium for oral communication

speech, accelerated recorded speech signals that have been temporally altered to increase the speed of playback

speech, cold-running connected or continuous discourse

speech, interrupted speech signals that have been altered by rapid periodic interruption

speech, time-compressed speech signals that have been accelerated by the process of time compression

speech and hearing sciences study of the processes and disorders related to the production and reception of speech and language

speech audiometer early term for an audiometer that had the capacity to deliver speech, via microphone, tape recorder, or turntable, with a controlled output level

speech audiometry measurement of the hearing of speech signals; includes measurement of speech awareness, speech reception, word and sentence recognition, sensitized speech processing, and dichotic listening

speech-awareness threshold SAT; lowest level at which a speech signal is audible; SYN: speech-detection threshold

speech conservation treatment designed to maintain speech-production ability following acquired hearing loss

speech detection perception of the presence of a speech signal

speech-detection threshold SDT; lowest level at which a speech signal is audible; SYN: speech-awareness threshold

speech discrimination SD; old term for word recognition

speech-discrimination score SDS; old term for word-recognition score, expressed as the percentage of words presented in a list that are correctly identified

speech frequencies audiometric frequencies at which a substantial amount of speech energy occurs, conventionally considered to be 500 Hz, 1000 Hz, and 2000 Hz

speech intelligibility speech-recognition ability

speech intelligibility in noise test SPIN test; measure of word-recognition ability in noise in which target words occur at the end of sentences with both low and high semantic predictability based on the content of the sentence

speech-intelligibility index SII; ANSI standard identifier of the articulation or audibility index; a measure of the proportion of speech cues that are audible

speech-interference level SIL; masking or interference effect of noise on the intelligibility of speech communication, originally expressed as the articulation index and later as sound pressure levels in various octave bands

speech-language pathologist SLP; healthcare professional who is credentialed in the practice of speech-language pathology to provide a comprehensive array of services related to prevention, evaluation, and rehabilitation of speech and language disorders

speech-language pathology branch of health care devoted to the study, diagnosis, and treatment of speech and language disorders

speech noise broad-band noise that is filtered to resemble the speech spectrum

speech perception awareness, recognition, and interpretation of speech signals received in the brain

speech perception, rapidly alternating RASP; test of sentence recognition in which the signal is alternated between ears at rates ranging from 200 msec to 400 msec, designed to assess auditory brainstem integrity

speech processor in a cochlear implant system, the component responsible for transforming acoustic speech signals into electrical impulses to be delivered to the implanted electrode

speech-reception threshold SRT; threshold level for speech recognition, expressed as the lowest intensity level at which 50% of spondaic words can be identified

speech recognition the ability to perceive and identify speech targets; SYN: speech intelligibility, speech discrimination

speech sound discrimination the ability to differentiate among speech sounds

speech spectrum, long-term LTSS; overall level and frequency composition of speech energy that represents everyday speech

speech Stenger modification of the Stenger test in which spondaic words are used in place of pure tones; SYN: modified Stenger test

speech target in speech audiometry, the speech signal of interest

speech threshold ST; generic term describing speech-reception threshold, as opposed to awareness or detection threshold

speech-transmission index, rapid RASTI; assessment of the integrity of signal transmission in a room, expressed as the reduction in signal modulation of amplitude-modulated broad-band noise centered at 500 Hz and 2000 Hz

speech-weighted composite signal complex sound that has a crest factor similar to that of speech

speech with alternating masking index SWAMI; early speech-recognition measure in which two signals—a target signal and noise of 20 dB greater intensity—were alternated rapidly between ears to assess dichotic integration at the level of the brainstem

speechreading the process of visual recognition of speech communication, combining lipreading with observation of facial expressions and gestures

spike in neurophysiology, a single nerve impulse or action potential

spillover the migration of electrical signals, usually from an FM transmitter, from one room to an adjoining room

SPIN test speech perception in noise test; measure of word-recognition ability in noise in which target words occur at the end of sentences with both low and high semantic predictability based on the content of the sentence

spiral bundles bundles of efferent nerve fibers from the uncrossed olivocochlear system that course immediately beneath the inner hair cells and synapse onto their afferent terminal endings

spiral ganglia cell bodies of the auditory nerve fibers, clustered in the modiolus; SYN: auditory ganglia

spiral lamina shelf of bone arising from the modiolar side of the cochlea, consisting of two thin plates of bones between which course the nerve fibers from the auditory nerve to and from the hair cells

spiral ligament band of connective tissue that affixes the basilar membrane to the outer bony wall, against which lies the stria vascularis within the scala media

spiral limbus   mound of connective tissue in the scala media, resting on the osseous spiral lamina, to which the medial end of the tectorial membrane is attached

spiral organ   hearing organ, composed of sensory and supporting cells, located on the basilar membrane in the cochlear duct; SYN: organ of Corti

spiral plate   spiral lamina

spiral prominence   shelflike bulge of the spiral ligament near the basilar membrane; SYN: basilar crest

spiral stria   stria vascularis

spiral sulcus   a furrow within the organ of Corti, formed by the concave surface of the spiral limbus, the tectorial membrane, and the medial surface of the inner hair cells; SYN: inner sulcus, inner spiral tunnel

spiral tunnel   spiral sulcus

SPL   sound pressure level; magnitude or quantity of sound energy relative to a reference pressure, 0.0002 dynes/cm^2 or 20 μPa

split-band amplification   seldom-used hearing aid fitting strategy in which a high-frequency response is fitted to the right ear and flat-frequency response to the left ear, in an effort to exploit the right-ear advantage for processing speech; SYN: dichotic amplification

spondaic   pertaining to spondees

spondaic threshold   speech-reception threshold

spondee   a two-syllable word spoken with equal emphasis on each syllable

spondee threshold   ST; speech-reception threshold

spontaneous nystagmus   ocular nystagmus that occurs in the absence of stimulation; ANT: induced nystagmus

spontaneous otoacoustic emission   SOAE; measurable low-level sound that is emitted by the cochlea in the absence of stimulation; related to the function of the outer hair cells; COM: evoked otoacoustic emissions

spread of masking   masking of a sound of one frequency by sound of another frequency, including upward spread of masking and downward or remote masking

spread of masking, downward   the masking of a low-frequency sound by an in-

tense level of high-frequency sound; SYN: remote masking

spread of masking, upward   the masking of high-frequency sound by low frequency sound, e.g., weaker high-frequency consonant sounds being masked by stronger low-frequency vowel sounds

SPV   slow phase velocity; commonly used measure of nystagmus strength, described as the size of the arc in degrees that the eyeball covers during the slow phase of nystagmus; SYN: vestibular eye speed

squamous   platelike or scaly

squamous cell carcinoma   most common malignant tumor of the auricle, characterized by a progression of skin thickening with scaling, painless out-growth, and formation of an ulcer with a raised edge

squamous portion of the temporal bone   thin, platelike section of the temporal bone, appearing as a fanlike projection superior and anterior to the external auditory meatus

square wave   periodic waveform consisting of a voltage that is constant in amplitude and that reverses polarity at regular intervals

squeal, hearing aid   shrill, high-pitched sound emitted from a hearing aid, resulting from acoustic feedback

squelch, binaural   improvement in speech intelligibility in noise of two ears over one because of interaural phase and intensity differences

SRT   speech-reception threshold; threshold level for speech recognition, expressed as lowest intensity level at which 50% of spondaic words can be identified

SSEP   steady-state evoked potential; auditory evoked potential in which the response waveform approximates the pattern of periodic stimulation, such as the stimulus rate or rate of stimulus modulation, e.g., 40-Hz response

SSI   synthetic sentence identification test; closed-set speech-recognition test in which approximations of sentences are presented in a background of single-talker competition in order to assess central auditory processing ability

SSI-CCM   SSI test in which the sentences are presented with a contralateral competing message (CCM) at various message-to-competition ratios

SSI-ICM   SSI test in which the sentences

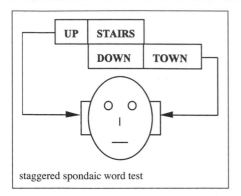

staggered spondaic word test

are presented with an ipsilateral competing message (ICM) at a message-to-competition ratio of 0 dB

SSPL90 saturation sound pressure level 90; electroacoustic assessment of a hearing aid's maximum output, expressed as a frequency response curve to a 90-dB input with the hearing aid gain control set to full on; SYN: maximum power output

SSPL90, HFA high-frequency average saturation sound pressure level; an ANSI hearing aid specification, derived by calculating the HFA output to a 90-dB-SPL input with the hearing aid adjusted to its full-on gain setting

SSW staggered spondaic word test; test of dichotic listening in which two spondaic words are presented so that the second syllable delivered to one ear is heard simultaneously with the first syllable delivered to the other ear.

ST 1. speech threshold; 2. spondee threshold

staggered spondaic word test SSW test; test of dichotic listening in which two spondaic words are presented so that the second syllable delivered to one ear is heard simultaneously with the first syllable delivered to the other ear.

standard deviation statistical measure of dispersion, expressed as the square root of the mean of the squares of the deviations from the mean of a distribution

standard earmold conventional type of earmold with a bowl completely filling the concha

standard threshold shift STS; change in hearing threshold in comparison to a baseline audiogram, defined as an average

change of 10 dB or more at 2000 Hz, 3000 Hz, and 4000 Hz in either ear

standing wave periodic waveform produced in a closed sound field resulting from the interference of progressive waves of the same frequency and kind that add and subtract, resulting in different amplitudes at various points in the room

stapedectomy surgical removal of the stapes footplate in whole or part, with prosthetic replacement, as treatment for stapes fixation

stapedial motoneurons single-celled column of neurons, responsible for stapedius muscle contraction, located medially to the motor nucleus of Cranial Nerve VII and extended anteriorly to the area between the superior olivary complex and the motor nucleus

stapedial reflex reflexive contraction of the stapedius muscle in response to loud sound; SYN: acoustic reflex

stapedial reflex decay decline in acoustic reflex amplitude over time in response to continuous stimulus presentation

stapediotenotomy surgical division of the tendon of the stapedius muscle.

stapedius muscle along with the tensor tympani, one of two striated muscles of the middle ear, classified as a pennate muscle, consisting of short fibers directed obliquely onto the stapedius tendon at the midline, innervated by the facial nerve

stapedius muscle reflex stapedial reflex

stapedius tendon round tendon projecting from the stapedius muscle through a small opening in the apex of the pyramidal eminence and attaching to the head of the stapes

stapedotomy surgical procedure used to correct stapes fixation in which the stapes crura are removed, a small fenestra is made in the stapes footplate, and a piston prosthesis is inserted in the fenestra and anchored to the incus

stapes smallest and medialmost bone of the ossicular chain, the head of which articulates to the lenticular process of the incus and the footplate of which fits into the oval window of the cochlea; COL: stirrup

stapes crura two struts that connect the head and neck of the stapes to the footplate

stapes fixation immobilization of the stapes at the oval window, often due to new bony growth resulting from otosclerosis

stapes mobilization surgical procedure

used to restore movement to a fixated stapes footplate

startle reflex normal reflexive extension and abduction of the limb and neck muscles in an infant when surprised by a sudden sound; SYN: Moro reflex

stat statim; at once; immediately

STAT suprathreshold adaptation test; procedure to measure auditory adaptation in which the signal is presented at a high-intensity level, and the patient responds to its presence for as long as it is audible

static at rest or in equilibrium

static acoustic compliance static acoustic immittance

static acoustic immittance measure of the contribution of the middle ear to acoustic impedance, calculated by subtracting the immittance measure of the external meatus, estimated by adding air pressure to decouple the middle ear, from the total immittance at its peak level

static acoustic impedance static acoustic immittance

static compliance static acoustic immittance

static immittance static acoustic immittance

stationary noise noise with negligible fluctuation of level

statoacoustic pertaining to equilibrium and hearing

statoacoustic nerve auditory and vestibular branches combined to form Cranial Nerve VIII

statoconia minute particles in the gelatinous membrane of the sacular and utricular maculae; SYN: otoconia

steady-state evoked potential SSEP; auditory evoked potential in which the response waveform approximates the pattern of periodic stimulation, such as the stimulus rate or rate of stimulus modulation, e.g., 40-Hz response

Stenger principle principle stating that when two tones of the same frequency are introduced simultaneously into both ears, only the louder tone will be perceived

Stenger test test for unilateral functional hearing loss based on the Stenger principle in which signals are presented to the normal ear at suprathreshold levels and the poorer ear at a higher level; lack of a response indicates nonorganicity

Stenger test, modified Stenger test in which spondaic words are used in place of pure tones; SYN: speech Stenger

Stenger test, speech modification of the Stenger test in which spondaic words are used in place of pure tones; SYN: modified Stenger test

stenosis narrowing in the diameter of an opening or canal

stenotic ear canal narrowed or constricted external auditory meatus

step size magnitude of change between adjacent electroacoustic settings

stereo three-dimensional spatial quality

stereocilia stiffened, hairlike microvilli that project from the apical end of the inner and outer hair cells

stethoscope, hearing aid stethoscope designed to auscultate a hearing instrument for the purposes of diagnostic listening

Stickler syndrome craniofacial disorder characterized by a flat facial profile, cleft palate, ocular changes, and joint disease, with conductive or mixed hearing loss associated with eustachian tube dysfunction secondary to cleft palate

stiffness rigidity, expressed as the amount of force required to change the displacement of an elastic medium; COM: compliance

stimulation, bipolar 1. delivery of an electrical signal across two poles of an electrode array; 2. cochlear implant stimulation in which both the active and indifferent electrodes are intracochlear

stimulation, caloric introduction of warm or cool water or air into the external auditory meatus to stimulate the vestibular system

stimulation, monopolar 1. delivery of an electrical signal to one pole of an electrode array; 2. cochlear implant stimulation in which the active electrode is intracochlear and the indifferent electrode is extracochlear

stimulation, promontory delivery of electrical stimulation to the promontory via a transtympanic electrode to elicit an electrically evoked action potential

stimulation, rotary vestibular system stimulation created by rotating a chair sinusoidally about its vertical axis, first in one direction and then the other, with variable velocity

stimulus anything that can elicit or evoke a response in an excitable receptor

stirrup colloquial term for stapes

stock earmold noncustomized earmold used mostly for demonstration or temporary use while a custom earmold is being made

stop consonant speech sound whose production requires a complete blocking of the breath stream, such as [p], [b], [t], [d], [k], and [g]

stop plosive stop consonant in which the breath, after being impounded, is released with a somewhat audible explosive puff, generally occurring when stops represent the initial consonant in a word; SYN: plosive

streptococcus pneumoniae common bacteriologic finding in middle ear aspirates

streptomycin aminoglycoside antibiotic, used in treating tuberculosis and other bacterial disease, which is ototoxic, particularly to the hair cells of the vestibular system

stria a narrow stripe or bandlike structure; used to describe longitudinal collections of nerve fibers in the brain

stria, dorsal acoustic DAS; nerve fiber bundle that emanates from the dorsal cochlear nucleus and synapses in the contralateral lateral lemniscus and inferior colliculus, bypassing the superior olivary complex

stria, intermediate acoustic IAS; nerve bundle, the fibers of which emanate from the posterior ventral cochlear nucleus and synapse on the ipsilateral and contralateral periolivary nuclei and the contralateral lateral lemniscus

stria, ventral acoustic second-order fiber bundle leaving the AVCN and projecting ventrally and medially to distribute fibers to the ipsilateral LSO and MSO and continuing across midline to distribute fibers to the contralateral MSO and MNTB; SYN: trapezoid body

stria of Held bundle of nerve fibers emanating from the posterior ventral cochlear nucleus and synapsing on the ipsilateral and contralateral periolivary nuclei and the contralateral lateral lemniscus; SYN: intermediate acoustic stria

stria of Monakow bundle of nerve fibers emanating from the dorsal cochlear nucleus and synapsing in the contralateral lateral lemniscus and inferior colliculus, bypassing the superior olivary complex; SYN: dorsal acoustic stria

stria vascularis highly vascularized band of cells on the internal surface of the spiral ligament within the scala media extending from the spiral prominence to Reissner's membrane

striae, acoustic second-order fiber bundles that leave the cochlear nucleus toward higher brainstem levels, the ventral acoustic stria from the AVCN, intermediate a.s. from the PVCN, and dorsal a.s. from the DCN

strial presbyacusis age-related hearing loss due to patchy atrophy of the stria vascularis in the middle and apical turns of the cochlea

striated muscle typically voluntary skeletal muscle with fibers divided by transverse bands into striations

stroke sudden cerebral vascular accident due to thrombosis, hemorrhage, or embolism

STS standard threshold shift; change in hearing threshold in comparison to a baseline audiogram, defined as an average change of 10 dB or more at 2000 Hz, 3000 Hz, and 4000 Hz in either ear

stylomastoid artery branch of the posterior auricular artery that supplies the facial nerve, bone and mucosa of adjacent mastoid region and otic capsule, and the stapedius muscle

stylomastoid foramen opening in the temporal bone through which the facial nerve and stylomastoid artery pass

styrene industrial solvent, which can be ototoxic if inhaled in high concentrations over extended periods

subacute otitis media inflammation of the middle ear having a duration ranging in duration from 22 days to 8 weeks

subclinical infantile meningogenic labyrinthitis labyrinthitis secondary to subclinical bacterial or viral meningitis in a young infant, resulting in mild to profound loss of auditory and vestibular function

subcutaneous fibroproliferative external otitis chronic diffuse external otitis characterized by stenosis of the lumen of the external auditory meatus

subdural abscess collection of purulent fluid between the dura mater and brain that can occur secondary to chronic otitis media

subjective not physically measurable, but perceived only by the individual involved; COM: objective

subjective tinnitus perception by an individual of ringing or other noise in the ear or head that is not evident to the examiner

subjective vertigo   a sensation that one is spinning or whirling; COM: objective vertigo

subluxation   an incomplete dislocation

subsonic   pertaining to frequencies below the audible range; COM: ultrasonic

sudden hearing loss   acute rapid-onset loss of hearing that is often idiopathic, unilateral, and substantial and that may or may not spontaneously resolve

sulcus   furrow or groove, especially on the surface of the brain

sulcus, tympanic   groove in the osseous wall of the external auditory meatus into which the annulus of the tympanic membrane fits

summating potential   SP; a direct-current electrical potential of cochlear origin that follows the envelope of acoustic stimulation and is measured with electrocochleography

summation   the aggregation of neuronal function resulting from the addition of energy along some parameter, such as the additional duration in temporal summation or the additional ear in binaural summation

summation, binaural   cumulative effect of sound reaching both ears, resulting in enhancement in hearing with both ears over one ear, characterized by binaural improvement in hearing sensitivity of approximately 3 dB over monaural sensitivity

summation, loudness   the addition of loudness by the expansion of bandwidth even when overall sound pressure level remains the same

summation, temporal   the aggregation of neuronal function resulting from additional duration of sound energy so that thresholds improve as durations increase up to about 200 msec

superficial   anatomical direction, referring to structures that are located away from the center of the body; ANT: deep

superior   anatomical direction, referring to structures that are located toward the top or upper surface; ANT: inferior

superior ampulla   bulging portion of the superior semicircular canal that contains the crista ampullaris

superior ampullary nerve   nerve fiber bundle from the hair cells of the crista ampullaris of the superior semicircular canal that joins with similar bundles from the other semicircular canals, the utricle, and

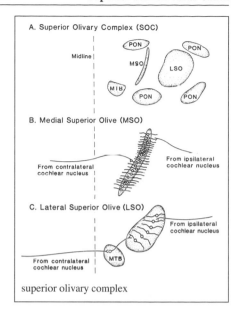

superior olivary complex

the saccule to form the vestibular branch of Cranial Nerve VIII

superior auricular muscle   one of four muscles attaching to the medial surface of the auricle

superior malleolar ligament   one of several ligaments responsible for maintaining the position of the ossicles, extending from the head of the malleus to tegmen tympani

superior olivary complex   SOC; collection of auditory nuclei in the hindbrain that relay information from the cochlear nucleus to the midbrain; these include the lateral superior olive, medial superior olive, medial nucleus of the trapezoid body, and periolivary nuclei

superior olive, lateral   LSO; one of the primary nuclei of the superior olivary complex, located in the hindbrain, receiving primary ascending projections directly from the ipsilateral AVCN and indirectly from the contralateral AVCN via the ipsilateral MTB

superior olive, medial   MSO; one of the primary nuclei of the superior olivary complex, located in the hindbrain, receiving primary ascending projections directly from both the ipsilateral and contralateral anterior ventral cochlear nuclei

superior semicircular canal   one of

three bony canals of the vestibular apparatus containing sensory epithelia that respond to angular motion

superior semicircular duct one of three membranous canals of the vestibular apparatus containing sensory epithelia that respond to angular motion

superior tympanic artery vessel arising from the middle meningeal artery and entering the middle ear to supply the tensor tympani muscle, the medial half of the roof, and the medial wall of the epitympanic space

superior vestibular nerve division of the vestibular portion of Cranial Nerve VIII, consisting of neurons from the cristae of the superior and lateral semicircular canals, the macula of the utricle, and the anterosuperior part of the macula of the saccule

supernumerary exceeding the normal number

supersonic pertaining to speeds greater than the speed of sound

supine lying on the back, face upward

suppression, fixation in ENG assessment, reduction or elimination of nystagmus by visual fixation

suppression of otoacoustic emissions reduction in the amplitude of transient otoacoustic emissions by the introduction of noise into the contralateral ear; SYN: contralateral suppression

suppurative pertaining to the formation of pus; SYN: purulent

suppurative labyrinthitis inflammation of the labyrinth caused by bacterial invasion of the cochlea by contiguous areas of the temporal bone, resulting in severe vertigo and hearing loss

suppurative otitis media inflammation of the middle ear with infected effusion containing pus

supra-aural above the ear

suprageniculate facial palsy facial nerve paralysis or paresis due to a lesion located between the geniculate ganglion and motor nucleus, affecting taste, lacrimation, and the stapedial reflex

supraliminal above the threshold of awareness

suprasegmentals variations in pitch, loudness, and duration that are superimposed on the phonemes of speech, resulting in intonation, stress, juncture, duration, etc.

suprastapedial facial palsy facial nerve paralysis or paresis due to a lesion located

between the stapedius muscle nerve and the geniculate ganglion, affecting taste and the stapedial reflex, but not lacrimation

supratentorial pertaining to a disorder that is "all in the head," or above the tentorium, such as functional hearing loss

suprathreshold pertaining to an intensity level above threshold

suprathreshold adaptation test STAT test; procedure to measure auditory adaptation in which the signal is presented at a high-intensity level, and the patient responds as long as it is audible

surface electrode noninvasive electrode attached by conductive paste or gel to the skin

susceptance B; energy flow associated with reactance; reciprocal of reactance

susurrus aurium murmur in the ear

SWAMI speech with alternating masking index; early speech-recognition measure in which two signals—a target signal and noise of 20 dB greater intensity—were alternated rapidly between ears to assess dichotic integration

sweep-frequency audiometry the use of Békésy or automatic audiometry to track sensitivity thresholds as the frequency of the signal slowly increases across the audiometric frequency range; COM: fixed-frequency audiometry

swim plugs custom earmolds without a bore, designed to protect the external auditory meatus from water and to protect the middle ears of children with PE tubes

swimmer's ear colloquial term for diffuse red, pustular lesions surrounding hair follicles, usually due to gram-negative bacterial infection during hot, humid weather and often initiated by swimming; SYN: acute diffuse external otitis

swinging story test early test of unilateral functional hearing loss in which portions of a story were presented to the better ear and portions to the poorer ear to ascertain which information the patient could recall

switched capacitor filter integrated circuit filter system that permits a variety of filtering characteristics, including low-pass, high-pass, band-pass, and notched

syllabic compression hearing aid compression algorithm that incorporates a low threshold of activation, short attack and release times, and a low compression ratio, resulting in a reduction of the dynamic range of the input

syllable, nonsense single-syllable speech utterance that has no meaning, used in speech audiometric measures

symmetric hearing loss hearing loss that is identical or nearly so in both ears

symphalangism autosomal dominant skeletal disorder, characterized by bony ankylosis of the finger and toe joints, with conductive hearing loss associated with stapes fixation

symptom any organic or physiologic manifestation of a disease that is experienced by the patient; COM: sign

synapse functional point of communication between neurons

synapse remodeling changes in innervation pattern that occur during embryologic development; e.g., early in development, both afferent and efferent fibers contact the inner hair cells, but with development, efferent fibers relocate onto the afferent terminals

synaptogenesis any embryonic development of synaptic connections

syncope a sudden loss of strength; a fainting or swooning

syndrome aggregate of symptoms and signs resulting from a single cause or occurring together commonly enough to constitute a distinct clinical entity

syndromic hearing loss hearing loss that occurs as part of a constellation of other medical and physical disorders; ANT: nonsyndromic hearing loss

synergic pertaining to synergy

synergism combined action of agents, such as drugs, that has a greater total effect than the sum of the individual effects, such as certain combinations of drugs having greater ototoxic effects than any of the drugs alone

synergistic pertaining to synergism

synergy correlated action or cooperation

syntax word order in a language

synthesis formation by combining or putting together

synthesis, auditory perceptual process by which discrete phonemes are integrated into syllables or whole words

synthesize to combine separate elements to form a whole

synthetic sentence-identification test SSI test; closed-set speech-recognition test in which approximations of sentences are presented in a background of single-talker competition in order to assess central auditory processing ability

syphilis specific congenital or acquired disease caused by the spirochete Treponema pallidum

syphilis, acquired venereal disease, caused by the spirochete Treponema pallidum, which in its secondary and tertiary stages may result in auditory and vestibular disorders due to membranous labyrinthitis

syphilis, secondary acquired secondary stage of a syphilis infection, which can result in membranous labyrinthitis associated with acute meningitis

syphilis, tertiary acquired late stage of development of syphilis infection, occurring within 3 years to 10 years of initial infection, often resulting in otosyphilis

syphilitic labyrinthitis acquired or congenital labyrinthitis, secondary to syphilis, that results in progressive, fluctuating sensorineural hearing loss due to endolymphatic hydrops and degenerative changes in sensory and neural structures

system consistent and functional whole made up of combined parts

systemic pertaining to or affecting an entire system or the body as a whole

T

T tympanogram; graph of middle ear immittance as a function of the amount of air pressure delivered to the ear canal

T & A tonsillectomy and adenoidectomy; surgical extraction of tonsils and adenoids to limit chronic upper respiratory infection

T coil telecoil; an induction coil often included in a hearing aid to receive electromagnetic signals from a telephone or a loop amplification system

T switch telecoil switch; switch circuit on some hearing aids that permits use of an induction coil to receive electromagnetic signals from a telephone or a loop amplification system

tack procedure procedure designed to treat endolymphatic hydrops by fistulizing the membranous labyrinth with a sharp tack placed permanently through the stapes footplate into the vestibule

tactile pertaining to the sense of touch

tactile device hearing aid that converts sound into vibration for tactual stimulation, designed as a replacement for auditory stimulation in cases of profound deafness; SYN: vibrotactile hearing aid

tactile response tactual threshold obtained during bone-conduction and occasionally air-conduction audiometry in a patient whose auditory threshold exceeds the transducer vibration level

tactual pertaining to or caused by touch

tag small flaplike or polypoid appendage

tag, preauricular craniofacial anomaly characterized by a small appendage, often containing cartilage, lying anterior to the auricle

tangible reinforcement operant conditioning audiometry TROCA; audiometric technique that uses a mechanical box from which the child or mentally disabled patient receives reinforcement, usually in the form of candy or cereal, for the correct identification of a signal presentation

target 1. in speech audiometry, the signal of interest; 2. in hearing aid fitting, the prescriptive gain and frequency response against which the actual hearing aid output is compared

target, speech in speech audiometry, the speech signal of interest

target signal in event-related potential measurement, the signal that occurs less frequently than a second signal, to which the patient is usually instructed to attend

task relevance in event-related potential measurement, the value attached to a certain stimulus or type of response

TB trapezoid body; second-order neural fiber bundle leaving the AVCN and projecting ventrally and medially to distribute fibers to the ipsilateral LSO and MSO and continuing across midline to distribute fibers to the contralateral MSO and MNTB

TC total communication; habilitative approach used in individuals with severe and profound hearing impairment consisting of the integration of oral/aural and manual communication strategies

TD threshold of discomfort; lowest intensity level at which sound is judged to be uncomfortably loud; SYN: uncomfortable loudness level

TDD telecommunication or telephone device for the deaf; telephone system used by those with significant hearing impairment in which a typewritten message is transmitted over telephone lines and is received as a printed message; SYN: TT, TTY, TTD

TDH telephonic dynamic headphone; standard earphone for audiometric testing, usually stated with numeric designator specifying the version, such as TDH-39 and TDH-49

tectorial membrane gelatinous membrane within the scala media projecting radially from the spiral limbus and overlying the organ of Corti, in which the cilia of the outer hair cells are embedded

tegmen tympani thin plate of bone from the petrous and squamous portions of the temporal bone forming the tegmental wall or roof of the tympanic cavity

tegmental wall superior wall or ceiling of the tympanic cavity

telecoil T coil; an induction coil often included in a hearing aid to receive electromagnetic signals from a telephone or a loop amplification system

telecoil switch T switch; switch circuit on some hearing aids that permits use of an induction coil to receive electromagnetic signals from a telephone or a loop amplification system

telecommunication device for the deaf TDD; telephone system used by those with significant hearing impairment in which a typewritten message is transmitted over telephone lines and is received as a printed message; SYN: text telephone (TT), TTY, TTD

telemagnetic loop system assistive listening device consisting of a microphone/amplifier that delivers signals to a loop of wire encircling a room, which are received by the telecoil of a hearing aid via magnetic induction

telephone amplifier any of several types of assistive devices designed to increase the intensity level output of a telephone receiver

telephone coil telecoil

telephone device for the deaf TDD; telecommunication device for the deaf

telereceptors sensory endorgans capable of receiving stimuli from a distance

Television Decoder Circuitry Act United States public law (PL) 101–336, a 1990 act requiring that all televisions with 13-inch diagonal screens or wider contain decoder circuitry for closed captioning

temporal 1. pertaining to time; 2. pertaining to the lateral portion of the upper part of the head

temporal acuity the ability to distinguish or resolve small time intervals or order of occurrence

temporal bone bilateral bones of the cranium that form most of the lateral base and sides of the skull, consisting of the squamous, mastoid, petrous and tympanic portions, and the styloid process

temporal envelope the time versus amplitude description of a signal represented as the smooth curve joining the peaks of the modulation function

temporal integration temporal summation

temporal lobe portion of the cerebrum, located below the lateral sulcus and above and adjacent to the temporal bone, containing the primary auditory cortex

temporal masking the interference of one sound with another that is not presented simultaneously, increasing systematically as the interval between the signal and masker decreases

temporal resolution ability to perceive or discriminate as separate events sound segments spaced closely in time

temporal summation the aggregation of neuronal function resulting from additional duration of sound energy so that thresholds improve as durations increase up to about 200 msec

temporary threshold shift TTS; transient or reversible hearing loss due to auditory fatigue following exposure to excessive levels of sound

temporary threshold shift, noise-induced NITTS; SYN: temporary threshold shift

temporomandibular joint TMJ; point of articulation of the mandible and temporal bone

temporomandibular joint syndrome TMJ syndrome; disorder of the temporomandibular joint, characterized by varying degrees of impaired movement, discomfort, headache, earache, tinnitus, stuffiness, and vertigo

10-20 International Electrode System conventional system for describing electrode location on the scalp in evoked potential measurement, so named because each electrode is 10% or 20% of the distance between the nasion, the inion, and left and right pre-auricular points

tendon, stapedius round tendon projecting from the stapedius muscle through a small opening in the apex of the pyramidal eminence and attaching to the head of the stapes

tendon, tensor tympani tendon projecting from the tensor tympani muscle through the cochleariform process and attaching to the upper portion of the manubrium of the malleus, drawing the malleus medially and anteriorly upon contraction of the muscle

tensor any muscle that makes a body structure firm or tight

tensor tympani muscle along with the stapedius, one of two striated muscles of the middle ear, classified as a pennate muscle, consisting of short fibers directed obliquely onto the stapedius tendon at the midline, innervated by the trigeminal nerve, Cranial Nerve V

tensor tympani semicanal canal in the temporal bone that opens into the carotid wall of the middle ear through which the tensor tympani muscle courses

tensor tympani tendon tendon projecting from the tensor tympani muscle through the cochleariform process and attaching to the upper portion of the manubrium of the malleus, drawing the malleus medially and anteriorly upon contraction of the muscle

tensor veli palatini along with the levator veli palatini, one of two muscles of the nasophyarynx responsible for opening the end of the eustachian tube by medial displacement of the tube membrane, innervated by the trigeminal nerve, Cranial Nerve V

tentorium membranous cover separating most of the lower portions of the brain from the cortex

TEOAE transient evoked otoacoustic emission; low-level acoustic echo emitted by the cochlea in response to a click or transient auditory stimulus; related to the integrity and function of the outer hair cells of the cochlea; COM: DPOAE; SOAE

teratogen a drug or other agent or influence that causes abnormal embryologic development

teratogenic pertaining to a teratogen

teratogenic drugs drugs such as thalidomide, quinine, dilantin, and accutane that if ingested by the mother during pregnancy have a substantial teratogenic effect on the developing embryo, including otic malformation

teratoma benign neoplasm, composed of various tissues, that occurs in an area foreign to the one in which the tissues normally reside; sometimes found in the temporal bone with associated hearing loss

tertiary third in order

tertiary acquired syphilis late stage of development of syphilis infection, occurring within 3 years to 10 years of initial infection, often resulting in otosyphilis

test-retest reliability measure of the consistency of test results from one trial to the next

tetanus antitoxin antibody formed in response to a specific neurotropic toxin, which when used prophylactically or therapeutically has been associated with bilateral profound sensorineural hearing loss

text telephone TT; telephone system used by those with significant hearing impairment in which a typewritten message is transmitted over telephone lines and is received as a printed message; SYN: TDD, telecommunication device for the deaf

thalamocortical projections bundles of efferent nerve fibers emanating from the cortex to the thalamus, including those from the primary auditory cortex to the medial geniculate body

thalamus large ovoid mass of gray matter located in the forebrain, including sensory relay nuclei such as the medial geniculate bodies

thalidomide tranquilizing drug that can have a teratogenic effect on the auditory system of the developing embryo when taken by the mother during pregnancy, resulting in congenital hearing loss

thermal noise broad-band noise having constant energy at all frequencies; SYN: white noise

third-octave filter filter that passes a frequency band with a width of one-third octave

3-dB rule time-intensity tradeoff stating that for every halving of noise-exposure time, a 3-dBA increase in noise is permitted without increasing the risk of noise-induced hearing loss

threshold level at which a stimulus or change in stimulus is just sufficient to produce a sensation or an effect

threshold, absolute 1. psychophysical term used to denote the value of stimulus magnitude that elicits a desired response and is often related to detection threshold of a signal; 2. in audiometry, the lowest intensity level at which an acoustic signal can be detected

threshold, acoustic reflex lowest intensity level of a stimulus at which an acoustic reflex is detected

threshold, aided lowest level at which a signal is audible to an individual wearing a hearing aid

threshold, air-conduction absolute threshold of hearing sensitivity to pure-tone stimuli delivered via earphone

threshold, audibility threshold of hearing sensitivity

threshold, auditory lowest intensity level at which a specified sound is perceptible

threshold, bone-conduction absolute threshold of hearing sensitivity to pure-tone stimuli delivered via bone-conduction oscillator

threshold, compression the minimum input decibel level at which compression circuitry is activated in a hearing aid

threshold, detectability detection threshold

threshold, detection   absolute threshold of hearing sensitivity

threshold, differential   the smallest difference that can be detected between two signals that vary in intensity, frequency, time, etc.; SYN: difference limen

threshold, elevated   absolute threshold that is poorer than normal and thus at a decibel level that is greater or elevated

threshold, hearing   absolute threshold of hearing sensitivity, or the lowest intensity level at which sound is perceived

threshold, masked   pure-tone or speech audiometric threshold obtained in one ear while the other ear was effectively masked

threshold, noise-detection   NDT; lowest intensity level at which a specified noise signal is audible

threshold, pure-tone   lowest level at which a pure-tone stimulus is audible

threshold, pure-tone air-conduction lowest level at which a pure-tone stimulus, presented through earphones, is audible

threshold, pure-tone bone-conduction lowest level at which a pure-tone stimulus, presented via a vibrating oscillator placed on the forehead or mastoid, is audible

threshold, raised   elevated or abnormal threshold of hearing sensitivity

threshold, sensitivity   lowest level at which a signal is detectable

threshold, speech   ST; generic term describing speech-reception threshold, as opposed to awareness or detection threshold

threshold, speech-awareness   SAT; lowest level at which a speech signal is audible; SYN: speech-detection threshold

threshold, speech-detection   SDT; SYN: speech-awareness threshold

threshold, speech-reception   SRT; threshold level for speech recognition, expressed as the lowest intensity level at which 50% of spondaic words can be identified

threshold, spondee   ST; speech-reception threshold

threshold, unmasked   pure-tone or speech audiometric threshold obtained without masking the nontest ear

threshold of audibility   lowest intensity level at which an auditory signal is perceptible

threshold of discomfort   TD; lowest intensity level at which sound is judged to be uncomfortably loud; SYN: uncomfortable loudness level

threshold of hearing sensitivity   lowest intensity level at which an auditory signal is audible

threshold shift   change in hearing sensitivity, usually a decrement, expressed in dB

threshold shift, permanent   PTS; irreversible hearing sensitivity loss following exposure to excessive noise levels; COM: temporary threshold shift

threshold shift, standard   STS; change in hearing threshold in comparison to a baseline audiogram, defined as an average change of 10 dB or more at 2000 Hz, 3000 Hz, and 4000 Hz in either ear

threshold shift, temporary   TTS; transient or reversible hearing loss due to auditory fatigue following exposure to excessive levels of sound

thrombosis   clotting within a blood vessel resulting in loss of blood flow to the tissues supplied by the vessel

thrombus   clot within a blood vessel

thymine   one of four chemical bases that make up the genetic alphabet

TIA   transient ischemic attack; sudden reversible loss of neurologic function due to cerebral vascular incident

Tietze syndrome   autosomal dominant hereditary disorder characterized by generalized pigment loss, absence of eyebrows, blue irises, and profound hearing loss

TILL   treble increases at low levels; type of automatic signal processing in a hearing aid that uses level-dependent control of frequency response, increasing high frequencies in response to low-intensity input

timbre   the characteristic quality of a sound

time-compressed speech   speech signals that have been accelerated by the process of time compression

time-compressed speech measures speech audiometric measures in which sensitized speech signals that have undergone time compression are used to assess the integrity of the central auditory nervous system

time compression   signal-processing technique designed to accelerate the speed of acoustic signals without altering their frequency characteristics by removing segments and compressing the remaining segments

time-intensity tradeoff   relationship of the permissible noise intensity level to the duration of exposure to that level

time-weighted average TWA; measure of daily noise exposure, expressed as the product of durations of exposure at particular sound levels relative to the allowable durations of exposure for those levels

tinnitus sensation of ringing or other sound in the head, without an external cause

tinnitus, clicking subjective and sometimes objective tinnitus, characterized by a clicking sound, present in cases of chronic middle-ear disorder presumably caused by an opening and closing of the eustachian tube

tinnitus, intractable ringing that is resistant to treatment

tinnitus, Leudet objective tinnitus, characterized by spasmodic dry clicking and caused by reflex spasm of the tensor palati muscle of the eustachian tube

tinnitus, objective ringing or other head noises that can be heard and measured by an examiner

tinnitus, pulsatile objective tinnitus, characterized by pulsing sound, that results from vascular abnormalities such as glomus tumor, arterial anomaly, and heart murmurs

tinnitus, subjective perception by an individual of ringing or other noise in the ear or head that is not evident to an examiner

tinnitus aurium subjective tinnitus localized to one or both ears

tinnitus cerebri subjective tinnitus localized generally in the head rather than the ears

tinnitus earmold open style of earmold for use with a tinnitus masker

tinnitus masker electronic hearing aid device that generates and emits broad-band or narrow-band noise at low levels, designed to mask the presence of tinnitus

TM tympanic membrane; thin, membranous vibrating tissue terminating the external auditory meatus and forming the major portion of the lateral wall of the middle ear cavity, onto which the malleus is attached; COL: eardrum

TMJ temporomandibular joint; point of articulation of the mandible and temporal bone

TMJ syndrome TMJ syndrome; disorder of the temporomandibular joint, characterized by varying degrees of impaired movement, discomfort, headache, earache, tinnitus, stuffiness, and vertigo

TOAE transient otoacoustic emission; transient evoked otoacoustic emission

tobramycin ototoxic aminoglycoside antibiotic that is active against gram-negative organisms

tolerance ability to endure, often over a sustained time period

tolerance level threshold of discomfort

toluene industrial solvent, which can be ototoxic if inhaled in high concentrations over extended periods

tomography the taking of sectional radiographs of specified areas of the brain

tonality having the subjective qualities of a tone

tone a periodic sound of distinct pitch

tone, combination harmonic perceived when two pure tones are presented simultaneously

tone, complex sound containing more than one frequency component

tone, difference a distinctive tone perceived at a frequency equal to the difference between the frequencies of two stimulating tones

tone, frequency-modulated sinusoidal signal whose frequency varies at a fixed rate; SYN: warble tone

tone, probe in immittance measurement, the pure tone that is held at a constant intensity level in the external auditory meatus; used to indirectly measure changes in energy flow through the middle ear mechanism

tone, pure sound wave having only one frequency of vibration

tone, warble frequency-modulated pure tone, often used in sound field audiometry

tone burst a brief pure tone having a rapid rise and fall time with a duration sufficient to be perceived as having tonality

tone control a potentiometer on a hearing aid that changes the frequency response of the device

tone deafness colloquial term for the condition of being unable to distinguish among different frequencies or carry a tune

tone decay perstimulatory adaptation, in which an audible sound becomes inaudible during prolonged stimulation

tone-decay test test of auditory adaptation in which a continuous tone is presented near threshold and the change in perception is monitored over a given time period, abnormal adaptation being consistent with retrocochlear site of disorder

tone pip tone burst with no more than 1 cycle at the maximum amplitude

tonotopic pertaining to structures in the peripheral and central auditory nervous system that are topograpically or spatially arranged according to tonal frequency

tonotopic organization topographic arrangement of structures within the peripheral and central auditory nervous system according to tonal frequency

tonotopicity condition of being topographically arranged according to frequency

tonsil normal collection of lymphoid tissue on the lateral walls of the pharynx

tonsillectomy surgical removal of the tonsils

tonsillectomy and adenoidectomy T & A; surgical extraction of tonsils and adenoids to limit chronic upper respiratory infection

tonus state of normal tension of tissues

topical pertaining to a particular location or region; local

topograph a detailed depiction of the surface features of an area or region

topographic mapping the display of the distribution of electrical activity of the brain measured and derived from multiple electrodes affixed to the scalp

TORCH infections congenital perinatal infections grouped as risk factors associated with hearing impairment and other disorders, including *t*oxoplasmosis, *o*ther infections, especially syphilis, *r*ubella, *c*ytomegalovirus infection, and *h*erpes simplex

total communication TC; habilitative approach used in individuals with severe and profound hearing impairment consisting of the integration of oral/aural and manual communication strategies

Townes-Brocks syndrome autosomal dominant disorder characterized by anomalies of the ear, hand, foot, anus, and kidney, with associated mixed or progressive sensorineural hearing loss

toxic pertaining to a toxin

toxic hearing loss loss in hearing sensitivity due to exposure to ototoxic drugs

toxic labyrinthitis inflammation of the labyrinth caused by degradation of the tissue fluid environment in the inner ear due to bacterial toxins or contamination of perilymph during surgery; SYN: serous labyrinthitis

toxicity the state of being toxic or poisonous

toxin poisonous substance

tracing, continuous C tracing; graph that results from threshold tracking in Békésy audiometry to a continuous pure tone at a fixed or swept frequency

tracing, interrupted I tracing; graph that results from threshold tracking in Békésy audiometry to an interrupted or pulsed tone at a fixed or swept frequency

tracking aural rehabilitation technique, used to train and evaluate reception of ongoing speech, in which the listener attempts to track or follow the ongoing speech of the talker; performance is expressed in number of words repeated per unit of time

tracking, pendular component of the electronystagmography test battery in which an object or spot of light moving sinusoidally is tracked horizontally and vertically to assess the smooth- or slow-pursuit eye movement system

tracking audiometry automatic or Békésy audiometry in which the patient controls signal attenuation with a switch and adjusts the intensity alternately from a level of audibility to inaudibility to audibility and so on

tract bundle of nerve fibers having a common origin, function, and termination

tragus small cartilaginous flap on the anterior wall of the external auditory meatus

tragus configuration earmold modification in which a lip is added that extends over the tragus for additional feedback control

transcanal tympanoplasty middle ear surgery in which the tympanic cavity is exposed via tympanomeatal flap

transcranial CROS contralateral routing of signal (CROS) strategy for unilateral hearing loss in which a high-gain in-the-ear hearing aid is fitted to the poor ear in an effort to transfer sound across the skull by bone conduction to the cochlea of the good ear

transduce to convert one form of energy to another

transducer a device that converts one form of energy to another, such as an earphone converting electrical energy to acoustic energy

transduction the conversion of energy from one form to another

transection surgical cutting across or through, as in a nerve transection

transfer function, modulation description of the ability of an acoustic or electronic transmission system to maintain

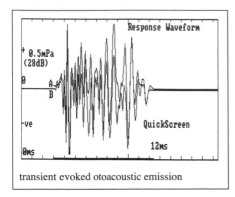

transient evoked otoacoustic emission

the amplitude characteristics of a signal envelope

transformer device that converts energy from one level to another

transient response of a transducer to the rapid onset or offset of an electrical signal, resulting in a short-duration, broad-band click characterized by a bandwidth that increases as the duration of the electrical signal decreases

transient distortion the inexact reproduction of a sound resulting from failure of an amplifier to process or follow sudden changes of voltage

transient evoked otoacoustic emission TEOAE; low-level acoustic echo emitted by the cochlea in response to a click or transient auditory stimulus; related to the integrity and function of the outer hair cells of the cochlea

transient evoked potential auditory evoked potential of brief duration, occurring in response to a stimulus and ending prior to the next stimulus presentation; examples are the ECochG, ABR, AMLR, LLAEP; COM: steady-state evoked potential

transient hearing loss temporary loss of hearing sensitivity

transient ischemic attack TIA; sudden reversible loss of neurologic function due to cerebral vascular incident

transient otoacoustic emission TOAE; transient evoked otoacoustic emission

transient response term usually used to refer to auditory evoked potentials elicited by click stimuli

transient stimulus rapid-onset, short-duration, broad-band sound produced by delivering an electric pulse to an earphone; used

to elicit an auditory brainstem response and transient evoked otoacoustic emissions; SYN: click

translabyrinthine pertaining to the surgical approach through the labyrinth in which the cochlea is obliterated in an effort to access the internal auditory meatus for tumor removal or nerve section

transmission loss loss of power as acoustic energy travels through a medium

transmitter in an FM amplification system, the device worn by the talker, coupled to a microphone, that transmits electrical energy to the FM receiver

transposer, frequency circuitry that converts frequency components of a waveform from one range into another range

transpositional hearing aid hearing aid that converts high-frequency acoustic energy into low-frequency signals for individuals with profound hearing loss who have measurable hearing only in the lower frequencies

transtympanic electrode needle electrode placed through the tympanic membrane onto the promontory of the middle ear cavity; used as a recording electrode in electrocochleography and stimulating electrode in promontory testing

transudate any fluid that has passed through a membrane

transudation passage of body fluid through a membrane or tissue surface

transverse auricular muscle one of four muscles attaching to the medial surface of the auricle

transverse fracture a break that traverses the temporal bone perpendicular to the long axis of the petrous pyramid; usually caused by a blow to the occipital region of the skull, resulting in extensive destruction of the membranous labyrinth; ANT: longitudinal fracture

transverse plane a slice in the horizontal plane, the anatomic plane of reference dividing the head into upper and lower portions

transverse wave wave in which the particles of the medium move at right angles to the direction of the wave movement; ANT: longitudinal wave

trapezoid body TB; second-order fiber bundle leaving the AVCN and projecting ventrally and medially to distribute fibers to the ipsilateral LSO and MSO and continuing across midline to distribute fibers to the contralateral MSO and MNTB; SYN: ventral acoustic stria

trapezoid body, medial nucleus of MNTB or MTB; a nucleus of the superior olivary complex that receives primary ascending projections from the contralateral anterior ventral cochlear nucleus and sends projections to the ipsilateral lateral superior olive and lateral lemniscus

trauma an injury produced by external force

trauma, acoustic 1. damage to hearing from a transient, high-intensity sound; 2. long-term insult to hearing from excessive noise exposure

trauma, noise SYN: acoustic trauma

trauma, penetrating damage to the ear as a result of any sharp object traversing the external auditory meatus, with auditory disorder ranging from minor perforation of the tympanic membrane to ossicular destruction and oval window fistula

traveling wave sound-induced displacement pattern along the basilar membrane that describes fundamental cochlear processing, characterized by maximum displacement at a location corresponding to the frequency of the signal

Treacher Collins syndrome autosomal dominant disorder of craniofacial morphogenesis, characterized by downward sloping palpebral fissures, depressed cheek bones, malformed pinna, receding chin, and large mouth, with associated atresia and ossicular malformation

treble increases at low levels TILL; type of automatic signal processing in a hearing aid that uses level-dependent control of frequency response, increasing high frequencies in response to low-intensity input

tremor involuntary trembling movement due to alternating contractions of opposing muscles

triangular fossa depression on the auricle, formed by a split in the antihelix

trichlorethylene industrial solvent which can be ototoxic if inhaled in high concentrations over extended periods

trigeminal nerve Cranial Nerve V; cranial nerve that provides efferent innervation to the mastication muscles, including the tensor tympani, and afferent innervation from the face

trimester period of 3 months, usually used to describe portions of a pregnancy

trimmer a variable control used to make adjustments to the output of a hearing aid

trisomy 13-15 syndrome chromosomal abnormality, characterized by microphthalmia, cleft lip and palate, and polydactyly, with associated outer, middle, and inner ear anomalies

trisomy 18 syndrome chromosomal abnormality, characterized by microcephaly, agenesis of bones of the extremities, congenital heart disease, craniofacial anomalies, and mental retardation, with associated outer, middle, and inner ear anomalies; SYN: Edward syndrome

trisomy 21 syndrome congenital genetic abnormality, characterized by mental retardation and characteristic facial features, with high incidence of chronic otitis media and associated conductive, mixed, and sensorineural hearing loss; SYN: Down syndrome

TROCA tangible reinforcement of operant conditioned audiometry; audiometric technique that uses tangible reinforcement, usually in the form of candy or cereal, for the correct identification of a signal presentation

trochaic word word of two syllables, the first of which is stressed

trochlear nerve Cranial Nerve IV; cranial nerve that provides efferent innervation to the superior oblique muscle involved in eye movement

TT text telephone; telephone system used by those with significant hearing impairment in which a typewritten message is transmitted over telephone lines and is received as a printed message; SYN: telecommunication device for the deaf, TDD

TTD teletypewriter for the deaf; early term for TDD or TT

TTS temporary threshold shift; transient or reversible hearing loss due to auditory fatigue following exposure to excessive levels of sound

TTY teletypewriter; early term for TDD or TT

tube, grommet ventilation or pressure-equalization tube

tube, pressure-equalization PE tube; small tube or grommet inserted in the tympanic membrane following myringotomy to provide equalization of air pressure within the middle ear space as a substitute for a nonfunctional eustachian tube; SYN: tympanostomy tube

tube, tympanotomy SYN: pressure-equalization tube

tube, ventilation SYN: pressure-equalization tube

tube lock metal cuff with a small flange that attaches to earmold tubing to secure it into an earmold, eliminating the need to cement the tubing in soft earmold material

tubercle small, rounded nodule, especially on bone

tuberculosis infectious bacterial disease characterized by formation of tubercles in the body tissues, especially the lungs

tuberculosis, miliary infectious bacterial disease characterized by formation of tubercles of millet-seed size in the central nervous system; involvement of the auditory pathways can result in retrocochlear disorder

tuberculous otitis media chronic inflammation of the middle ear and mastoid secondary to tuberculosis, resulting in early perforation and suppurative otorrhea

tubing tubelike portion of a hearing aid that serves as the transmission line from the receiver to the tip of the earmold

tubing, extended receiver extension of the receiver tubing beyond a hearing aid casing to reduce feedback and to prevent cerumen accumulation

tubotympanic pertaining to the eustachian tube and the middle ear cavity

tubotympanitis inflammation of the middle ear cavity and eustachian tube

Tullio phenomenon transient vertigo and nystagmus caused by substantial movement of the inner ear fluid in response to a high-intensity sound, occurring commonly in congenital syphilis

tumor abnormal growth of tissue, resulting from an excessively rapid proliferation of cells; SYN: neoplasm

tumor, acoustic generic term referring to a neoplasm of Cranial Nerve VIII, most often a cochleovestibular Schwannoma; SYN: acoustic neuroma

tumor, cerebellopontine angle CPA tumor; most often a cochleovestibular Schwannoma located or growing outside the internal auditory canal at the juncture of the cerebellum and pons

tumor, eighth nerve generic term referring to a neoplasm of Cranial Nerve VIII, most often a cochleovestibular Schwannoma; SYN: acoustic tumor

tumor, extra-axial lesion that originates outside the brainstem, e.g., cochleovestibular Schwannoma

tumor, glomus small neoplasm of paraganglionic tissue with a rich vascular supply located near or within the jugular bulb

tumor, intra-axial tumor that originates within the brainstem

tumor, pineal neoplasm derived from the pineal gland; SYN: pinealoma

tuning, mechanical in hearing, the amount of frequency resolution or tuning attributable to the cochlea from the displacement caused by Békésy's traveling wave

tuning curve graph of the frequency-resolving properties of the auditory system showing the lowest sound level at which a nerve fiber will respond as a function of frequency, or the SPL of a stimulus that just masks a probe as a function of masker frequency

tuning curve, psychophysical psychophysically determined plot of the level of a variable-frequency masking tone that just masks a fixed-frequency probe tone as a function of the frequency of the masker

tuning fork a two-pronged metal fork that, when struck, produces a specific tonal frequency

tuning fork test any of several tests in which a tuning fork is used to estimate hearing sensitivity or to assess the presence of a conductive hearing loss

tunnel of Corti triangular space formed by the inner and outer pillars of the organ of Corti

Turner syndrome chromosomal abnormality in females characterized by a missing X chromosome, resulting in small stature, lack of ovarian tissue, and eye, heart, and ear anomalies with associated conductive and sensorineural hearing loss; SYN: XO syndrome

TWA time-weighted average; measure of daily noise exposure, expressed as the product of durations of exposure at particular sound levels relative to the allowable durations of exposure for those levels

2-cc coupler metal cylinder with a 2-cc air space, designed to represent the average amount of air enclosed in an ear canal by an earmold; used to connect a hearing aid receiver to the microphone of a sound level meter to measure output characteristics

two-channel compression process in which a hearing aid separates the input signal into two frequency bands, each having independently controlled compression circuitry

Tx therapy or treatment

tympanectomy surgical excision of the tympanic membrane

tympanic pertaining to the middle ear cavity

tympanic aditus orifice in the posterior wall of the epitympanic recess that serves as passage from the tympanic cavity to the tympanic antrum

tympanic annulus incomplete cartilaginous ring from which the osseous portion of the external auditory meatus develops during infancy and early childhood

tympanic antrum enlarged space in the mastoid portion of the temporal lobe extending posteriorly from the epitympanic recess and connected via the aditus

tympanic cavity one of three regions of the middle ear cavity lying directly between the tympanic membrane and the inner ear, containing the ossicular chain; SYN: tympanum

tympanic membrane TM; thin, membranous vibrating tissue terminating the external auditory meatus and forming the major portion of the lateral wall of the middle ear cavity, onto which the malleus is attached; COL: eardrum

tympanic membrane, dimeric thin area of the tympanic membrane, secondary to the healing of a perforation; consists of epidermis and mucous membrane

tympanic membrane, monomeric eardrum membrane that is missing a portion of the fibrous layer

tympanic membrane, secondary round window membrane

tympanic membrane fibroproliferation proliferation of fibrous tissue growth in the submucosal and subcutaneous layers of the tympanic membrane, resulting from chronic inflammation, causing thickening and stiffness

tympanic membrane retraction a drawing back of the eardrum into the middle ear space due to negative pressure formed in the cavity secondary to eustachian tube dysfunction

tympanic muscles stapedius and tensor tympanic muscles of the middle ear, which serve to suspend the ossicles of the middle ear, thereby reducing the effective mass of the ossicular chain

tympanic nerve nerve branch arising from the inferior ganglion of Cranial Nerve IX, providing the main sensory fibers to the mucosa of the tympanum and eustachian tube; SYN: Jacobson's nerve

tympanic portion of the temporal bone portion of the temporal bone forming the floor and part of the anterior and posterior walls of the external auditory meatus

tympanic sulcus groove in the osseous wall of the external auditory meatus into which the annulus of the tympanic membrane fits

tympanitis inflammation of the tympanic membrane; SYN: myringitis

tympanocentesis aspiration of middle ear fluid with a needle through the tympanic membrane; SYN: tympanotomy

tympanogram T; graph of middle ear immittance as a function of the amount of air pressure delivered to the ear canal

tympanogram, Type A normal tympanogram with maximum immittance at atmospheric pressure

tympanogram, Type A$_d$ deep (d) Type A tympanogram associated with a flaccid middle ear mechanism, characterized by excessive immittance that is maximum at atmospheric pressure

tympanogram, Type A$_s$ shallow (s) Type A tympanogram associated with ossicular fixation, characterized by reduced immittance that is maximum at atmospheric pressure

tympanogram, Type B flat tympanogram associated with increase in the mass of the middle ear system, characterized by little change in immittance as ear canal air pressure is varied

tympanogram, Type C tympanogram associated with significant negative pressure in the middle ear space, characterized by immittance that is maximum at a negative ear-canal pressure equal to that of the middle ear cavity

tympanomastoid pertaining to the tympanic cavity and mastoid air cells

tympanomastoid septum bony partition separating the facial recess from the mastoid air cells

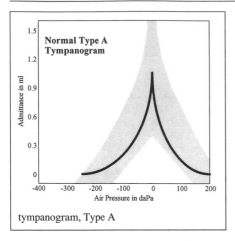

tympanogram, Type A

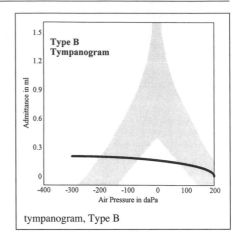

tympanogram, Type B

tympanomastoiditis inflammation of the mucosal linings of the middle ear and mastoid cavities

tympanomeatal flap flap of skin created in the external auditory meatus during transcanal tympanoplasty surgery

tympanometry procedure used in the assessment of middle ear function in which the immittance of the tympanic membrane and middle ear is measured as air pressure delivered to the ear canal is varied

tympanometry, multifrequency tympanometric assessment of middle ear function with a conventional 220-Hz probe tone and with one or more additional probe-tone frequencies

tympanoplasty reconstructive surgery of

the middle ear, usually classified in types according to the magnitude of the reconstructive process

tympanosclerosis formation of whitish plaques in the tympanic membrane and nodular deposits in the mucosa of the middle ear, secondary to chronic otitis media, that may result in ossicular fixation

tympanostomy tube tympanotomy tube

tympanotomy passage of a needle through the tympanic membrane to remove effusion from the middle ear; SYN: myringotomy, tympanocentesis

tympanotomy tube small tube or grommet inserted in the tympanic membrane following myringotomy to equalize air pressure within the middle ear space as a substitute for

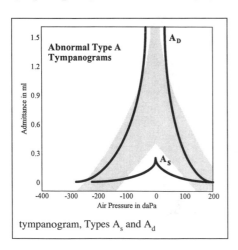

tympanogram, Types A$_s$ and A$_d$

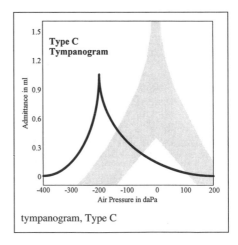

tympanogram, Type C

a nonfunctional eustachian tube; SYN: pressure-equalization tube

tympanum   the region of the middle ear cavity lying directly between the tympanic membrane and the inner ear, containing the ossicular chain; SYN: tympanic cavity

Type I hearing loss   type of hearing loss based on loudness growth, classified for the purpose of hearing aid fitting; caused by outer hair cell loss, and characterized by a loss of sensitivity for soft sound, but little or no hearing loss for loud sounds

Type II hearing loss   type of hearing loss based on loudness growth, classified for the purpose of hearing aid fitting; caused by outer hair cell loss and some inner hair cell loss, and characterized by a loss of hearing for soft sound and a loss of some loud speech cues

Type III hearing loss   type of hearing loss based on loudness growth, classified for the purpose of hearing aid fitting; caused by inner and outer hair cell loss, and characterized by a loss of sensitivity for soft and loud sounds

U

U-shaped curve   description of an audiometric configuration with poorest thresholds in the middle frequencies, often associated with congenital hearing loss

UCL   uncomfortable loudness

UL   uncomfortable level; level at which sound is judged to be uncomfortably loud by a listener

ULBW   ultra-low birth weight; classification of newborns based on birth weight, specifically any infant with a birth weight less than 1000 grams

ULCL   upper limits of comfortable loudness; measure of loudness comfort level describing the highest intensity level at which the loudness of sound remains comfortable

ULL   uncomfortable loudness level; intensity level at which sound is perceived to be uncomfortably loud; SYN: loudness discomfort level

ultrasonic   pertaining to ultrasound

ultrasound   sound having a frequency above the range of human hearing, approximately 20,000 Hz

umbo   projecting center of a rounded surface, such as the end of the cone of the tympanic membrane at the tip of the manubrium of the malleus

unaided   not fitted with or assisted by the use of a hearing aid

unaided gain, real-ear   REUG; probe-microphone measurement of the difference, in dB as a function of frequency, between the SPL in an unoccluded ear canal and the SPL at the field reference point for a specified sound field

unaided response, real-ear   REUR; probe-microphone measurement of the sound pressure level, as a function of frequency, at a specified point near the tympanic membrane in an unoccluded ear canal

uncomfortable level   UL; level at which sound is judged to be uncomfortably loud by a listener

uncomfortable loudness level   ULL; UCL; intensity level at which sound is perceived to be uncomfortably loud; SYN: loudness discomfort level

uncrossed acoustic reflex   acoustic reflex occurring in one ear as a result of stimulation of the same ear; SYN: ipsilateral acoustic reflex

undermasking   condition during audiometric masking in which the intensity level of the masker in the nontest ear is insufficient to mask the signal that has contralateralized from the opposite test ear, thereby resulting in an underestimate of the test-ear threshold

unidirectional microphone   microphone that is responsive predominantly to sound incident from a single position; SYN: directional microphone

unilateral   pertaining to one side only

unilateral hearing loss   hearing sensitivity loss in one ear only

unilateral weakness   UW; measure in percentage of the difference in magnitude of nystagmus from right-ear versus left-ear bithermal caloric stimulation; a difference exceeding 20% is considered to be abnormal

unimodal   pertaining to the use of only one sensory modality

unintelligible speech   oral language that is so degraded that it cannot be understood by the listener

unisensory   unimodal

unity gain   gain of 1 dB of output for every 1 dB of input

unmasked   pertaining to a response obtained with no masking in the nontest ear

unmasked threshold   pure-tone or speech audiometric threshold obtained without masking the nontest ear

unoccluded   open, as the normal external auditory meatus

unresponsive otitis media   middle ear inflammation that persists after 48 hours of initial antibiotic therapy, occurring more frequently in children with recurrent otitis media

up-beating nystagmus   vertical nystagmus in which the fast movement is upward, enhanced by upward or downward gaze, consistent with central vestibular pathology

uplift earmold   specialized earmold for use by individuals with normal hearing and prolapsed ear canals, designed with a funnel-shaped bore for acoustic enhancement

upper limits of comfortable loudness   ULCL; measure of loudness comfort level describing the highest intensity level at which the loudness of sound remains comfortable

upward spread of masking the masking of high-frequency sound by low-frequency sound, e.g., weaker high-frequency consonant sounds being masked by stronger low-frequency vowel sounds

use gain amount of gain provided by a hearing aid with the volume control adjusted to the setting at which it is typically worn

Usher syndrome autosomal recessive disorder characterized by congenital sensorineural hearing loss and progressive loss of vision due to retinitis pigmentosa

utero, in within the uterus; not yet born

utilization factors epidemiologic factors of a defined population that influence use of healthcare services; SYN: frequency factors

utilization review evaluation of the efficacy and appropriateness of any healthcare service, with particular emphasis on how it uses resources

utricle larger of the two sac like structures in the vestibule containing a macula that is responsive to linear acceleration

utricular macula sensory epithelium of the utricle, which is responsive to linear acceleration, particularly to the accelerative forces of gravity experienced during body or head tilt

utricular nerve nerve fiber bundle from the hair cells of the utricular macula that joins with similar bundles from the semicircular canals and the saccule to form the vestibular branch of Cranial Nerve VIII

utricular sensory epithelium macula, consisting of Type I and Type II hair cells embedded in a gelatinous otolithic membrane

utriculitis inflammation of the utricle

utriculoendolymphatic valve small valve in the utricle that permits controlled drainage of endolymph toward the endolymphatic sac

utriculofugal deviation deflection of the kinocilia in the semicircular canals away from the utricle, associated with decreased electrical activity in the horizontal canal and increased activity in the superior and posterior canals; SYN: ampullofugal deviation

utriculopetal deviation deflection of the kinocilia in the semicircular canals toward the utricle, associated with increased electrical activity in the horizontal canal and decreased activity in the superior and posterior canals; SYN: ampullopetal deviation

UW unilateral weakness; measure in percentage of the difference in magnitude of nystagmus from right-ear versus left-ear bithermal caloric stimulation; a difference exceeding 20% is considered to be abnormal

V

V volt; unit of electromotive force producing a current of 1 ampere through a resistance of 1 ohm

VAB VI vinblastine, actinomycin D, bleomycin, cisplatin, cylcophosphamide; potentially ototoxic chemotherapy regimen used in the treatment of testicular cancer

vagus nerve Cranial Nerve X; cranial nerve that provides efferent and afferent innervation to the thoracic and abdominal viscera, pharynx, and larynx

validity the extent to which a test measures what it is intended to measure

validity, concurrent extent to which test results agree with a specified criterion

validity, construct extent to which a test measures the nature of a trait

validity, content extent to which a test represents an appropriate sampling of the trait it is intended to measure

Valsalva Valsalva maneuver

Valsalva maneuver attempt to force open the eustachian tube by blowing with the nostrils and mouth closed

Van Buchem syndrome autosomal recessive craniofacial disorder characterized by childhood-onset generalized osteosclerotic narrowing of the skull foramen, resulting in cranial nerve paresis, including sensorineural hearing loss

Van Der Hoeve syndrome autosomal dominant disorder, characterized by symptoms related to having brittle bones, including multiple fractures at birth, weak joints, bone deformities, nerve-root compression, and temporal bone malformation; SYN: osteogenesis imperfecta

variable release time a characteristic of some compression circuits in which the compression release time changes in direct relation to duration of the input, e.g., the shorter the compression-activating input, the shorter the release time

variable venting valve insert that can be used to modify the diameter of an earmold vent

varicella acute contagious viral disease occurring in children; COL: chicken pox

vascular pertaining to blood vessels

vasculitis inflammation of a blood vessel

vasoconstriction narrowing of the blood vessels

vasodilation widening of the blood vessels

vasomotor pertaining to constriction or dilation of the blood vessels

VBP vinblastine, bleomycin, cisplatin (platinol); potentially ototoxic chemotherapy regimen used in the treatment of testicular cancer and malignant melanoma

VC volume control; manual or automatic control designed to adjust the output level of a hearing instrument

VDP vinblastine, dacarbazine, cisplatin (platinol); potentially ototoxic chemotherapy regimen used in the treatment of malignant melanoma

vein, anterior vestibular vessel that drains the utricle and the ampullae of the superior and lateral semicircular canals

vein, common modiolar vessel providing venous drainage of the cochlea

vein, mastoid emissary vein through the mastoid that carries blood from the scalp, entering the lateral venous sinus in its sigmoid portion

velocity speed of movement of an object, expressed as distance traveled per unit time

velocity, slow-phase SPV; commonly used measure of nystagmus strength, described as the size of the arc in degrees that the eyeball covers during the slow phase of nystagmus; SYN: vestibular eye speed

venous sinuses collecting veins from the brain, temporal bone, and orbit located in the dura mater

vent bore made in an earmold that permits the passage of sound and air into the otherwise blocked external auditory meatus; used for aeration of the canal and/or acoustic alteration

vent inserts small inserts, with holes of graduated diameter, that fit in the lateral end of an carmold vent to permit alteration of vent size

vent, external type of earmold vent characterized by an external channel that runs along the length of the canal portion into the body of the mold

vent, parallel vent that runs parallel to the bore for the entire length of an earmold

vent, pressure small vent in an earmold or hearing aid to provide pressure equalization in the external auditory meatus

ventilation tube small tube or grommet inserted in the tympanic membrane following myringotomy to equalize air pressure within the middle ear space as a substitute for a nonfunctional eustachian tube; SYN: pressure-equalization tube

venting valve, positive PVV; series of small inserts, with holes of graduated diameter, that fit in the lateral end of an earmold vent to permit alteration of vent size

ventral anatomical direction, referring to structures that are located toward the front or away from the backbone; SYN: anterior; ANT: posterior

ventral acoustic stria second-order fiber bundle leaving the AVCN and projecting ventrally and medially to distribute fibers to the ipsilateral LSO and MSO and continuing across midline to distribute fibers to the contralateral MSO and MNTB; SYN: trapezoid body

ventral cochlear nucleus anterior ventral cochlear nucleus; portion of the cochlear nucleus that receives primary afferent projections from Cranial Nerve VIII and sends second-order fibers via the ventral acoustic stria to the superior olivary complex

ventral nucleus of the lateral lemniscus LLV; one of three fiber tracts constituting auditory nuclei of the pons that serves as a relay for ascending auditory fibers from the AVCN, LSO, and MSO in the hindbrain to the inferior colliculus

ventricle a normal cavity in the brain

ventrolateral inferior colliculus afferent portion of the central nucleus of the inferior colliculus that receives ascending input from the cochlear nucleus and superior olivary complex

VEP visual evoked potential; electrophysiologic responses to light changes

verbotonal method a program designed to enhance speech and language development in children who are severely hearing impaired by maximizing input at those frequencies at which they have residual hearing

vermis wormlike structure, usually referring to the median portion between the two hemispheres of the cerebellum

vernix fatty substance covering the skin of a fetus

vertebrobasilar ischemia reduced blood flow or mechanical compression of the vertebral or basilar arteries, often resulting in transient episodes of vertigo due to ischemia involving the vestibular nuclei

vertex summit, top, or crown of the head

vertex electrode electrode that is placed at the top and center of the head; the noninverting or active electrode in conventional auditory brainstem response recordings; SYN: Cz electrode

vertex negative denoting the negative polarity of an evoked potential peak when the vertex is designated as the noninverting electrode

vertex positive denoting the positive polarity of an evoked potential peak when the vertex is designated as the noninverting electrode

vertex potential any evoked potential that is most prominent when recorded at the vertex

vertex response, auditory late vertex response

vertex response, late auditory evoked potential, having two main waveform peaks—a vertex negative peak at approximately 90 msec following signal presentation and a vertex positive peak at approximately 180 msec following signal presentation; SYN: long-latency auditory evoked potential

vertex response, slow late vertex response

vertical gaze nystagmus nystagmus in upward or downward gaze directions, consistent with central nervous system pathology

vertical localization identification of the direction of a sound source in the vertical plane

vertical spontaneous nystagmus normal nystagmus in the vertical direction with eyes closed

vertiginous pertaining to or experiencing vertigo

vertigo a form of dizziness, describing a definite sensation of spinning or whirling

vertigo, apoplectiform single or recurring, sudden, severe attack of vertigo accompanied by nausea and vomiting, often caused by vestibular neuritis

vertigo, aural nonspecific term for sensation of motion caused by labyrinthine disorders

vertigo, benign paroxysmal positioning BPPV; a recurrent, acute form of vertigo occurring in clusters in response to positional changes

vertigo, objective a sensation of external objects spinning or whirling around the person

vertigo, paroxysmal sudden, brief episodes of dizziness and nystagmus, often accompanied by nausea and vomiting

vertigo, paroxysmal positioning a recurrent, acute form of vertigo due to semicircular canal dysfunction, occurring in clusters in response to positional changes; SYN: benign paroxysmal positioning vertigo

vertigo, positional dizziness that occurs when the head is placed in a certain position and that does not involve head movement

vertigo, reflexogenic nystagmus and vertigo resulting from stimulation of the utricular macula when positive pressure is placed on the stapes footplate, via pneumatic otoscopy, tympanometry, stapedius muscle contraction, etc.,

vertigo, subjective a sensation that one is spinning or whirling

VES vestibular eye speed; measure of nystagmus expressed as the speed of the slow phase: SYN: slow-phase velocity

vesicle small sac containing fluid

vesicle, auditory otic vesicle

vesicle, otic saclike cavity formed by closure of the auditory pit in the human embryo from which the cochlea develops

vessel channel or duct conveying body fluid

vestibular pertaining to the vestibule

vestibular aqueduct small canal in the medial wall of the vestibule containing the endolymphatic duct

vestibular atelectasis collapse of the walls of the utricle and ampullae, compressing the sensory epithelia, resulting in acute severe vertiginous episodes with nausea and vomiting

vestibular autorotation test VAT; vestibular assessment in which the patient wears a headband containing a sensor to measure the rotational velocity of the head as it moves in synchrony with stimuli in vertical and horizontal direction; EOG is also used to record eye movement

vestibular eye speed VES; measure of nystagmus expressed as the speed of the slow phase: SYN: slow-phase velocity

vestibular fibrosis fibrous tissue proliferation within the vestibule secondary to endolymphatic hydrops

vestibular ganglia two adjacent cell-body masses of the peripheral vestibular neurons, located in the internal auditory canal, associated with the superior and infe-

rior divisions of the vestibular nerve portion of Cranial Nerve VIII; SYN: Scarpa's ganglia

vestibular membrane Reissner's membrane, separating the scala vestibuli and scala media

vestibular Ménière's disease atypical form of Ménière's disease in which only the characteristic vestibular symptoms are present without hearing loss

vestibular nerve portion of Cranial Nerve VIII consisting of nerve fibers from the maculae of the utricle and saccule and the cristae of the superior, lateral, and posterior semicircular canals

vestibular neuritis inflammation of the vestibular nerve, often of a viral nature, resulting in a single episode of severe vertigo that is prolonged and gradually subsides over a period of days or weeks

vestibular neuronitis inflammation of the vestibular nerve characterized by recurring episodes of disequilibrium and persistent or intermittent unsteadiness

vestibular neurons, peripheral neurons of the superior and inferior division of the vestibular portion of Cranial Nerve VIII, located in the internal auditory meatus

vestibular nuclei superior, lateral, medial, and inferior nuclei of the vestibular system, located in the upper medulla oblongata, and serving as the initial obligatory stop for vestibular nerve fibers

vestibular system biological system that, in conjunction with the ocular and proprioceptive systems, functions to maintain equilibrium

vestibular window oval window opening in the labyrinthine wall of the middle ear space leading into the scala vestibuli of the cochlea, into which the footplate of the stapes fits; SYN: oval window, fenestra vestibuli

vestibule ovoid cavity forming the central portion of the bony labyrinth continuous with the semicircular canals and cochlea, that contains the utricle and saccule and communicates with the tympanum through the oval window

vestibulocochlear artery branch of the common cochlear artery that divides into the posterior vestibular artery and the cochlear ramus, supplying the saccule, posterior semicircular canal, and the basal end of the cochlea

vestibulocochlear nerve Cranial Nerve VIII, consisting of a vestibular and a cochlear branch

vestibulofacial anastomosis joining of a small bundle of fibers from the superior vestibular nerve with the sensory portion of the facial nerve in the internal auditory meatus

vestibulo-ocular reflex VOR; reflex arc between the vestibular system and extraocular muscles, activated by asymmetric neural firing rate of the vestibular nerve, serving to maintain gaze stability by generating compensatory eye movements in response to head rotation

vestibulopathy degeneration of the vestibular labyrinth, particularly with aging, resulting in motion-induced vertigo

vestibulospinal tract neural pathway from the vestibular nuclei to the spinal cord for postural reflexes

vestibulotoxic having a poisonous action on the hair cells of the cristae and macullae of the vestibular labyrinth; COM: cochleotoxic, ototoxic

vestibulotoxicity the property of being vestibulotoxic; COM: cochleotoxicity, ototoxicity

vibration vibratory motion

vibratory motion oscillation of an object between two points

vibrotactile pertaining to the detection of vibrations via the sense of touch

vibrotactile hearing aid device designed for profound hearing loss in which acoustic energy is converted to vibratory energy and delivered to the skin

vibrotactile response in bone-conduction audiometry, a response to a signal that was perceived by tactile stimulation rather than auditory stimulation

video otoscopy endoscopic examination of the external auditory meatus and tympanic membrane displayed on a video monitor

VIOLA Visual Input/Output Locator Algorithm; computer-assisted method for selection of hearing aid parameters based on the determination of loudness growth

viomycin aminoglycoside antibiotic, used extensively for the treatment of tuberculosis, which is ototoxic, particularly to the vestibular system

VIP VePesid, ifosfamide, cisplatin (platinol), mesna; potentially ototoxic chemotherapy regimen used in the treatment of testicular cancer

viral labyrinthitis inflammation of the labyrinth due to viral infections, including mumps, measles, rubella, and herpes zoster oticus

viscera organs of the digestive, respiratory, urogenital, and endocrine systems

viscid sticky; adhesive

viscosity the property of fluid that resists change in shape during its flow

viscous viscid

viseme one in a group of speech sounds that appear identically on the lips, e.g., [p], [b], [m]

visual alerting systems household devices such as alarm clocks, doorbells, and fire alarms in which the alerting sound is replaced by flashing light

visual cue any gesture, posture, or facial expression that adds meaning to spoken language

Visual Input/Output Locator Algorithm VIOLA; computer-assisted method for selection of hearing aid parameters based on the determination of loudness growth

visual reinforcement audiometry VRA; audiometric technique used in pediatric assessment in which a correct response to signal presentation, such as a head turn toward the speaker, is rewarded by the activation of a light or lighted toy

VLBW very low birth weight; classification of newborns based on birth weight, specifically any infant with a birth weight less than 1500 grams

Voit's nerve saccular branch of the vestibular nerve

volley principle theory of cochlear function stating that nerve impulses resulting from low-frequency stimulation are grouped together in successive bursts or volleys

volt V; unit of electromotive force producing a current of 1 ampere through a resistance of 1 ohm

voltmeter instrument for measuring electromotive force

volume generic term for magnitude or loudness of sound

volume, equivalent in immittance measurement, the translation of changes in probe-tone SPL into volume changes, so that an increase in SPL would appear as a decrease in equivalent volume of a cavity and a decrease in SPL would appear as a increase in equivalent volume

volume control   VC; manual or automatic control designed to adjust the output level of a hearing instrument

volume test, physical   PVT; subtest of immittance audiometry in which the volume of the ear canal is estimated; e.g., a large volume is found in the case of a tympanic membrane perforation or a patent PE tube and a small volume in the case of impacted cerumen

volume unit meter   VU meter; visual indicator on an audiometer showing intensity of an input signal in dB, where 0 dB is equal to the attenuator output setting

von Recklinghausen's disease   autosomal dominant disease characterized by café-au-lait spots and multiple cutaneous tumors, with associated optic gliomas, peripheral and spinal neurofibromas, and, rarely, acoustic neuromas; SYN: neurofibromatosis I

VOR   vestibulo-ocular reflex; reflex arc between the vestibular system and extraocular muscles, activated by asymmetric neural firing rate of the vestibular nerve, serving to generate compensatory eye movements in response to head rotation

VRA   visual reinforcement audiometry; audiometric technique used in pediatric assessment in which a correct response to signal presentation, such as a head turn toward the speaker, is rewarded by the activation of a light or lighted toy

VU meter   volume unit meter; visual indicator on an audiometer showing intensity of an input signal in dB, where 0 dB is equal to the attenuator output setting

W

W watt; unit of electrical power with a current of 1 ampere and an electromotive force of 1 volt

W-1 list of 36 spondaic words, developed at the Central Institute for the Deaf, commonly used in the determination of speech-reception threshold; SYN: CID Auditory Test W-1

W-2 version of the CID Auditory Test W-1 in which the 36 spondees were recorded with 3 dB of attenuation for every three words; SYN: CID Auditory Test W-2

W-22 word-recognition test developed at the Central Institute for the Deaf consisting of four lists of 50 monosyllabic words; SYN: CID Auditory Test W-22

Waardenburg syndrome autosomal dominant disorder characterized by lateral displacement of the medial canthi, increased width of the root of the nose, multicolored iris, white forelock, and mild to severe sensorineural hearing loss

Waldenstrom's macroglobulinemia vascular disorder characterized by increased blood viscosity and increased resistance to blood flow, one neurological manifestation of which is sudden, bilateral, progressive sensorineural hearing loss

Walsh-Healey noise standard noise-exposure standard, promulgated in 1969 as part of the Walsh-Healey Public Contracts Act, that recommended limiting exposure to steady-state noise to a level of 90 dBA over an 8-hour work day

Walsh-Healey Public Contracts Act act that authorized the U.S. Department of Labor to impose certain regulations on employers who have contracts with the government, including the regulation of employee exposure to noise

warble tone frequency-modulated pure tone, often used in sound field audiometry

watch tick test crude assessment of high-frequency hearing sensitivity in which a patient's ability to hear the ticking of a time piece is evaluated

watt W; unit of electrical power with a current of 1 ampere and an electromotive force of 1 volt

wave orderly disturbance of the molecules of a medium caused by the vibratory motion of an object; propagated disturbance in a medium

wave, longitudinal type of pressure wave movement, such as a sound wave, in which particle movement is parallel to the wave movement

wave, transverse wave in which the particles of the medium move at right angles to the direction of the wave movement

wave, traveling sound-induced displacement pattern along the basilar membrane that describes fundamental cochlear processing, characterized by maximum displacement at a location corresponding to the frequency of the signal

waveform form or shape of a wave, represented graphically as magnitude as a function of time

wavelength length of a sound wave, defined as the distance in space that 1 cycle occupies

wax colloquial term for cerumen, or the waxy secretion of the ceruminous glands in the external auditory meatus

wax guard shield placed over the end of a custom hearing aid, designed to prevent or reduce accumulation of cerumen in the receiver

WDRC wide-dynamic-range compression; hearing aid compression algorithm, with a low threshold of activation, designed to distribute signals between a listener's thresholds of sensitivity and discomfort in a manner that matches loudness growth

WDS word-discrimination score; word-recognition score

weakness, bilateral BW; hypoactivity of vestibular system to caloric stimulation in both ears, consistent with bilateral peripheral vestibular disorder

weakness, unilateral UW; measure in percentage of the difference in magnitude of nystagmus from right-ear versus left-ear bithermal caloric stimulation; a difference exceeding 20% is considered to be abnormal

Weber test test in which a tuning fork or bone vibrator is placed on the midline of the forehead; lateralization to the poorer-hearing ear suggests the presence of a conductive hearing loss, lateralization to the better ear suggests sensorineural hearing loss

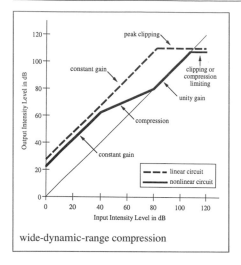

wide-dynamic-range compression

Weber test, audiometric Weber test in which the bone-conduction vibrator of an audiometer (rather than a tuning fork) is placed on the forehead at midline, and the patient indicates the location of sound in the head

Wegener granulomatosis syndrome of necrotizing granulomatous vasculitis of the airway and kidneys, which can result in otitis media with effusion, and occasional secondary sensorineural loss, due to encroachment on the eustachian tube by the granuloma

weighting scale sound level meter filtering network, such as the dBA scale, that is based on emphasizing the measurement of one band of frequencies over another

well-baby nursery hospital unit designed to provide care for healthy newborns

Wernicke's area in early classification system, term for the cortical region in the temporal lobe responsible for reception of oral language

WFL within functional limits

WFR wearer frequency response; early term for real-ear unaided response

white noise broad-band noise having similar energy at all frequencies

whole-nerve action potential 1. synchronous change in electrical potential of the fibers of a nerve; 2. in auditory-evoked potential measures, compound action potential of Cranial Nerve VIII, represented as the main component of the ECochG and Wave I of the ABR

wide-band noise white noise

wide-dynamic-range compression WDRC; hearing aid compression algorithm, with a low threshold of activation, designed to deliver signals between a listener's thresholds of sensitivity and discomfort in a manner that matches loudness growth; SYN: full-dynamic-range compression

wide-range having a broader than conventional frequency response or other capability

wide-range audiometer early term describing an audiometer with a full range of audiometric frequencies and air- and bone-conduction capabilities

wide-range earmold earmold designed with the specific function of providing maximum acoustic enhancement at the higher frequencies around 5000 Hz

Wildervanck syndrome congenital branchial arch syndrome, occurring primarily in females, characterized by fusion of two or more cervical vertebrae, similar to Klippel-Feil syndrome, with retraction of eyeballs, lateral gaze weakness, and hearing loss; SYN: cervico-oculo-acoustic syndrome

window, cochlear SYN: round window; fenestra rotunda

window, oval oval window opening in the labyrinthine wall of the middle ear space leading into the scala vestibuli of the cochlea, into which the footplate of the stapes fits; SYN: vestibular window, fenestra vestibuli

window, round membrane-covered opening in the labyrinthine wall of the middle ear space, leading into the scala tympani of the cochlea; SYN: cochlear window; fenestra rotunda

window, vestibular SYN: oval window, fenestra vestibuli

windscreen shield placed around a microphone, designed to reduce wind-related noise

WIPI word intelligibility by picture identification test; pediatric test of monosyllabic word-recognition ability in which a closed-set picture-pointing task is used to identify the target word

WNL within normal limits

word, monosyllabic word of one syllable

word deafness inexact term describing

the inability to understand spoken language, as in fluent or receptive aphasia

word discrimination   word recognition

word intelligibility   word recognition

word intelligibility by picture identification test   WIPI; pediatric test of monosyllabic word-recognition ability in which a closed-set picture-pointing task is used to identify the target word

word list, NU-6   Northwestern University Auditory Test Number 6; monosyllabic word-recognition measure, designed to be phonetically balanced within a word list

word list, PAL PB-50   Psycho-Acoustic Laboratory (Harvard University) phonetically balanced 50 (word list); one of the earliest word-recognition measures, designed to be phonetically balanced within a word list

word list, PB   phonetically balanced word list; list of words used in word-recognition testing that contain speech sounds that oc-

cur with the same frequency as those of conversational speech

word list, PBK   phonetically balanced kindergarten word lists; lists of words used in word-recognition testing, designed both to be phonetically balanced and to contain words that are at a vocabulary level appropriate for use with young school children

word list, W-22   word-recognition test developed at the Central Institute for the Deaf consisting of four lists of 50 monosyllabic words; SYN: CID Auditory Test W-22

word recognition   the ability to perceive and identify a word; SYN: word discrimination, word intelligibility

word-recognition score   WRS; percentage of correctly identified words

word-recognition test   speech audiometric measure of the ability to identify monosyllabic words, usually presented in quiet

WRS   word-recognition score

X

X reactance; opposition to energy flow due to storage

X-linked hearing disorder hereditary hearing disorder due to a faulty gene located on the X chromosome, such as that found in Alport syndrome or Hunter syndrome

X-linked inheritance any genetic trait related to the X chromosome; transmitted by a mother to 50% of her sons, who will be affected, and 50% of her daughters, who will be carriers; transmitted by a father to 100% of his daughters

x-ray electromagnetic radiation of very short wavelength

x-ray irradiation injury atrophy of the membranous labyrinth, particularly the spiral and annular ligaments, secondary to x-ray irradiation, resulting in delayed-onset, progressive, sensorineural hearing loss

x-y recorder graphic display device that draws the relation between two variables on the x and y axes

xanthoma soft tissue tumor, containing lipid infiltrate, which may occur anywhere in the temporal bone in association with a metabolic disorder or ear infection

XO syndrome chromosomal abnormality leading to an XO configuration with 45 chromosomes; results in small stature, obesity, low hairline, webbing of digits, narrow palate, and anomalous auricles, with associated conductive and sensorineural hearing loss; SYN: Turner syndrome

Y

Y admittance; total energy flow through a system, expressed in mhos; reciprocal of impedance

Y-cord hearing aid early body-worn hearing aid with the output of the amplifier directed to both ears by a Y-shaped cord

yes-no audiometry technique for establishing auditory thresholds in children or others who are exaggerating hearing loss by asking them to respond by saying "yes" when they hear the tone that is presented and "no" when they do not hear the tone that is presented

Z

Z impedance; total opposition to energy flow or resistance to the absorption of energy, expressed in ohms

Zeta noise blocker early digital signal-processing noise-reduction algorithm in which signals were separated by temporal characteristics, with attenuation of the frequency bands containing longer time constants assumed to be noise

zona arcuata medial portion of the basilar membrane with a single fibrous layer, ranging from the inner hair cells medially to the outer pillars laterally

zona pectinata portion of the basilar membrane with two fibrous layers, ranging from the outer pillars medially to the medial tip of the spiral ligament laterally

Zwislocki coupler Zwislocki ear simulator

Zwislocki ear simulator a hard-wall cylindrical cavity that connects a hearing aid receiver to the microphone of a sound level meter, with acoustic impedances designed to be more like those of a human ear across the frequency range than the conventional 2-cc coupler

zygote cell formed by the union of male and female gametes

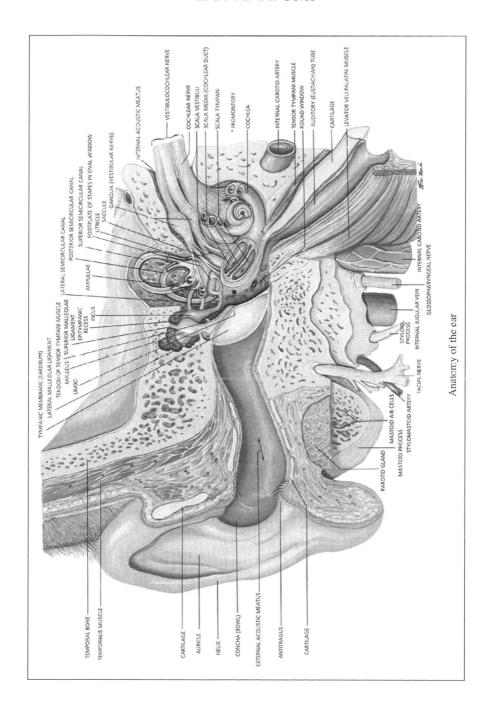

Anatomy of the ear

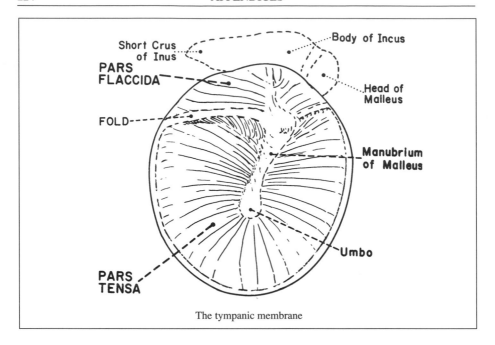

The tympanic membrane

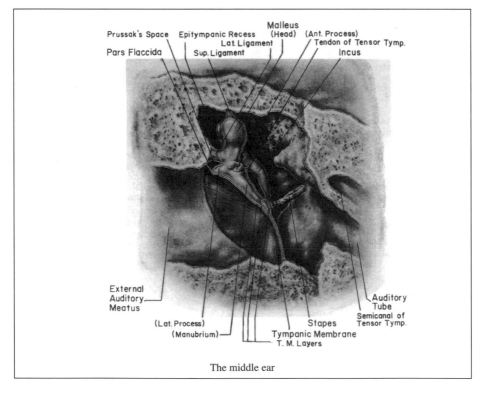

The middle ear

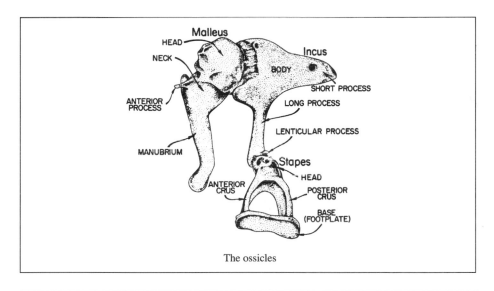

The ossicles

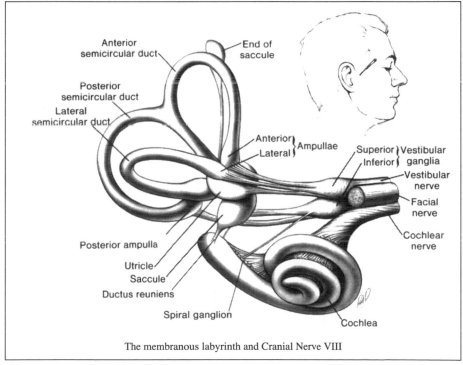

The membranous labyrinth and Cranial Nerve VIII

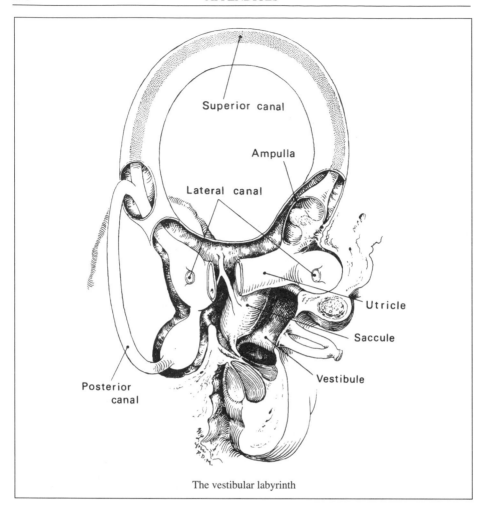

The vestibular labyrinth

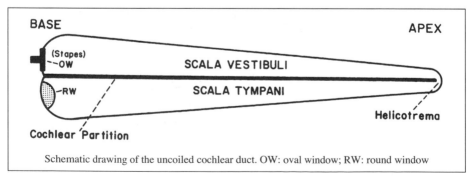

Schematic drawing of the uncoiled cochlear duct. OW: oval window; RW: round window

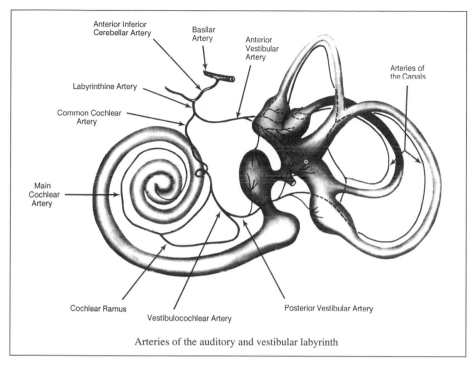

Arteries of the auditory and vestibular labyrinth

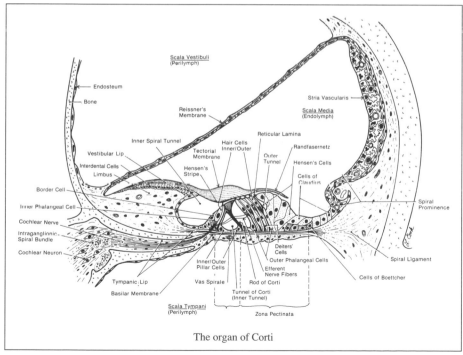

The organ of Corti

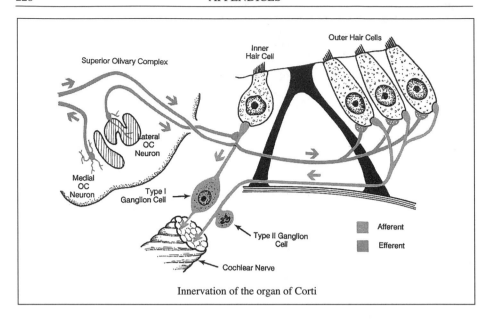

Innervation of the organ of Corti

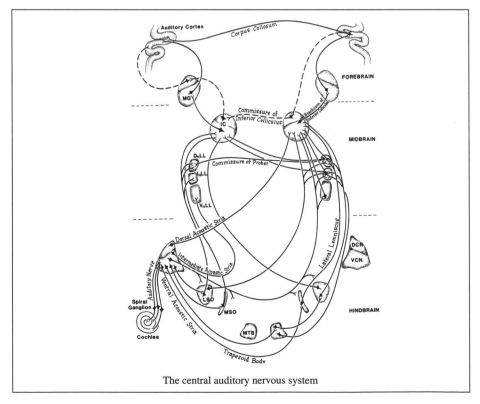

The central auditory nervous system

AUDIOMETRIC SYMBOLS

The figures below are standard for audiometric use, according to the Guidelines for Audiometric Symbols of the American Speech-Language-Hearing Association. Colors may also be used to distinguish ears, with red representing the right ear and blue representing the left ear. If a response is not present at equipment limits, the symbol is plotted at that limit with a small arrow extending downward from the symbol to the right for the left ear and the left for the right ear. The shaded area represents the limits of normal hearing based on convention.

The figures below are often used in scientific publications and have found widespread clinical acceptance. Ears are plotted separately. If a response is not present at equipment limits, no symbol is plotted. The shaded area represents audiometric zero plus and minus two standard deviations.

Representative audiograms plotted with the two symbol systems are presented on the following pages for normal hearing, mild conductive hearing loss, severe mixed hearing loss, and high-frequency sensorineural hearing loss.

Key to Symbols	Ear		
	Left	Unspecified	Right
AC			
Unmasked	✕		◯
Masked	☐		△
BC - mastoid			
Unmasked	>	^	<
Masked	⊐		⊏
BC - forehead			
Unmasked		⌄	
Masked	Γ		⌐
Sound Field		S	
Acoustic Reflex			
Contralateral	>-		-<
Ipsilateral	⊢		⊣

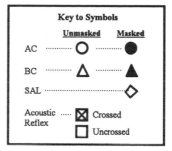

229

Normal Hearing Sensivitivity

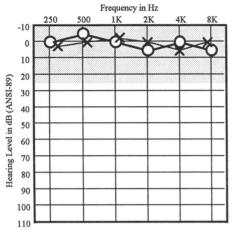

Mild Conductive Hearing Loss

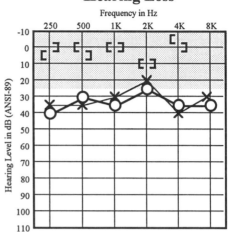

Severe Mixed Hearing Loss

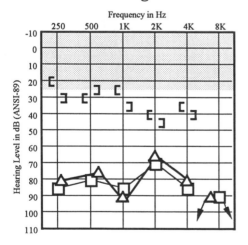

High-Frequency Sensorineural Hearing Loss

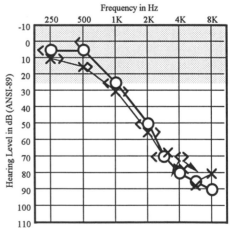

Normal Hearing Sensivitivity

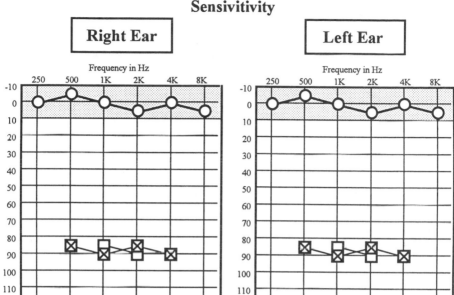

Mild Conductive Hearing Loss

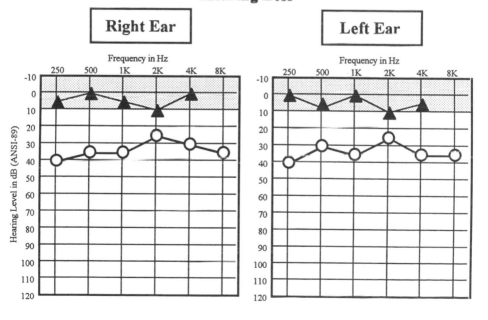

Severe Mixed
Hearing Loss

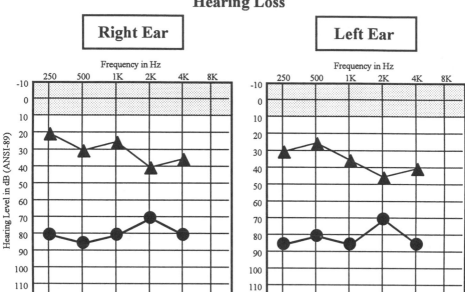

High-Frequency
Sensorineural
Hearing Loss

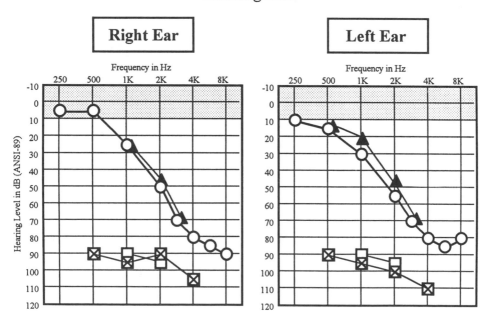

ACRONYMS, ABBREVIATIONS, AND SYMBOLS

A1   left (1) earlobe (a) electrode location, typically used for inverting-electrode placement in auditory evoked potential testing, according to the 10 20 International Electrode System nomenclature

A2   right (2) earlobe (a) electrode location, typically used for inverting-electrode placement in auditory evoked potential testing, according to the 10–20 International Electrode System nomenclature

AAA   American Academy of Audiology; professional association of audiologists founded in 1988

AAMD   American Association on Mental Deficiency; professional organization of specialists from many fields who provide care for individuals with mental retardation

AAO-HNS   American Academy of Otolaryngology—Head and Neck Surgery; professional organization of otolaryngologists

AAOHN   American Association of Occupational Health Nurses

AAOO   American Academy of Ophthalmology and Otolaryngology; former professional association that divided into two organization, the American Academy of Ophthalmology and the AAO-HNS

AAP   American Academy of Pediatrics; professional organization of pediatricians

AARP   American Association of Retired Persons; consumer organization of people over the age of 55

AAS   American Auditory Society; multidisciplinary association of professionals in audiology, otolaryngology, hearing science, and the hearing industry; formerly American Audiology Society

ABESPA   American Board of Examiners in Speech-Language Pathology and Audiology; independent organization responsible for the national examination in audiology and speech-language pathology

ABI   1. auditory behavior index; classification of expected behavioral responses from infants and young children; 2. auditory brainstem implant; electrode implanted at the juncture of Cranial Nerve VIII and the cochlear nucleus that receives signals from an external processor and sends electrical impulses directly to the brainstem

ABLB   alternate binaural loudness balance test; auditory test designed to measure loudness growth or recruitment in the impaired ear of a patient with unilateral hearing loss

ABO   American Board of Otolaryngology

ABR   auditory brainstem response; auditory evoked potential, originating from Cranial Nerve VIII and auditory brainstem structures, consisting of five to seven identifiable peaks that represent neural function of auditory pathways and nuclei

AC   air conduction; transmission of sound, delivered by an earphone, through the outer and middle ear to the cochlea; COM: BC
alternating current; electric current that periodically changes its value or direction of flow

ACE   Award for Continuing Education; certificate given by the American Speech-Language-Hearing Association for completion of a prescribed number of continuing education units

ACh   acetylcholine; excitatory neurotransmitter, released in synaptic regions, that controls the action of muscles and nervous system receptors

ACOEM   American College of Occupational and Environmental Medicine

AD   [L. *auris dextra*] right ear

ADA   1. Academy of Dispensing Audiologists; organization of audiologists with a particular interest in dispensing hearing aids; 2. Americans with Disabilities Act; United States law enacted to provide equal access for individuals with disabilities

ADC   analog-to-digital conversion; the process of turning a continuously varying (analog) waveform into a numerical (digital) representation of the waveform

ADD   attention deficit disorder; SYN: ADHD

ADHD   attention deficit hyperactivity disorder; cognitive disorder involving reduced ability to focus on an activity, task, or sensory stimulus, characterized by restlessness and distractibility; SYN: ADD

AEF auditory evoked field; electromagnetic response of the auditory nervous system

AEP auditory evoked potential; SYN: AER

AER auditory evoked response; electrophysiologic response to sound, usually distinguished according to latency, including ECoG, ABR, MLR, LVR, SSEP, P3

AERA averaged evoked response audiometry; audiometry using auditory evoked potentials to predict hearing sensitivity

AFR adaptive frequency response; hearing aid circuitry technique in which frequency response changes as input level changes

AGC automatic gain control; nonlinear hearing aid compression circuitry designed to automatically change gain as signal level changes or limit output when signal level reaches a specified criterion; SYN: automatic volume control

AGC−I automatic gain control−input; circuitry of a hearing aid in which the volume control follows the AGC

AGC−O automatic gain control−output; circuitry of a hearing aid in which the AGC follows the volume control

AI articulation index or audibility index; measure of the proportion of speech cues that are audible; SYN: SII

AICA anterior inferior cerebellar artery; large vessel arising from the basilar artery, a branch of which is the labyrinthine artery, which supplies blood to the cochlea

AIDS acquired immunodeficiency syndrome; disease compromising the efficacy of the immune system, characterized by opportunistic infectious diseases

ALD assistive listening device; hearing instrument or class of hearing instruments, usually with a remote microphone for improving signal-to-noise ratio, including FM systems, personal amplifiers, telephone amplifiers, television listeners

ALR auditory late response; evoked potential, originating from the cortex and having two main waveform peaks, a vertex negative peak at approximately 90 msec and a vertex positive peak at approximately 180 msec following signal presentation; SYN: LLAEP

AM amplitude modulation; the process of varying the magnitude of a radio wave or sound wave in relation to the strength of the carrier wave; COM: FM

AMA American Medical Association

Ameslan American Sign Language; common form of manual communication used in the United States

amg amgaminoglycoside; any of a group of bacteriocidal antibiotics, which are often cochleotoxic and/or vestibulotoxic, derived from streptomyces or micromonosporum used primarily against gram-negative bacteria, including streptomycin, neomycin, kanamycin, and gentamicin

AMLB alternate monaural loudness balance test; auditory test designed to measure loudness growth or recruitment in an ear with normal hearing sensitivity at some frequencies and sensorineural hearing loss at others

AMLR auditory middle latency response; auditory evoked potential, originating from the region of the auditory radiations and cortex, having as a primary component a vertex positive peak at 25 msec to 40 msec following signal presentation; SYN: MLR

AN 1. acoustic neuroma; generic term referring to a neoplasm of Cranial Nerve VIII, most often a cochleovestibular Schwannoma; SYN: acoustic tumor; 2. auditory nerve; Cranial Nerve VIII, consisting of a vestibular and cochlear branch; SYN: vestibulocochlear nerve

ANC adaptive noise canceler; multiple microphone instrument that attempts to reduce background noise by changing the hearing aid microphone's directionality adaptively

ANS 1. American Neurotology Society; professional organization of otolaryngologists who have a special interest in neurotology; 2. autonomic nervous system; that portion of the nervous system that regulates glandular and visceral responses

ANSI American National Standards Institute; association of specialists, manufacturers, and consumers that determines standards for measuring instruments, including audiometers; formerly ASA

AOM acute otitis media; inflammation of the middle ear having a duration of fewer than 21 days

AOR   audito-oculogyric reflex; rapid turning of the eyes toward the source of a sudden sound

AP   action potential; 1. synchronous change in electrical potential of nerve or muscle tissue; 2. in auditory evoked potential measures, whole-nerve or compound action potential of Cranial Nerve VIII, the main component of ECochG and Wave I of the ABR

APD   auditory processing disorder; reduction in the ability to manipulate acoustic signals, despite normal hearing sensitivity and regardless of language, attention, and cognition ability; SYN: central auditory processing disorder

APHAB   Abbreviated Profile of Hearing Aid Benefit; self-assessment questionnaire consisting of four subscales used for evaluating benefit received from amplification

APR   auropalpebral reflex; eyeblink or twitch at the canthus caused by a sudden loud sound

AR   acoustic reflex; reflexive contraction of the intra-aural muscles in response to loud sound, dominated by the stapedius muscle in humans; SYN: acoustic stapedial reflex

ARA   Academy of Rehabilitative Audiology; association of audiologists with a particular interest in rehabilitation issues

ARO   Association for Research in Otolaryngology; professional organization devoted to research related to ear, nose, and throat diseases and functions

ART   acoustic reflex threshold; lowest intensity level of a stimulus at which an acoustic reflex is detected

AS   [L. *auris sinistra*] left ear

ASA   Acoustical Society of America
American Standards Association; former name of American National Standards Institute

ASHA   American Speech-Language-Hearing Association; professional organization of audiologists and speech-language pathologists; formerly American Speech and Hearing Association

ASL   American Sign Language; common form of manual communication used in the United States

ASNHL   asymmetric sensorineural hearing loss

ASP   1. adaptive signal processing; SYN: automatic signal processing; 2. automatic signal processing; hearing aid circuitry that adjusts some parameter of the amplified output automatically or adaptively as the input signal reaches a certain criterion

ATA   American Tinnitus Association; consumer organization of people with tinnitus

ATP   adenosine triphosphate; neurochemical substance produced by the stria vascularis

AU   [L. *auris uterque*] each ear; [L. *aures unitas*] both ears together

AuD   Doctor of Audiology; designator for professional doctorate degree in audiology

AVC   automatic volume control

AVCN   anterior ventral cochlear nucleus; portion of the cochlear nucleus that receives primary afferent projections from Cranial Nerve VIII and sends second-order fibers via the ventral acoustic stria to the superior olivary complex

B   susceptance; energy flow associated with reactance; reciprocal of reactance

BADGE   Békésy ascending descending gap evaluation test; variation of Békésy audiometry, used to detect functional hearing loss, in which the tracking levels obtained with an ascending and descending approach are compared for discrepancies

BAEP   brainstem auditory evoked potential; SYN: auditory brainstem response

BAER   brainstem auditory evoked response; SYN auditory brainstem response

BBN   broad-band noise; sound with a wide bandwidth, containing a continuous spectrum of frequencies, with equal energy per cycle throughout the band

BC   bone conduction; transmission of sound to the cochlea by vibration of the skull; COM: AC

BC-HIS   board-certified in hearing instrument sciences; credential awarded to qualifying hearing instrument specialists by the National Board for Certification in Hearing Instrument Sciences

BCL   Békésy comfortable loudness test; variant of Bekesy audiometry, used to detect functional hearing loss, in which pulsed and continuous tracings are obtained at comfortable loudness rather than threshold

BERA   brainstem evoked response audiometry; brainstem electric response audiometry

BHI   Better Hearing Institute

BICROS bilateral contralateral routing of signals; a hearing aid system with one microphone contained in a hearing aid at each ear; the microphones lead to a single amplifier and receiver in the better hearing ear of a person with bilateral asymmetric hearing loss

BIFROS bilateral frontal routing of signals; hearing aid system with microphones placed in the front of eyeglass hearing aids

BILL bass increase at low levels; type of automatic signal processing in a hearing aid that uses level-dependent control of the frequency response, reducing low frequencies in response to high-intensity input

BMLD binaural masking level difference; measure of binaural release from masking in which binaural thresholds are determined in noise for tones that are in phase and 180° out of phase

BMT bilateral myringotomy tube

BOA behavioral observation audiometry; pediatric assessment of hearing by observation of a child's unconditioned responses to sounds

BOE bilateral otitis externa

BOM bilateral otitis media

BOMA bilateral otitis media, acute

BP bipolar; pertaining to an electrode array with two poles

BPPN benign paroxysmal positioning nystagmus; sudden, transient burst of nystagmus during the Dix-Hallpike maneuver, which disappears within 10 seconds once the head position is achieved

BPPV benign paroxysmal positional vertigo; a recurrent, acute form of vertigo occurring in clusters in response to positional changes

BRA brainstem response audiometry

BSAER brainstem auditory evoked response; SYN: auditory brainstem response

BSER brainstem evoked response; SYN: auditory brainstem response

BSERA brainstem evoked response audiometry

BSOM bilateral serous otitis media

BTA brief-tone audiometry; test developed to identify cochlear site of lesion, in which thresholds are obtained for 100-msec tone bursts and 10-msec tone bursts; normal threshold reduction is 10 dB for a tenfold decrease in duration

BTE behind-the-ear hearing aid; a hearing aid that fits over the ear and is coupled to the ear canal via an earmold; SYN: postauricular hearing aid

BW bilateral weakness; hypoactivity of vestibular system to caloric stimulation in both ears, consistent with bilateral peripheral vestibular disorder

C compliance; measure of the ease of energy transfer through the outer and middle ear; reciprocal of stiffness

C tracing continuous tracing; graph that results from threshold tracking in Békésy audiometry to a continuous pure tone at a fixed or swept frequency; ANT: interrupted tracing

C8 Cranial Nerve VIII; auditory nerve, consisting of a vestibular and a cochlear branch; SYN: vestibulocochlear nerve

CA chronological age; age of an individual from date of birth

CA processing compressed analog processing; cochlear implant processing strategy in which speech signals are divided into frequency bands and delivered to corresponding implant electrodes

Ca++ chemical symbol for calcium

CAD central auditory disorder; functional disorder resulting from diseases of or trauma to the central auditory nervous system

cal tone calibration tone; a 1000-Hz tone preceding recorded speech materials that is used to adjust an audiometer's VU meter to insure identical output calibration of speech signals from one test session to the next

CANS central auditory nervous system; portion from Cranial Nerve VIII to the auditory cortex that involves hearing, including the cochlear nucleus, superior olivary complex, lateral lemniscus, inferior colliculus, medial geniculate, and auditory cortex

CAOHC Council for Accreditation in Occupational Hearing Conservation; multidisciplinary coordinating body involved in the training and certification of occupational hearing conservationists

CAP 1. central auditory processing; function of the central auditory nervous system, including sound localization, lateralization, binaural processes, speech perception, etc.; 2. compound action potential; a. synchronous change in electrical potential of nerve or muscle tissue; b. in auditory evoked potential measures, whole-nerve potential of Cranial Nerve VIII, the main component of ECochG and Wave I of the ABR

CAPD central auditory processing disorder; disorder in function of central auditory structures, characterized by impaired ability of the central auditory nervous system to manipulate and use acoustic signals

CAPS communication assessment procedure for seniors; a self-assessment inventory used for evaluating the communication needs of aging patients

CAT scan computerized axial tomography scan; sectional radiographs of specified areas of the brain presented as a computer-generated image representing a synthesis of x-rays obtained from different directions on a given plane

cc cubic centimeter; measure of volume; 1 cc equals 1 ml

CC closed captioning; printed text of the dialogue or narrative on television or video that is available only with an adapter or special circuitry

CCC-A Certificate of Clinical Competence in Audiology; certification awarded by the American Speech-Language-Hearing Association to individuals who have met the academic and clinical requirements necessary to become audiologists

CCM contralateral competing message; in speech audiometry, noise or other competing signal that is delivered to the ear opposite the ear receiving the target signal; ANT: ICM

CCS Crippled Children's Services; state-funded organization that provides financial assistance for healthcare and other services to children with disabilities

CCT California Consonant Test; adult speech audiometric test of monosyllabic word recognition that is particularly useful in assessing the influence of high-frequency hearing loss on speech recognition

CD communication disorder; impairment in communication ability, resulting from speech, language, and/or hearing disorders

CDP computerized dynamic posturography; quantitative assessment of integrated function of the balance system for postural stability during quiet and perturbed stance, using a computer-based moving platform and motion transducers

CEC Council on Exceptional Children

CERA 1. cardiac evoked response audiometry; electrophysiologic technique for predicting hearing sensitivity by measuring changes in heart rate in response to auditory stimulation; 2. cortical evoked response audiometry; electrophysiologic technique for predicting hearing sensitivity by measuring late-latency auditory evoked responses to auditory stimulation

CES Competing Environmental Sounds; test of dichotic processing of familiar nonspeech sounds

CF characteristic frequency; the frequency to which an auditory neuron is most sensitive

CFA continuous flow adapter; earmold with a constant interior tubing diameter designed to permit high-frequency amplification with a smooth frequency response

CHAMPUS Civilian Health and Medical Programs of the Uniformed Services

CHARGE association genetic association featuring *c*oloboma, *h*eart disease, *a*tresia choanae (nasal cavity), *r*etarded growth and development, *g*enital hypoplasia, and *e*ar anomalies and/or hearing loss that can be conductive, sensorineural, or mixed

CHI closed head injury; brain injury in which the primary cause is blunt trauma, rather than penetrating wound, CVA, neoplasms, etc.

CIC 1. commissure of the inferior colliculus; bundle of nerve fibers passing from the dorsomedial portion of the inferior colliculus on one side of the brain to that on the other side of the brain; 2. completely-in-the-canal hearing aid; small amplification device, extending from 1 mm to 2 mm inside the meatal opening to near the tympanic membrane, that allows greater gain with less power due to the proximity of the receiver to the membrane

CID Central Institute for the Deaf; residential school for the deaf in St. Louis, founded in 1914

CIS processing   continuous interleaved sampling processing; cochlear implant processing strategy designed to deliver nonsimultaneous pulses at a high rate of stimulation to multiple implant electrodes

CM   cochlear microphonic; minute alternating-current electrical potential of the hair cells of the cochlea that resembles the input signal

CMOS   complementary metal oxide semiconductor; integrated circuitry used in hearing aid design

CMR   common mode rejection; noise-rejection strategy used in electrophysiologic measurement in which noise that is identical (common) at two electrodes is subtracted by a differential amplifier

CMRR   common mode rejection ratio; amount of reduction in dB of signals determined to be common at two electrodes

CMV   cytomegalovirus; intrauterine-prenatal or postnatal herpetoviral infection, usually transmitted in utero, that can cause central nervous system disorder, including brain damage, hearing loss, vision loss, and seizures

CN   1. cochlear nucleus; cluster of cell bodies of second order neurons on the lateral edge of the hindbrain in the central auditory nervous system at which fibers from Cranial Nerve VIII have an obligatory synapse; 2. cranial nerve; any of 12 pairs of neuron bundles exiting the brainstem above the first cervical vertebra

CN-VIII   Cranial Nerve VIII; auditory nerve, consisting of a vestibular and a cochlear branch; SYN: vestibulocochlear nerve

CNAP   cochlear nerve action potential; compound action potential recorded from an electrode placed directly on Cranial Nerve VIII

CNC   consonant-nucleus-consonant; a word or syllable used in speech-recognition testing, consisting of a vowel or diphthong (nucleus) between two consonants; SYN: CVC

CNE   could not evaluate; could not establish

CNR   composite noise rating; a scale used to rate and predict the total noise environment in a specified geographic area, such as around an airport, for evaluating compatible land use

CNS   central nervous system; that portion of the nervous system to which sensory impulses and from which motor impulses are transmitted, including the cortex, brainstem, and spinal cord

CNT   could not test

CNV   contingent negative variation; evoked potential, characterized by a low-frequency negative-voltage electrophysiologic response occurring in the 300 msec to 500 msec latency region; associated with anticipation of a stimulus condition

COCB   crossed olivocochlear bundle; group of efferent nerve fibers of the medial olivocochlear bundle, coursing from the periolivary nuclei near the medial superior olive, across the brainstem, to the outer hair cells of the contralateral cochlea

COG   center of gravity; point in a body around which weight is evenly balanced

COM   chronic otitis media; persistent inflammation of the middle ear having a duration of greater than 8 weeks

COME   chronic otitis media with effusion; persistent inflammation of the middle ear, accompanied by fluid in the middle ear space

COR   conditioned orientation reflex; behavioral audiometry, designed to assess hearing sensitivity in a young child, in which an orienting head-turn response to a sound source is conditioned by visual reinforcement

CORA   conditioned orientation reflex audiometry

CORFIG   coupler response for flat insertion gain; frequency response that is added to a real-ear insertion response to obtain a prescribed 2-cc coupler response

COT   critical off time; interval between pulsed tones at which threshold or loudness is equal to that of a continuous tone

COWS   cold-opposite warm-same; mnemonic acronym that describes the direction of nystagmus beating in response to caloric stimulation; stimulation of an ear with cold water results in nystagmus that beats in the direction of the opposite ear

CP   cerebral palsy; motor-control disorder caused by damage to the motor cortex of the brain

CPA cerebellopontine angle; anatomical angle formed by the proximity of the cerebellum and the pons from which Cranial Nerve VIII exits into the brainstem

CPA tumor cerebellopontine angle tumor; most often a cochleovestibular Schwannoma located or growing outside the internal auditory canal at the juncture of the cerebellum and pons

CPHI communication profile for the hearing impaired; self-assessment questionnaire designed to quantify a patient's perception of the communication disorder and acceptance of the hearing loss

CPR cochleopalpebral reflex; eyeblink or twitch at the canthus caused by a sudden loud sound; SYN: auropalpebral reflex

cps cycles per second; measurement of sound frequency in terms of the number of complete cycles of a sinusoid that occur within a second; SYN: Hz

CPT codes current procedural terminology codes; numeric codes assigned to diagnostic and treatment procedures, used primarily for billing purposes

CROS contralateral routing of signals; hearing aid configuration designed for unilateral hearing loss, in which a microphone is placed on the poor ear and the signal is routed to a hearing aid on the better ear

CRP corneoretinal potential; electrical potential generated by the voltage difference between the relatively positive cornea and the relatively negative retina

CSF cerebrospinal fluid; liquid filling the ventricles and the subarachnoid space surrounding the brain and spinal cord that supports and cushions the central nervous system against trauma and may serve to remove waste products of neuronal metabolism

CSOM chronic suppurative otitis media; persistent inflammation of the middle ear with infected effusion containing pus

CST Competing Sentence Test; test of dichotic processing of simple sentences

CT computed tomography; sectional radiographs of specified areas of the brain presented as a computer-generated image representing a synthesis of x-rays obtained from different directions on a given plane; SYN: computerized axial tomography

CTP caloric test position; conventional head position for caloric testing in which the patient lies in a supine position with the head angled at 30°

CV consonant vowel; syllable used in speech audiometric measures that consists of a consonant followed by a vowel

CVA cerebrovascular accident; interruption of blood supply to the brain due to aneurysm, embolism, or clot, resulting in sudden loss of function related to the affected portion of the brain; COL: stroke

CVC consonant-vowel-consonant; a word or syllable used in speech-recognition testing, consisting of a vowel or diphthong between two consonants; SYN: CNC

CVIII Cranial Nerve VIII; auditory nerve, consisting of a vestibular and a cochlear branch; SYN: vestibulocochlear nerve

Cz coronal (C) midline (z) electrode location, or vertex electrode, typically used for noninverting-electrode placement in auditory evoked potential testing, according to the 10–20 International Electrode System nomenclature

DAC digital-to-analog conversion; the process of turning numerical (digital) representation of a waveform into a continuously varying (analog) signal

DAF delayed auditory feedback; condition in which a listener's speech is delayed by a controlled amount of time and delivered back to the listener's ears, interfering with the rate and fluency of the speech

DAI direct audio input; direct input of sound into a hearing aid by means of a hard-wire connection between the hearing aid and an assistive listening devices or other sound source

daPa decaPascal; unit of pressure in which 1 daPa equals 10 Pascals

DAS dorsal acoustic stria; nerve fiber bundle that emanates from the dorsal cochlear nucleus and synapses in the contralateral lateral lemniscus and inferior colliculus, bypassing the superior olivary complex

DAT digital audio tape; type of magnetic tape used with tape recorder/player employing digital conversion of acoustic signals

dB   decibel; one-tenth of a bel; unit of sound intensity, based on a logarithmic relationship of one intensity to a reference intensity

dB gain   decibels of gain; the difference between the input SPL and the output SPL of an amplifier or hearing aid

dB HL   decibels hearing level; decibel notation used on the audiogram that is referenced to audiometric zero

dB HTL   decibels hearing threshold level; decibel notation used to refer to a patient's threshold of hearing sensitivity

dB nHL   decibels normalized hearing level; decibel notation referenced to behavioral thresholds of a sample of normal-hearing persons, used most often to describe the intensity level of click stimuli used in evoked potential audiometry

dB SL   decibels sensation level; decibel notation that refers to the number of dB above a person's threshold for a given acoustic signal

dB SPL   decibels sound pressure level; dB SPL equals 20 times the log of the ratio of an observed sound pressure level to the reference sound pressure level of 20 microPascals (or 0.0002 dynes/cm^2, 0.0002 microbar, 20 microNewtons/meter^2)

dBA   decibels expressed in sound pressure level as measured on the A-weighted scale of a sound level meter filtering network, used in the measurement of environmental noise in the workplace

dBB   decibels expressed in sound pressure level as measured on the B-weighted scale of a sound level meter filtering network

dBC   decibels expressed in sound pressure level as measured on the C-weighted scale of a sound level meter filtering network

dBm   decibels referenced to 1 milliwatt

dc   direct current; electric current of a fixed value that flows continuously in one direction

DCA hearing aid   digitally controlled analog hearing aid; hybrid hearing device in which microphone-amplifier-loudspeaker functions are analog, but their parameters are under digital control

DCN   dorsal cochlear nucleus; dorsal portion of the cochlear nucleus that receives nerve fibers from the posterior branch of Cranial Nerve VIII after it bifurcates

DCPN   direction-changing positional nystagmus; abnormal nystagmus that changes direction either with head position changes or with the head kept in the same position

DDx   differential diagnosis; diagnosis of a disease or disorder in a patient from among two or more diseases or disorders with similar symptoms or findings

df   degrees of freedom; in statistics, the number of data points that are free to vary if the statistic is known; e.g., if the mean of a set of 10 numbers is known, then 9 of the numbers are free to vary, because the 10th will be determinable from knowing the rest

DFA   delayed feedback audiometry; the use of delayed auditory feedback in assessing the organicity of a suspected functional hearing loss; the delayed delivery of speech, if audible, interferes with fluency or rate of speech

DI   directivity index; quantification of the directional properties of a hearing aid microphone, expressed as the decibel improvement in signal-to-noise ratio over that expected for an omnidirectional microphone

DIP switch   dual in-line package switch; a row of integrated circuit switches that allows the same electronic instrument to be configured in different ways

DL   difference limen; the smallest difference that can be detected between two signals that vary in intensity, frequency, time, etc.; SYN: differential threshold, just-noticeable difference

DLF   difference limen for frequency; smallest difference in frequency of a signal that can be detected

DLI   difference limen for intensity; smallest difference in intensity of a signal that can be detected

DMQ   deafness management quotient; formula used to predict success in an oral education program, based on weighted factors related to residual hearing, central function, intellect, family support, and socioeconomics

DNA   deoxyribonucleic acid; large and complex molecules carrying genetic instructions

DNE   did not evaluate

DNT   did not test

DP   1. directional preponderance; superiority in one direction or the other of the slow phase velocity of nystagmus; e.g. for caloric labyrinthine stimulation, right beating nystagmus is compared to left beating nystagmus; 2. distortion product; acoustic energy resulting from cochlear nonlinearity that occurs at frequencies that are a combination of two stimulating frequencies, created when two pure tones are presented simultaneously to the cochlea

DPHL   dominant progressive hearing loss; genetic condition in which sensorineural hearing loss gradually worsens over a period of years, caused by dominant inheritance

DPOAE   distortion-product otoacoustic emission; otoacoustic emission, measured as the cubic distortion product that occurs at the frequency represented by $2f_1$-f_2, resulting from the simultaneous presentation of two pure tones (f_1 and f_2)

DPT   Demerol, Phenergan, and Thorazine; drug mixture used for sedation of children undergoing evoked potential audiometry

DRC   damage risk criterion; amount of exposure time to sound of a specified frequency and intensity that is associated with a defined risk of hearing loss

DRF   Deafness Research Foundation; foundation that funds scientific research in hearing and deafness

DRG   diagnosis-related groups; major diagnostic categories into which patients are classified for the purpose of determining reimbursement levels

DS   discrimination score; early term for word-recognition score, expressed as the percentage of words correctly perceived and identified

DSI   dichotic sentence identification test; speech audiometric test of central auditory function in which different synthetic sentences are presented simultaneously to each ear

DSL   desired sensation level; number of decibels above behavioral threshold necessary to amplify the long-term speech spectrum to a prescribed level across the frequency range

DSP   digital signal processing; manipulation by mathematical algorithms of a signal that has been converted from analog to digital form

DSP hearing aid   digital signal processing hearing aid that converts output from the microphone from analog to digital form, uses software algorithms to manipulate gain characteristics, and converts the signal back to analog form for delivery to the loudspeaker

Dx   diagnosis; determination of the nature of disease or disorder

E wave   expectancy wave; event-related potential occurring between a warning stimulus and an imperative stimulus, associated with readiness to respond

E&E   eyes and ears

EA   educational age; grade-level-equivalent age of a student based on standardized achievement tests

EAA   Educational Audiology Association; professional association of audiologists with a particular interest in providing audiologic services in the schools

EABR   electrically evoked auditory brainstem response; ABR generated by electrical stimulation of the cochlea with either an extracochlear promontory electrode or a cochlear implant

EAC   external auditory canal

EAM   external auditory meatus; canal extending from the auricle to the tympanic membrane

EAP   electrically evoked action potential; compound action potential generated by electrical stimulation of the cochlea with either an extracochlear promontory electrode or a cochlear implant

EAR plugs   Etymotic Applied Research plugs; ear inserts made of an expandable material, designed to attenuate excessive noise levels

ECMO   extracorporeal membrane oxygenation; therapeutic technique for augmenting ventilation in high-risk infants

ECochG, ECoG   electrocochleography; method of recording transient AEPs from the cochlea and Cranial Nerve VIII, including the cochlear microphonic, summating potential, and compound action potential, with a promontory or ear canal electrode

EDA   electrodermal audiometry; method of determining hearing sensitivity in cases of suspected functional hearing loss by measuring psychogalvanic skin response to sound, following conditioning to the sound paired with a mild shock

EE external ear; outer ear consisting of the auricle, external auditory meatus, and lateral surface of the tympanic membrane

EEA electroencephalic audiometry; earliest use of electrophysiologic responses to predict hearing sensitivity, involving observation of changes in EEG patterns in response to auditory stimulation

EEE external ear effect; influence of outer ear structures on the acoustic characteristics of sounds reaching the tympanic membrane

EEG electroencephalogram; record obtained by electroencephalography
electroencephalography; the recording of electrical potentials of the brain from scalp electrodes

EENT eye, ear, nose, and throat; early term used to denote a physician with a specialty in diagnosis and treatment of diseases of the eye, ear, nose, and throat

EEPROM electrically erasable programmable read-only memory; computer memory used in many hearing devices for storing electroacoustic configurations

EM effective masking; condition in which noise is just sufficient to mask a given signal when the signal and noise are presented to the same ear simultaneously
environmental microphone; the microphone on a hearing aid that transduces airborne sound

EMG electromyography; recording of electrical activity generated by muscles

EMLR electrically evoked middle latency response; auditory middle latency response generated by electrical stimulation of the cochlea with either an extracochlear promontory electrode or with a cochlear implant

ENG electronystagmography; a method of measuring eye movements, especially nystagmus, via electro-oculography, to assess the integrity of the vestibular mechanism

ENT ear, nose, and throat

ENT physician ear, nose, and throat physician; medical specialist in the diagnosis and treatment of diseases of the ear, nose, and throat; SYN: otorhinolaryngologist, otolaryngologist

EOAE evoked otoacoustic emission; otoacoustic emission that occurs in response to acoustic stimulation; COM: spontaneous otoacoustic emission

EOG electro-oculography; electrical recording of corneoretinal potentials related to eye movement used in electronystagmography testing

EP endocochlear potential; electrical potential or voltage of endolymph in the scala media
evoked potential; electrical activity of the brain responding to sensory stimulation

ER-3A *Etymotic Research insert earphones used in audiometry

ERA electric, electrophysiologic, or evoked response audiometry

ERP event-related potential; evoked potential elicited by an endogenous response to an external event, such as the P3 or CNV

ESP Early Speech Perception test; test battery designed to assess the speech-perception ability of young children; includes a standard and low-verbal version with subtests for pattern perception, spondee identification, and word identification

ET eustachian tube; passageway leading from the nasopharynx to the middle ear, which opens to equalize middle ear air pressure

et al. [L. *et alii*] and others

ETD eustachian tube dysfunction; failure of the eustachian tube to open, usually due to edema in the nasopharynx

eust. eustachian

EWOK either way, okay; hearing aid circuit that automatically senses the polarity of a battery and reverses it if the battery has been inserted incorrectly

f frequency; the number of times a repetitive event occurs in a specified time period; e.g. for a sine wave, the number of periods occurring in 1 second, expressed as cycles per seconds or Hertz (Hz)

f_0 fundamental frequency; principal or lowest component frequency of pattern repetition in the acoustic spectrum of a speech sound

$f_0/f_1/f_2$ processing   cochlear implant processing strategy designed to extract frequency and amplitude estimates of f_1 and f_2 from a speech signal and deliver them to an electrode corresponding to each frequency band at a pulse rate equal to f_0

f_1   formant 1 or first formant; first frequency region above f_0 of prominent energy in the acoustic spectrum of a speech sound

f_2   formant 2 or second formant; second frequency region above f_0 of prominent energy in the acoustic spectrum of a speech sound

f_3   formant 3 or third formant; third frequency region above f_0 of prominent energy in the acoustic spectrum of a speech sound

FAAA   Fellow of the American Academy of Audiology

FACP   Fellow of the American College of Physicians

FACS   Fellow of the American College of Surgeons

FBL   fitting by loudness; fitting strategy for hearing aids with dynamic-range compression, based on measures of loudness growth, prediction of loudness growth, or assumption of average loudness growth

FCC   Federal Communication Commission; U.S. government agency whose responsibilities include regulating radio waves over which FM systems broadcast

FDA   Food and Drug Administration; U.S. government agency whose responsibilities include regulating medical devices such as hearing aids

FDL   frequency difference limen; smallest difference in frequency of a signal that can be detected

FFR   1. fixed frequency response; subgroup of ASP techniques that includes compression limiting and wide-dynamic-range compression, wherein gain is automatically increased or decreased in response to input, regardless of input frequency; 2. frequency following response; short-latency auditory evoked potential of the same frequency as the low-frequency tone burst used to elicit the response

FFS   failure of fixation suppression; failure of visual fixation to suppress nystagmus in ENG measurement

FFT   fast Fourier transformation; rapid algorithm for determining the Fourier transform, or spectrum of frequency components of a waveform

FG   functional gain; difference in decibels between aided and unaided hearing sensitivity thresholds

FHL   functional hearing loss; hearing loss that is exaggerated or feigned

Fig6   figure 6; algorithm for fitting nonlinear hearing aids that have wide-dynamic-range compression, in which fitting curves are calculated for low, moderate, and high-level sounds based on a patient's audiometric thresholds

FIM   functional independence measures; collective assessment of an individual's capacity to function independently

FM   frequency modulation; the process of creating a complex signal by sinusoidally varying the frequency of a carrier wave; COM: AM

FN   facial nerve; Cranial Nerve VII; cranial nerve that provides efferent innervation to the facial muscles and afferent innervation from the soft palate and tongue
false negative; SYN: F_{neg}

F_{neg}   false negative; test outcome indicating the absence of a disease or condition when, in fact, that disease or condition exists

FOG   full-on gain; hearing aid setting that produces maximum acoustic output

FP   false positive; SYN: F_{pos}

F_{pos}   false positive; test outcome indicating the presence of a disease or condition when, in fact, that disease or condition is not present

Fpz   frontoproximal (Fp) midline (z) electrode location, or forehead electrode, typically used for ground-electrode placement in auditory evoked potential testing, according to the 10–20 International Electrode System nomenclature

FROS   front routing of signals; eyeglass hearing aid in which the microphone is placed near the front of the glasses and routed back to the amplifier at the ear

F_{sp}   algorithm used to estimate the likelihood of the presence of an auditory evoked potential, based on the F distribution of the variance of the averaged evoked potential divided by the variance of a single point (sp) in time across successive samples

FTLB full-term live birth; of a normal length of pregnancy

FTNB full-term newborn

FTND full-term normal delivery

FTNSD full-term normal spontaneous delivery

FU follow up

Fx fracture; breaking of a bone or cartilage

G conductance; ease of energy flow associated with resistance; reciprocal of resistance

GABA gamma-aminobutyric acid; inhibitory neurotransmitter present throughout the auditory system

GAD glutamic acid decarboxylase; amino acid neurotransmitter, which synthesizes GABA and is concentrated in the dorsal cochlear nucleus

GCS Glasgow coma score; method for grading depth of coma and severity of brain injury, based on eye opening, verbal response, and motor response

gent gentamicin; ototoxic aminoglycoside antibiotic that is an important agent in the treatment of gram-negative infections

GFW battery Goldman-Fristoe-Woodcock auditory skills test battery; diagnostic measure of auditory skills, including auditory selective attention, discrimination, memory, and sound-symbol tests

GIFROC frequency response that is added to a prescribed 2-cc coupler response to predict real-ear insertion response; inverse of CORFIG

GME graduate medical education

GRE graduate record examination

GSR galvanic skin response; change in skin resistance as a result of an emotional response to a stimulus; SYN: PGSR

H&P history and physical; preliminary examination in medical assessment

H$_0$ null hypothesis; in statistics, the hypothesis that no difference exists between two or more sets of data

HA hearing aid; any electronic device designed to amplify and deliver sound to the ear, consisting of a microphone, amplifier, and receiver

HAE hearing aid evaluation; process of choosing suitable hearing aid amplification for an individual, based on measurement of acoustic properties of the amplification and perceptual response to the amplified sound

HAIC Hearing Aid Industry Conference; organization of hearing instrument manufacturers and other companies in the hearing industry; predecessor to the Hearing Industries Association

HAPI Hearing Aid Performance Inventory; self-assessment questionnaire of a patient's perceived benefit from hearing aid use

HBP high blood pressure

HC hair cell; sensory cell of the organ of Corti to which nerve endings from Cranial Nerve VIII are attached, so named because of the hairlike stereocilia that project from the apical end

HCL highest comfortable level; the maximum level of gain at which loudness comfort can be achieved, used in the fitting of hearing aids to assist in determining output-limiting levels

HCP hearing conservation program; occupational program designed to quantify the nature and extent of hazardous noise exposure, monitor the effects of exposure on hearing, provide abatement of sound, and provide hearing protection when necessary

HD hearing device; SYN: HA

HEENT head, eyes, ears, nose, and throat

HF high frequency; nonspecific term referring to frequencies above approximately 2000 Hz

HFA high-frequency average; an ANSI hearing aid specification, expressed as the average of decibel response values at 1000 Hz, 1600 Hz, and 2500 Hz

HFA full-on gain high-frequency average full-on gain; an ANSI hearing aid specification, derived by calculating the HFA output to a 50-dB-SPL or 60-dB-SPL input with the hearing aid adjusted to its full-on gain setting

HFA SSPL90 high-frequency average saturation sound pressure level; an ANSI hearing aid specification, derived by calculating the HFA output to a 90-dB-SPL input with the hearing aid adjusted to its full-on gain setting

HHI Hearing Handicap Inventory; self-assessment scale designed to yield information about an individual's perceived social and emotional consequences of hearing impairment

HHIA Hearing Handicap Inventory for Adults; modification of the HHIE designed to yield information about a non-elderly adult's perceived social and emotional consequences of hearing impairment

HHIE Hearing Handicap Inventory for the Elderly; self-assessment scale designed to yield information about an elderly individual's perceived social and emotional consequences of hearing impairment

HI hearing impairment; abnormal or reduced function in hearing resulting from auditory disorder

HIA Hearing Industries Association; trade association of manufacturers of hearing aids and other companies in the hearing industry

HICROS high-frequency contralateral routing of signals; conventional CROS hearing aid configuration, but with a high-frequency emphasis on the aided ear

HINT hearing in noise test; speech-audiometric measure of sentence-recognition ability in background noise

HIS health information system; computer database system designed specifically for healthcare institutions for information processing of patient demographic data, diagnosis, payer source, etc.

HIV human immunodeficiency virus; cytopathic retrovirus that causes AIDS and can result in infectious diseases of the middle ear and mastoid as well as peripheral and central auditory nervous system disorder; SYN: HTLV-III

HL hearing level; the decibel level of sound referenced to audiometric zero that is used on audiograms and audiometers, expressed as dB HL
hearing loss; reduction in hearing sensitivity

HML indices high, medium, low indices; method of expressing attenuation capabilities of hearing protection devices based on octave band measures

HMO health maintenance organization; managed care organization in which groups of professionals, along with a specified facility, provide enrollees with health care at fixed reimbursement rates

HNS head and neck surgery

HOH hard of hearing; having a hearing impairment that is mild to severe

HPD hearing protection device; any of a number of devices used to attenuate excessive environmental noise to protect hearing, including those that block the ear canal or cover the external ear

HPI Hearing Performance Inventory; self-assessment scale used to assess subjective impression of hearing performance in everyday communication situations

HRA heart-rate audiometry; electrophysiologic technique for predicting hearing sensitivity by measuring changes in heart rate in response to auditory stimulation; SYN: cardiac evoked response audiometry

HTL hearing threshold level; an individual's threshold, or the number of dB by which an individual's hearing threshold exceeds the normal threshold, expressed as dB HTL

HTLV-III human T-cell lymphotropic virus-III; cytopathic retrovirus that causes AIDS and can result in infectious diseases of the middle ear and mastoid as well as peripheral and central auditory nervous system disorder; SYN: HIV

Hx history

Hz Hertz; unit of measure of frequency, representing cycles per second

HZO herpes zoster oticus; herpes zoster infection, which lingers in the ganglia and can be activated by systemic disease, resulting in vesicular eruptions of the auricle, facial nerve palsy, and sensorineural hearing loss; SYN: Ramsey-Hunt syndrome

I tracing   interrupted tracing; graph that results from threshold tracking in Békésy audiometry to an interrupted or pulsed tone at a fixed or swept frequency; ANT: C tracing

I/O function   input/output function; curve that plots output intensity level as a function of input intensity level; used to describe the gain characteristics of an amplifier

IA   interaural attenuation; reduction in the sound energy of a signal as it is transmitted by bone conduction from one side of the head to the opposite ear

IAC   internal auditory canal; SYN: IAM

IAM   internal auditory meatus; an opening on the posterior surface of the petrous portion of the temporal bone through which the auditory and facial nerves pass

IAS   intermediate acoustic stria; nerve bundle, the fibers of which emanate from the posterior ventral cochlear nucleus and synapse on the ipsilateral and contralateral periolivary nuclei and the contralateral lateral lemniscus

IC   inferior colliculus; central auditory nucleus the midbrain; its central nucleus receives ascending input from the cochlear nucleus and superior olivary complex, and its pericentral nucleus receives descending input from the cortex
integrated circuit; electronic circuit with its many interconnected elements formed on a single body of semiconductor material

ICD   International Classification of Diseases; classification system developed by the World Health Organization

ICD-9 codes   codes representing ICD classifications of surgical, therapeutic, and diagnostic procedures

ICM   ipsilateral competing message; in speech audiometry, noise or other competing signal that is delivered to the same ear as the target signal; ANT: CCM

ICN   1. intensive care nursery; hospital unit designed to provide care for newborns needing extensive support and monitoring; 2. intermediate care nursery; hospital unit designed as a step-down facility for newborns leaving the intensive care unit prior to discharge

ICU   intensive care unit; hospital unit designed to provide care for those needing extensive support and monitoring

IDE   investigational device exemption; status granted by the U.S. Food and Drug Administration to permit clinical trials of new medical devices that have not yet been approved for clinical use

IDEA   Individuals with Disabilities Education Act; U.S. public laws 94–142 and 99–457 mandating free and appropriate public education for all children, age 3 and older, who have handicapping conditions; also encourages services to infants and toddlers

IDL   intensity difference limen; smallest difference in intensity of a signal that can be detected

IEP   individualized educational plan; federally mandated, annually updated plan for the education of children with handicapping conditions

IFSP   individualized family service plan; federally mandated, annually updated plan for the education of preschool children with handicapping conditions and their families

IHAFF   Independent Hearing Aid Fitting Forum; group of audiologists who developed recommendations for the selection and fitting of nonlinear hearing aids

IHC   inner hair cells; sensory hair cells arranged in a single row in the organ of Corti to which the primary afferent nerve endings of Cranial Nerve VIII are attached

IHS   International Hearing Society; organization of hearing professionals, primarily hearing instrument specialists

IL   intensity level; acoustic intensity in decibels; the IL of a sound is equal to 10 times the common log of the ratio of the measured acoustic intensity to a reference intensity

ILD   interaural latency difference; the difference in latency of a component wave of an auditory evoked potential, usually ABR wave V, for right-ear versus left-ear stimulation, expressed in msec

IM   intramuscularly; within the muscle, usually referring to a method of delivering drugs into the system

IPA   international phonetic alphabet; alphabet of symbols representing sounds of speech

IRIS Intelligibility Rating Improvement Scale; patient estimation of the proportion of speech that can be understood in various listening situations

IROS ipsilateral routing of signals; method of monaural hearing aid fitting for mild hearing loss, in which a high-frequency-emphasis hearing aid is coupled to the ear with an open earmold or tube fitting; COM: CROS

ISI interstimulus interval; the time between successive stimulus presentations

ISO International Organization for Standardization; association of specialists that determines standards for measuring instruments

ITC hearing aid in-the-canal hearing aid; custom hearing aid that fits mostly in the external auditory meatus with a small portion extending into the concha; SYN: canal hearing aid

ITE hearing aid in-the-ear hearing aid; custom hearing aid that fits entirely in the concha of the ear

IV intravenous; within the vein, usually referring to a method of delivering drugs into the system

j joule; unit of energy, expressed as the energy expended by an ampere flowing against 1 ohm for 1 sec; equal to 1 Newton/meter

JCAHO Joint Commission on Accreditation of Healthcare Organizations; voluntary organization that provides support and accreditation to its member organizations, which are hospitals and other healthcare facilities; formerly JCAH

JCIH Joint Committee on Infant Hearing; organization formed to promote infant hearing health care with representation from AAA, AAO, AAP, ASHA, and others

JND just noticeable difference; the smallest change in a stimulus that is detectable; SYN: difference limen

k kilo; one thousand

K+ potassium; chemical found in low concentration in perilymph and high concentration in endolymph

K-AMP Killion amplifier; hearing aid circuit with TILL processing that provides substantial gain for low-intensity sound, reduced gain for moderate-level sound, no gain for high-intensity sound, and compression limiting for the highest-level sound

kc kilocycle; 1000 cycles/sec; SYN: kHz

KEMAR Knowles electronics mannequin for acoustic research; model used in the measurement of hearing aid performance that simulates the acoustic properties of an average adult head and torso

kg kilogram

kHz kilohertz; 1000 Hz

LAER late auditory evoked response; SYN: LLAER

LD learning disability; lack of skill in one or more areas of learning that is inconsistent with the person's intellectual capacity and is not the result of visual, hearing, motor, or emotional disorder

LDFR level-dependent frequency response; automatic signal processing that alters the frequency response of a hearing aid as a function of input level

LDL loudness discomfort level; intensity level at which sound is perceived to be uncomfortably loud, determined under earphones and expressed in dB HL or with probe microphone in dB SPL; SYN: uncomfortable loudness level

LED light-emitting diode; a small light on a device, often used to indicate that the device is on or activated

Leq equivalent sound level; measurement of a time-varying sound, expressed as a time-weighted energy average, representing the total sound energy experienced over a given time period as if the sound were unvarying

LF low frequency or frequencies; nonspecific term referring to frequencies below around 1000 Hz

LGOB loudness growth by octave bands; psychophysical technique in which loudness level is determined for various frequency bands, used as a fitting-by-loudness strategy for wide-dynamic-range-compression hearing aids

LL lateral lemniscus; large fiber tract, formed by dorsal, intermediate, and ventral nuclei and consisting of ascending auditory fibers from the CN and SOC, that runs along the lateral edge of the pons and carries information to the inferior colliculus

LLAER long-latency auditory evoked response; auditory evoked potential, having two main waveform peaks—a vertex negative peak at approximately 90 msec and a vertex positive peak at approximately 180 msec following signal presentation; SYN: ALR

LLD dorsal nucleus of the lateral lemniscus; one of three fiber tracts, constituting auditory nuclei of the pons, that serves as a relay for ascending auditory fibers from the DCN, LSO, and MSO in the hindbrain to the inferior colliculus

LLI intermediate nucleus of the lateral lemniscus; one of three fiber tracts, constituting auditory nuclei of the pons, that serves as a relay for ascending auditory fibers from the PVCN and LSO in the hindbrain to the inferior colliculus

LLR late-latency response; SYN: LLAER

LLV ventral nucleus of the lateral lemniscus; one of three fiber tracts, constituting auditory nuclei of the pons, that serves as a relay for ascending auditory fibers from the AVCN, LSO, and MSO in the hindbrain to the inferior colliculus

log logarithm; the exponent expressing the power to which a fixed number, the base, must be raised to produce a given number

LPFS test low-pass filtered speech test; word-recognition measure, consisting of monosyllabic words that have been bandpass filtered above approximately 800 Hz

LSO lateral superior olive; one of the primary nuclei of the superior olivary complex, located in the hindbrain, receiving primary ascending projections directly from the ipsilateral AVCN and indirectly from the contralateral AVCN via the ipsilateral MTB

LTSS long-term speech spectrum; overall level and frequency composition of speech energy that represents everyday speech

M1 left (1) mastoid (M) electrode location, typically used for inverting-electrode placement in auditory evoked potential testing, according to the 10–20 International Electrode System nomenclature

M2 right (2) mastoid (M) electrode location, typically used for inverting-electrode placement in auditory evoked potential testing, according to the 10–20 International Electrode System nomenclature

MA mental age; intellectual age, as measured on standardized tests

MAC battery minimum auditory capabilities battery; group of tests designed to assess auditory perception of persons with profound hearing loss

MAF minimum audible field; binaural threshold of sensitivity to sound presented in a sound field via loudspeaker placed at 0° azimuth; COM: MAP

MAIS Meaningful Auditory Integration Scale; assessment scale, completed by parents of children with hearing impairment, that assesses the effectiveness of hearing aids or cochlear implants

MAP minimum audible pressure; monaural threshold of sensitivity to sound presented via earphones; COM: MAF

MBD minimal brain dysfunction; early term used to describe a constellation of idiopathic behavioral, language, and learning disorders

MCL most comfortable loudness; intensity level at which sound is perceived to be most comfortable, usually expressed in dB HL

MCOs managed care organizations; HMOs, PPOs, insurance companies, and other organizations that participate in managed care

MCR message-to-competition ratio; in speech audiometry, the ratio in dB of the presentation level of a speech target to that of background competition; SYN: S/N

MCT earmold minimal contact technology earmold; earmold designed to reduce the occlusion effect by limiting contact with the cartilaginous portion of the external auditory meatus and instead sealing around its perimeter at the medial tip

ME middle ear; portion of the hearing mechanism extending from the medial membrane of the tympanic membrane to the oval window of the cochlea, including the ossicles and middle ear cavity; serves as an impedance matching device of the outer and inner ears

MEDLARS   medical literature analysis and retrieval system; computer-based index system of the U.S. National Library of Medicine

MEDLINE   MEDLARS on-line; computer network of U.S. medical libraries and MEDLARS for rapid literature searches

MEE   middle ear effusion; exudation of fluid from the membranous walls of the middle ear cavity, secondary to inflammation

MEG   magnoencephalography; noninvasive technique, using scalp recordings, designed to measure spontaneous or sensory-evoked changes in magnetic fields of the cortex

MEP   multimodality evoked potentials; collective term referring to the sensory evoked potentials, including auditory, visual, and somatosensory electrophysiologic measures

mg   milligram; one-thousandth of a gram

MG   medial geniculate; auditory nucleus of the thalamus, divided into central and surrounding pericentral nuclei, that receives primary ascending fibers from the inferior colliculus and sends fibers, via the auditory radiations, to the auditory cortex

mg per kg   milligrams per kilogram; method of expressing dosage of a drug in terms of quantity per measure of body weight

MGB   medial geniculate body; SYN: MG

MHz   megahertz; 1 million cycles per second

μV   microvolt; one-millionth of a volt

MLAER   middle latency auditory evoked response; auditory evoked potential, originating from the region of the auditory radiations and cortex, having as a primary component a vertex positive peak at 25 msec to 40 msec following signal presentation; SYN: AMLR

MLB   monaural loudness balance test; test of loudness recruitment that compares loudness growth at a frequency at which the patient has normal hearing to loudness growth at a frequency at which the patient has hearing loss in the same ear

MLD   masking level difference; measure of binaural release from masking in which binaural thresholds are tracked in noise for tones that are in phase and 180° out of phase

MLR   middle latency response; SYN: MLAER

MLS   maximum length sequence; signal processing technique of interleaved sampling in groups or patterns that permits the presentation of stimuli at very high rates

MLV   monitored live voice; outdated speech audiometric technique in which speech signals were presented via a microphone with controlled vocal output; SYN: live-voice testing

mm H₂0   millimeter of water; unit of air pressure used in tympanometry

mmho   millimho; one-thousandth of a mho

MMN   mismatched negativity; auditory evoked potential recorded using an oddball paradigm, characterized by a negative peak at 100 msec to 200 msec, reflecting discrimination ability for different simple and complex sound features

MNTB   medial nucleus of the trapezoid body; nucleus of the superior olivary complex that receives primary ascending projections from the contralateral AVCN and sends projections to the ipsilateral lateral superior olive and lateral lemniscus; SYN: MTB

MPO   maximum power output; highest intensity level that a hearing aid can produce, regardless of input level; SYN: saturation sound pressure level

MR   mental retardation; intellectual function below normal range

MRI   magnetic resonance imaging; radiographic technique used to provide precise structural images

MS   multiple sclerosis; demyelinating disease involving the white matter of the brainstem, resulting in diffuse neurologic symptoms, including hearing loss, speech-understanding deficits, and abnormalities of the acoustic reflexes and ABR

msec   millisecond; one-thousandth of a second

MSO   medial superior olive; one of the primary nuclei of the superior olivary complex, located in the hindbrain, receiving primary ascending projections directly from both the ipsilateral and contralateral anterior ventral cochlear nuclei

MSU prescriptive procedure   Memphis State University procedure; gain and frequency response selection algorithm based on the theory that a hearing aid should amplify the long-term speech spectrum to a point halfway between threshold and ULCL

MTB medial nucleus of the trapezoid body; a nucleus of the superior olivary complex, receiving primary ascending projections from the contralateral anterior ventral cochlear nucleus and sending projections to the ipsilateral LSO and lateral lemniscus; SYN: MNTB

MTS monosyllable-trochee-spondee test; speech-audiometric measure of word recognition and stress-pattern identification in children

μ mu; micro-; one-millionth

N Newton; unit of physical force

N/m² Newton per square meter; unit of measure of pressure used as a reference for sound measurement

N₁ major negative peak of the late-latency auditory evoked potential, occurring at around 90 msec following stimulus onset

N₁-P₂ major peak complex of the late-latency auditory evoked potential, occurring at around 90 msec and 180 msec following stimulus onset

Nₐ major negative peak of the auditory middle latency response

Na+ chemical symbol for sodium, a substance found in high concentration in perilymph and low concentration in endolymph

NAD National Association of the Deaf

NAL National Acoustic Laboratories in Australia; laboratory responsible for developing the widely used NAL prescriptive hearing aid fitting technique

NAL prescriptive procedure National Acoustic Laboratories procedure; gain and frequency response prescriptive strategy based on the theory that a hearing aid should amplify the long-term spectrum of speech so that it is equally and comfortably loud across frequency

NAL-R procedure revised NAL procedure

NAL-RM procedure modification of the revised NAL procedure for use in prescribing gain and frequency response in cases of severe and profound hearing loss

Nᵦ secondary negative peak of the auditory middle latency response

NBC-HIS National Board for Certification in Hearing Instrument Sciences; organization that sets standards for and awards certification in hearing instrument sciences

NBN narrow-band noise; bandpass-filtered noise that is centered at one of the audiometric frequencies, used for masking in pure-tone audiometry

NDT noise-detection threshold; lowest intensity level at which a specified noise signal is audible

NF1 neurofibromatosis 1; autosomal dominant disorder, characterized by childhood-onset multiple neurofibromas, located on any nerve, with associated sequelae; SYN: von Recklinghausen's disease

NF2 neurofibromatosis II; autosomal dominant disorder characterized by bilateral cochleovestibular Schwannomas, which are faster growing and more virulent than the unilateral type; associated with secondary hearing loss and other intracranial tumors

NHAS National Hearing Aid Society; former name of the International Hearing Society

NHCA National Hearing Conservation Association; professional association of specialists in hearing conservation

NHHHI Nursing Home Hearing Handicap Index; self- and staff-assessment scale designed to evaluate the handicapping influence of hearing impairment on aging residents of nursing homes

nHL normalized hearing level; the decibel level of a sound that lacks a standardized reference, referred to behaviorally determined normative levels, expressed as dB nHL

NICU neonatal intensive care nursery; hospital unit designed to provide care for newborns needing extensive support and monitoring

NIDCD National Institute on Deafness and other Communication Disorders

NIHL noise-induced hearing loss; permanent sensorineural hearing loss caused by acoustic trauma from exposure to excessive sound levels

NIHIS National Institute for Hearing Instrument Sciences; educational wing of the International Hearing Society

NIOSH   National Institute for Occupational Safety and Health; organization developed under the Occupational Safety and Health Act to fund and conduct research on occupational hazards and to develop criteria and recommend standards

NIPTS   noise-induced permanent threshold shift; permanent change in hearing sensitivity that occurs as a result of acoustic trauma from exposure to excessive levels of sound

NITTS   noise-induced temporary threshold shift; transient change in hearing sensitivity that occurs as a result of exposure to excessive levels of sound; SYN: temporary threshold shift

NLL   nuclei or nucleus of the lateral lemniscus

NPO   non per os; nothing by mouth; referring to instructions given to patients or parents before certain procedures, such as those requiring sedation

NR   no response

NRR   noise-reduction rating; standardized specifications of the attenuation properties of hearing-protection devices, expressed as the number of decibels of attenuation at specified frequencies throughout the frequency range

NST   nonsense syllable test; speech-audiometric measure of nonsense-syllable recognition

NU-6   Northwestern University Auditory Test Number 6; monosyllabic word-recognition measure, designed to be phonetically balanced within a word list

OAE   otoacoustic emission; low-level sound emitted by the cochlea, either spontaneously or as an echo or other sound evoked by an auditory stimulus, related to the function of the outer hair cells of the cochlea

OCB   olivocochlear bundle; crossed and uncrossed bundles of efferent fibers coursing from the periolivary nuclei surrounding the medial and lateral superior olives directly to the outer hair cells or to nerve fiber dendrites leading to the inner hair cells

OHC   occupational hearing conservationist; person who is certified by CAOHC to provide a comprehensive array of services related to hearing conservation
outer hair cell; motile cells within the organ of Corti with rich efferent innervation that appear to be responsible for fine-tuning frequency resolution and potentiating the sensitivity of the inner hair cells

OHCP   occupational hearing conservation program; industrial program designed to quantify the nature and extent of hazardous noise exposure, monitor the effects of exposure on hearing, provide abatement of sound, and provide hearing protection if necessary

OKN   optokinetic nystagmus; normally symmetric ocular nystagmus that occurs during optokinetic stimulation, reflecting the eye's attempt at smooth pursuit of alternating vertical stripes

OM   otitis media; inflammation of the middle ear, resulting predominantly from eustachian tube dysfunction

OME   otitis media with effusion; inflammation of the middle ear with an accumulation of any of several types of effusion in the middle ear cavity

OPK   optokinetic; pertaining to ocular tracking of repetitive moving targets

OR   operating room
orienting reflex; reflexive head turn toward the source of a sound

ORL   otorhinolaryngology; branch of medicine specializing in the diagnosis and treatment of diseases of the ear, nose, and throat

ORL—HNS   otorhinolaryngology—head and neck surgery; branch of medicine specializing in the diagnosis and treatment of diseases of the ear, nose, and throat, including diseases of related structures of the head and neck

OSHA   Occupational Safety and Health Administration; agency responsible for regulating occupational health and safety hazards, including the setting of minimum standards for industrial hearing conservation programs, and for enforcing the regulations

OSHRC   Occupational Safety and Health Review Commission; organization developed under the Occupational Safety and Health Act to adjudicate disputes that arise between OSHA and employers over the enforcement of regulations

OSPL90   output sound pressure level for 90-dB input; ANSI standard term for saturation sound pressure level

OTE hearing aid   over-the-ear; seldom used term for behind-the-ear hearing aid

OTO otolaryngology; branch of medicine specializing in the diagnosis and treatment of diseases of the ear, nose, and throat; SYN: otorhinolaryngology

P_2 major positive peak of the late-latency auditory evoked potential, occurring around 180 msec following stimulus onset

P_3 major peak of the endogenous event-related potential, occurring around 300 msec following acoustic stimulus onset; SYN: P300

P300 SYN: P_3

P_a major positive peak of the auditory middle latency response occurring 25 msec to 40 msec following stimulus onset

Pa Pascal; unit of measure of pressure; reference sound pressure for 0 dB SPL is 0.00002 Pa or 20 μPa

paed pediatrics; branch of medicine concerned with the development and care of children and in the diagnosis and treatment of their diseases

PAL PB-50 Psycho-Acoustic Laboratory (Harvard University) phonetically balanced 50 (word list); one of the earliest word-recognition measures, designed to be phonetically balanced within a word list

PAM postauricular muscle or myogenic potential; electrical potential generated from muscles of the neck that occurs around 20 msec and can be of sufficient magnitude to obscure the neurogenic auditory middle latency response

P_b secondary positive peak of the auditory middle latency response occurring 50 msec to 75 msec following stimulus onset

PB phonetically balanced; descriptive of a list of words containing speech sounds that occur with the same frequency as in conversational speech

PB max highest percentage-correct score obtained on monosyllabic word-recognition measures (PB word lists) presented at several intensity levels

PB min the lowest percentage-correct score obtained on monosyllabic word-recognition measures (PB word lists) at an intensity level above that at which PB max occurs

PB word list phonetically balanced word list; list of words used in word-recognition testing that contain speech sounds that occur with the same frequency as those of conversational speech

PB words phonetically balanced words; misnomer for PB word list

PBK word lists phonetically balanced kindergarten word lists; lists of words used in word-recognition testing, designed both to be phonetically balanced and to contain words that are at a vocabulary level appropriate for use with young school children

pe SPL peak equivalent sound pressure level: decibel level of a 1000-Hz tone at an amplitude equivalent to the peak of a transient signal; used to express the intensity level of click stimuli used in auditory evoked potential testing

PE tube pressure-equalization tube; small tube or grommet inserted in the tympanic membrane following myringotomy to provide equalization of air pressure within the middle ear space as a substitute for a nonfunctional eustachian tube

PGR psychogalvanic response; SYN: PGSR

PGSR psychogalvanic skin response; change in skin resistance resulting from an emotional response to a stimulus; SYN: GSR

PGSR audiometry method of determining hearing sensitivity in suspected functional hearing loss by measuring psychogalvanic skin response to sound, following conditioning of the patient to the sound paired with a mild shock; SYN: electrodermal audiometry

PHAB Profile of Hearing Aid Benefit; self-assessment inventory designed to evaluate perceived benefit from the use of hearing aids

PHAP Profile of Hearing Aid Performance; self-assessment inventory designed to assess the perceived performance received from the use of hearing aid amplification

PI function performance-intensity function; graph of percentage-correct speech-recognition scores as a function of presentation level of the target signals

PI-PB performance intensity (PI) function for phonetically balanced (PB) word lists

PI-SSI performance intensity (PI) function for the synthetic sentence identification (SSI) test

PICU pediatric intensive care unit; hospital unit designed to provide care for young children needing extensive support and monitoring

PILL programmable increases at low levels; type of automatic signal processing in a hearing aid that uses level-dependent control of frequency response, reducing either low-frequency or high-frequency gain as input level increases

PLL preferred loudness level; signal level at which speech is rated as most comfortable

POGO prescriptive procedure prescription of gain and output; hearing aid selection algorithm designed to prescribe a gain and frequency response that is based on a half-gain rule at frequencies above 500 Hz and reductions from half gain of -5 dB and -10 dB at 500 Hz and 250 Hz

POGO II prescriptive procedure prescription of gain and output II; modification of the POGO gain rule in which the gain is increased at each frequency by one-half the decibel amount that the hearing loss exceeds 65 dB HL

PON periolivary nuclei; group of nuclei of the superior olivary complex surrounding the lateral and medial superior olives that receive projections from the intermediate acoustic stria

pot potentiometer; a resistor connected across a voltage that permits variable change of a current or circuit

PPO preferred provider organization; managed care organization in which providers and employers or third-party administrators contract to provide services to a defined population at agreed-upon, usually discounted, fees

PPRF pontine paramedian reticular formation; nucleus in the pons that carries afferent information from the contralateral semicircular canal and vestibular nucleus to the motor nucleus of Cranial Nerve VI

prelim preliminary; used colloquially to refer to an initial draft of a patient report

PSI pediatric speech intelligibility test; closed-set test of word and sentence recognition, in quiet and in a background of speech competition, designed to assess speech perception ability of children ages 2.5 to 6 years

PTA pure-tone average; average of hearing sensitivity thresholds to pure-tone signals at 500 Hz, 1000 Hz, and 2000 Hz

PTA0 pure-tone average 0; low-frequency average of hearing sensitivity thresholds to pure-tone signals at 250 Hz, 500 Hz, and 1000 Hz

PTA2 pure-tone average 2; high-frequency average of hearing sensitivity thresholds to pure-tone signals at 1000 Hz, 2000 Hz, and 4000 Hz

PTS permanent threshold shift; irreversible hearing sensitivity loss following exposure to excessive noise levels; COM: TTS

PVCN posterior ventral cochlear nucleus; portion of the cochlear nucleus that receives nerve fibers from the posterior branch of Cranial Nerve VIII and sends fibers, via the intermediate acoustic stria, to the PON and contralateral lateral lemniscus

PVT physical volume test; subtest of immittance audiometry in which the volume of the ear canal is estimated; e.g., a large volume is found in the case of a tympanic membrane perforation and a small volume in the case of impacted cerumen

PVV positive venting valve; series of small inserts, with holes of graduated diameter, that fit in the lateral end of an earmold vent to permit alteration of vent size

R resistance; opposition to energy flow due to dissipation

RASP rapidly alternating speech perception; test of sentence recognition in which the signal is alternated between ears at rates ranging from 200 msec to 400 msec, designed to assess auditory brainstem integrity

RASTI rapid speech transmission index; assessment of the integrity of signal transmission in a room, expressed as the reduction in signal modulation of amplitude-modulated broadband noise centered at 500 Hz and 2000 Hz

RCT rotary chair testing; test of vestibular function, in which a computer-driven chair rotates in regulated variable-velocity clockwise and counterclockwise motion, with simultaneous electronystagmographic recording

REAG real-ear aided gain; measurement of the difference, in dB as a function of frequency, between the SPL in the ear canal and the SPL at a field reference point for a specified sound field with the hearing aid in place and turned on

REAR real-ear aided response; probe-microphone measurement of the sound pressure level, as a function of frequency, at a specified point near the tympanic membrane with a hearing aid in place and turned on

RECD   real-ear coupler difference; measurement of the difference, in dB as a function of frequency, between the output of a hearing aid measured by a probe microphone in the ear canal and the output measured in a 2-cc coupler

REDD   real-ear dial difference; measurement of the difference, in dB, between a signal measured by a probe microphone in the ear canal and the dial reading of that signal on the audiometer

REIG   real-ear insertion gain; probe-microphone measurement of the difference, in dB as a function of frequency, between the real-ear unaided gain and the real-ear aided gain at the same point near the tympanic membrane

REIR   real-ear insertion response; probe-microphone measurement of the difference, in dB as a function of frequency, between the real-ear unaided response and the real-ear aided response at the same point near the tympanic membrane

REMR   real-ear masker response; probe-microphone measurement of tinnitus masker output

REOG   real-ear occluded gain; probe-microphone measurement of the difference in dB between the SPL in the ear canal and the SPL at a field reference point for a specified sound field with a hearing aid in place and turned off

REOR   real-ear occluded response; probe-microphone measurement of the sound pressure level, as a function of frequency, at a specified point near the tympanic membrane with a hearing aid in place and turned off

RESR   real-ear saturation response; probe-microphone measurement of the SPL at a specified point near the tympanic membrane, with a hearing aid in place and turned on and with sufficient stimulus level to drive the hearing aid at its maximum output

RETSPL   reference equivalent threshold sound pressure level; ANSI standard specification of the sound-pressure levels that correspond to audiometric zero for a specific earphone

REUG   real-ear unaided gain; probe-microphone measurement of the difference, in dB as a function of frequency, between the SPL in an unoccluded ear canal and the SPL at the field reference point for a specified sound field

REUR   real-ear unaided response; probe-microphone measurement of the sound pressure level, as a function of frequency, at a specified point near the tympanic membrane in an unoccluded ear canal

RMS   root mean square; overall effective level of a signal, expressed as the square root of the mean of the squared values of a signal integrated over a time period sufficient to characterize the signal

ROC curve   receiver-operating characteristic curve; graph used in signal detection theory in which the hit rate, or probability of a positive response to a signal, is plotted as a function of the false-alarm rate, or probability of a positive response to noise

Rx   prescription

S/N   signal-to-noise ratio; relative difference in dB between a sound of interest and a background of noise

SAC   Self Assessment of Communication; a self-assessment questionnaire designed to assess perceived communication ability of adults with hearing impairment

SAL   sensorineural acuity level; method for quantifying the size of an air-bone gap by establishing air-conduction thresholds under earphones in quiet and in the presence of bone-conducted noise and comparing the shift in threshold to normative values

SAT   speech-awareness threshold; lowest level at which a speech signal is audible; SYN: SDT

SBMPL   simultaneous binaural median plane localization; early test of lateralization in which the intensity level of identical tones delivered simultaneously to the two ears was adjusted until a fused tone at the midline of the head was perceived

SD   speech discrimination; old term for word recognition

SDS   speech-discrimination score; old term for word-recognition score, expressed as the percentage of words presented in a list that are correctly identified

SDT   speech-detection threshold; lowest level at which a speech signal is just audible; SYN: SAT

SEE1 Seeing Essential English; contrived manual communication dialect based on American Sign Language that has been modified so that its syntax more closely resembles that of English

SEE2 Signing Exact English; manual communication dialect based on a simplification of Seeing Essential English

SEP somatosensory evoked potential; evoked electrical activity of the brain created by stimulation of the somatosensory system, usually by electrical stimulation over a peripheral nerve or the spinal cord

SHHH Self Help for Hard of Hearing People; organization for persons with hearing impairment

SIFTER Screening Instrument For Targeting Educational Risk; formalized teacher checklist designed to assess communication performance in the classroom of a child with hearing impairment

SII speech intelligibility index; ANSI standard identifier of the articulation or audibility index; a measure of the proportion of speech cues that are audible

SIL speech-interference level; masking or interference effect of noise on the intelligibility of speech communication, originally expressed as the articulation index and later as sound pressure levels in various octave bands

SIP Sickness Impact Profile; standardized questionnaire designed to assess the physical and psychosocial impact of impairment on an individual

SISI short increment sensitivity index; early test used in differential diagnosis based on differential sensitivity to 1-dB increments superimposed on a pure tone; the ability to perceive the increments is related to a cochlear site of disorder

SL sensation level; the intensity level of a sound in dB above an individual's threshold; usually used to refer to the intensity level of a signal presentation above a specified threshold, such as pure-tone threshold or acoustic reflex threshold

SLP speech-language pathologist; healthcare professional who is credentialed in the practice of speech-language pathology to provide a comprehensive array of services related to prevention, evaluation, and rehabilitation of speech and language disorders

SMSP spectral maxima sound processor; cochlear implant signal-processing strategy in which the highest six amplitudes of 16 processed bands are delivered in a nonoverlapping sequence to electrode locations mapped to the identified channels

SN10 slow negative (auditory evoked response occurring at) 10 msec; averaged auditory electrical potential evoked by tone bursts, characterized as a broad vertex negative peak occurring around 10 msec following signal onset

SNHL sensorineural hearing loss; cochlear or retrocochlear loss in hearing sensitivity due to disorders involving the cochlea and/or the auditory nerves fibers of Cranial Nerve VIII

SOAE spontaneous otoacoustic emission; measurable low-level sound that is emitted by the cochlea in the absence of stimulation; related to the function of the outer hair cells; COM: EOAE

SOC superior olivary complex; auditory nuclei in the hindbrain that relay information from the cochlear nucleus to the midbrain, including the lateral superior olive, medial superior olive, medial nucleus of the trapezoid body, and periolivary nuclei

SOM serous otitis media; inflammation of middle ear mucosa, with serous effusion

SOT sensory organization test; component of computerized dynamic posturography designed to assess equilibrium with six different combinations of sensory input

SP summating potential; a direct-current electrical potential of cochlear origin that follows the envelope of acoustic stimulation and is measured with electrocochleography

SPAR sensitivity prediction from the acoustic reflex; test designed to predict the presence or absence of cochlear hearing loss by determining the difference between acoustic reflex thresholds elicited by pure tones and by broad-band noise

SPIN speech perception in noise test; measure of word-recognition ability in noise in which target words occur at the end of sentences with both low and high semantic predictability based on the content of the sentence

SPL   sound pressure level; magnitude or quantity of sound energy relative to a reference pressure, 0.0002 dynes/cm^2 or 20 μPa

SPV   slow phase velocity; commonly used measure of nystagmus strength, described as the size of the arc in degrees that the eyeball covers during the slow phase of nystagmus; SYN: VES

SRT   speech-reception threshold; threshold level for speech recognition, expressed as lowest intensity level at which 50% of spondaic words can be identified; SYN: ST

SSEP   steady-state evoked potential; auditory evoked potential in which the response waveform approximates the pattern of periodic stimulation, such as the stimulus rate or rate of stimulus modulation, e.g., 40-Hz response

SSI   synthetic sentence identification test; closed-set speech-recognition test in which approximations of sentences are presented in a background of single-talker competition in order to assess central auditory processing ability

SSI-CCM   SSI test in which the sentences are presented with a contralateral competing message (CCM) at various message-to-competition ratios

SSI-ICM   SSI test in which the sentences are presented with an ipsilateral competing message (ICM) at a message-to-competition ratio of 0 dB

SSPL90   saturation sound pressure level 90; electroacoustic assessment of a hearing aid's maximum output, expressed as a frequency response curve to a 90-dB input with the hearing aid gain control set to full on; SYN: MPO

SSW   staggered spondaic word test; test of dichotic listening in which two spondaic words are presented so that the second syllable delivered to one ear is heard simultaneously with the first syllable delivered to the other ear.

ST   1. speech threshold; generic term describing speech-reception threshold, as opposed to awareness or detection threshold; 2. spondee threshold; SYN: SRT

stat   statum; at once; immediately

STAT   suprathreshold adaptation test; procedure to measure auditory adaptation in which the signal is presented at a high-intensity level, and the patient responds to its presence for as long as it is audible

STS   standard threshold shift; change in hearing threshold in comparison to a baseline audiogram, defined as an average change of 10 dB or more at 2000 Hz, 3000 Hz, and 4000 Hz in either ear

SWAMI   speech with alternating masking index; early speech-recognition measure in which two signals—a target signal and noise of 20 dB greater intensity—were alternated rapidly between ears to assess dichotic integration

T   tympanogram; graph of middle ear immittance as a function of the amount of air pressure delivered to the ear canal

T&A   tonsillectomy and adenoidectomy; surgical extraction of tonsils and adenoids to limit chronic upper respiratory infection

T coil   telecoil; an induction coil often included in a hearing aid to receive electromagnetic signals from a telephone or a loop amplification system

T switch   telecoil switch; switch circuit on some hearing aids that permits use of an induction coil to receive electromagnetic signals from a telephone or a loop amplification system

TB   trapezoid body; second-order neural fiber bundle leaving the AVCN and projecting ventrally and medially to distribute fibers to the ipsilateral LSO and MSO and continuing across midline to distribute fibers to the contralateral MSO and MNTB

TC   total communication; habilitative approach used in individuals with severe and profound hearing impairment consisting of the integration of oral/aural and manual communication strategies

TD   threshold of discomfort; lowest intensity level at which sound is judged to be uncomfortably loud; SYN: ULL

TDD   telecommunication or telephone device for the deaf; telephone system used by those with significant hearing impairment in which a typewritten message is transmitted over telephone lines and is received as a printed message; SYN: TT, TTY, TTD

TDH   telephonic dynamic headphone; standard earphone for audiometric testing, usually stated with numeric designator specifying the version, such as TDH-39 and TDH-49

TEOAE   transient evoked otoacoustic emission; low-level acoustic echo emitted by the cochlea in response to a click or transient auditory stimulus; related to the integrity and function of the outer hair cells of the cochlea; COM: DPOAE; SOAE

TIA   transient ischemic attack; sudden reversible loss of neurologic function due to cerebral vascular incident

TILL   treble increases at low levels; type of automatic signal processing in a hearing aid that uses level-dependent control of frequency response, increasing high frequencies in response to low-intensity input

TM   tympanic membrane; thin, membranous vibrating tissue terminating the external auditory meatus and forming the major portion of the lateral wall of the middle ear cavity, onto which the malleus is attached

TMJ   temporomandibular joint; point of articulation of the mandible and temporal bone

TMJ syndrome   temporomandibular joint syndrome; disorder of the temporomandibular joint, characterized by varying degrees of impaired movement, discomfort, headache, earache, tinnitus, stuffiness, and vertigo

TOAE   transient otoacoustic emission; SYN: TEOAE

TORCH infections   congenital perinatal infections grouped as risk factors associated with hearing impairment and other disorders, including *t*oxoplasmosis, *o*ther infections, especially syphilis, *r*ubella, *c*ytomegalovirus infection, and *h*erpes simplex

TROCA   tangible reinforcement of operant conditioned audiometry; audiometric technique that uses tangible reinforcement, usually in the form of candy or cereal, for the correct identification of a signal presentation

TT   text telephone; telephone system used by those with significant hearing impairment in which a typewritten message is transmitted over telephone lines and is received as a printed message; SYN: TDD

TTD   teletypewriter for the deaf; early term for TDD or TT

TTS   temporary threshold shift; transient or reversible hearing loss due to auditory fatigue following exposure to excessive levels of sound

TTY   teletypewriter; early term for TDD or TT

TWA   time-weighted average; measure of daily noise exposure, expressed as the product of durations of exposure at particular sound levels to the allowable durations of exposure for those levels

Tx   therapy or treatment

UCL   uncomfortable loudness; SYN: ULL

UL   uncomfortable level; level at which sound is judged to be uncomfortably loud by a listener

ULBW   ultra-low birth weight; classification of newborns based on birth weight, specifically any infant with a birth weight less than 1000 grams

ULCL   upper limits of comfortable loudness; measure of loudness comfort level describing the highest intensity level at which the loudness of sound remains comfortable

ULL   uncomfortable loudness level; intensity level at which sound is perceived to be uncomfortably loud; SYN: LDL

UW   unilateral weakness; measure in percentage of the difference in magnitude of nystagmus from right-ear versus left-ear bithermal caloric stimulation; a difference exceeding 20% is considered to be abnormal

V   volt; unit of electromotive force producing a current of 1 ampere through a resistance of 1 ohm

VC   volume control; manual or automatic control designed to adjust the output level of a hearing instrument

VEP   visual evoked potential; electrophysiologic responses to light changes

VES   vestibular eye speed; measure of nystagmus expressed as the speed of the slow phase; SYN: slow-phase velocity

VIOLA   Visual Input/Output Locator Algorithm; computer-assisted method for selection of hearing aid parameters based on the determination of loudness growth

VLBW   very low birth weight; classification of newborns based on birth weight, specifically any infant with a birth weight less than 1500 grams

VOR   vestibulo-ocular reflex; reflex arc between the vestibular system and extraocular muscles, activated by asymmetric neural firing rate of the vestibular nerve, serving to generate compensatory eye movements in response to head rotation

VRA   visual reinforcement audiometry; audiometric technique used in pediatric assessment in which a correct response to signal presentation, such as a head turn toward the speaker, is rewarded by the activation of a light or lighted toy

VU meter   volume unit meter; visual indicator on an audiometer showing intensity of an input signal in dB, where 0 dB is equal to the attenuator output setting

W   watt; unit of electrical power with a current of 1 ampere and an electromotive force of 1 volt

WDRC   wide-dynamic-range compression; hearing aid compression algorithm, with a low threshold of activation, designed to distribute signals between a listener's thresholds of sensitivity and discomfort in a manner that matches loudness growth

WDS   word-discrimination score; SYN: WRS

WFL   within functional limits

WFR   wearer frequency response; early term for real-ear unaided response

WIPI   word intelligibility by picture identification test; pediatric test of monosyllabic word-recognition ability in which a closed-set picture-pointing task is used to identify the target word

WNL   within normal limits

WRS   word-recognition score; percent correct identification of words

X   reactance; opposition to energy flow due to storage

Y   admittance; total energy flow through a system, expressed in mhos; reciprocal of impedance

Z   impedance; total opposition to energy flow or resistance to the absorption of energy, expressed in ohms

OTOTOXICITY

Iatrogenic Toxins

The **aminoglycosides** are a group of bacteriocidal antibiotics, which are often cochleotoxic and/or vestibulotoxic, derived from streptomyces or micromonosporum used primarily against gram-negative bacteria. Hearing loss is usually bilateral, sensorineural, and permanent.

> **amikacin**
> **dihydrostreptomycin**
> **garamycin**
> **gentamicin; gentamycin**
> **kanamycin**
> **neomycin**
> **netilmicin**
> **streptomycin**
> **tobramycin**
> **viomycin**

The following **antimalarial drugs** have been associated with ototoxicity that may be temporary, but can be permanent in large doses.

> **chloroquine**
> **quinine**

Drugs known as **salicylates** are used in large quantities as therapeutic agents in the treatment of arthritis and other connective tissue disorders. Hearing loss is usually reversible and accompanied by tinnitus.

> **acetylsalicylic acid**
> **aspirin**

Agents known as **loop diuretic** are used to promote the excretion of urine by inhibiting resorption of sodium and water in the kidneys. Hearing loss due to ototoxicity may be reversible or permanent.

> **ethacrynic acid**
> **furosemide**
> **lasix**

Other drugs that have been associated with ototoxicity include:

ampicillin	used in the treatment of meningitis and urinary tract infections
arsacetin	used in the treatment of syphilis and parasitic infections
atoxyl	used in the treatment of syphilis and parasitic infections
bumetanide	used in the treatment of edema associated with cardiac and renal disease
carboplatin	used as chemotherapy treatment for cancer
cisplatin	antimitotic and antineoplastic drug often used in cancer treatment
erythromycin lactobionate	used to treat gram-positive bacterial infections

glucocorticoids	steroidlike compound with an anti-inflammatory effect
naproxen	anti-inflammatory analgesic drug used to treat rheumatoid arthritis
nitrogen mustard	chemotherapeutic anticancer agent
practolol	beta blocker used for management of cardiac arhythmia
sisomicin	an antibiotic with a spectrum and application similar to gentamicin
tetanus antitoxin	antibody formed in response to a specific neurotropic toxin

Teratogenic Toxins

The following drugs are among those that may have a teratogenic effect on the auditory system of the developing embryo when taken by the mother during pregnancy:

accutane
dilantin
diphenyl hydantoin
isotretinoin
quinine
thalidomide

Environmental Toxins

The following substances are among those that have been associated with ototoxicity:

potassium bromate	colorless, odorless, tasteless neutralizer used in hair-styling solutions, food preservatives, and other commercial applications, associated with nephrotoxicity and ototoxicity
styrene	industrial solvent which can be ototoxic if inhaled in high concentrations over extended periods
toluene	industrial solvent which can be ototoxic if inhaled in high concentrations over extended periods
trichlorethylene	industrial solvent which can be ototoxic if inhaled in high concentrations over extended periods

Chemotherapy Regimens

The following chemotherapy regimens, as commonly specified by their abbreviations, contain cisplatin or carboplatin, which have been associated with ototoxicity.

BAPP	used in the treatment of malignant thymoma
BEP	used in the treatment of testicular cancer
BMC	used in the treatment of head and neck cancer
BOMP	used in the treatment of cervical cancer
CAP	used in the treatment of various cancers
CBM	used in the treatment of head and neck cancer
CHAP	used in the treatment of ovarian cancer
CISCA	used in the treatment of genito-urinary cancer

CMB	used in the treatment of cervical cancer
COB	used in the treatment of head and neck cancer
CVB	used in the treatment of esophageal cancer
DHAP	used in the treatment of non-Hodgkin's lymphoma
FAP	used in the treatment of esophageal cancer
FCE	used in the treatment of gastric cancer
FDC	used in the treatment of gastric cancer
IMAC	used in the treatment of bony sarcoma
MAP	used in the treatment of head and neck cancer
MBC	used in the treatment of cervical cancer
MVAC	used in the treatment of bladder cancer
PAC	used in the treatment of ovarian cancer
PE	used in the treatment of testicular cancer
PFL	used in the treatment of head and neck cancer
PT	used in the treatment of ovarian cancer
VAB VI	used in the treatment of testicular cancer
VBP	used in the treatment of testicular cancer and malignant melanoma
VDP	used in the treatment of malignant melanoma
VIP	used in the treatment of testicular cancer

AUDITORY DISORDERS

Syndromes and Inherited Disorders

Abruzzo-Erickson syndrome orofacial clefting syndrome, characterized by cleft palate, eye anomalies, short stature, and mixed or sensorineural hearing loss

achondroplasia autosomal dominant disorder characterized by short stature, short limbs, large head, and middle and inner ear anomalies with associated hearing loss; SYN: chondrodystrophia fetalis

acrocephalosyndactyly, Type I congenital syndrome characterized by a peaked head, fused digits, low-set ears, otitis media, stapes fixation, and associated conductive hearing loss; SYN: Apert syndrome

acrodysostosis skeletal dysplasia syndrome with recurrent otitis media and associated conductive hearing loss

acrofacial dysostosis syndrome of mandibulofacial dysostosis, or Treacher Collins syndrome, with absence of thumbs, often associated with ear and facial anomalies similar to those in Treacher Collins; SYN: Nager syndrome

Albers-Schönberg disease autosomal recessive craniofacial and skeletal disorder characterized by brittle bones; may include disarticulated ossicular chain and progressive sensorineural hearing loss; SYN: osteopetrosis

albinism syndrome autosomal recessive deficiency or absence of pigment in the skin, hair, and eyes often associated with sensorineural hearing loss of varying severity

Albrecht syndrome hereditary, sensorineural hearing loss occurring during childhood, with progression that is suggestive of early presbyacusis

Alport syndrome egenetic syndrome characterized by progressive kidney disease and sensorineural hearing loss, probably resulting from X-linked inheritance through a gene that codes for collagen, identified as COL4A5

Alstrom syndrome autosomal recessive metabolic disorder with delayed-onset progressive sensorineural hearing lossa-

nencephalycongenital malformation of the brain, characterized by the absence of cerebral and cerebellar hemispheres, often associated with malformed temporal bones and severe anomalies of the outer, middle, and inner ear

Antley-Bixler syndrome craniosynostosis syndrome that can include dysplastic ears, low-set protruding ears, external canal atresia, and associated conductive hearing loss

Apert syndrome congenital syndrome characterized by a peaked head, fused digits, low-set ears, otitis media, stapes fixation, and associated conductive hearing loss; SYN: acrocephalosyndactyly, Type 1

ataxia-hypogonadism syndrome autosomal recessive nervous system disorder, characterized by ataxia, muscle wasting, and severe mental retardation, with early-onset, progressive sensorineural hearing loss; SYN: Richards-Rundle syndrome

athreotic cretinism type of congenital hypothyroidism resulting from failure of thyroid embryogenesis, often accompanied by sensorineural hearing loss

Baller-Gerold syndrome craniosynostosis syndrome that may include auricular malformation, characterized by low-set dysplastic auricles

Beckwith-Weidemann syndrome overgrowth syndrome, which may include auricular malformations, characterized by earlobe grooves and indented lesions on the helix or concha and associated conductive hearing loss

Björnstad syndrome autosomal dominant disorder with low penetrance, characterized by congenital sensorineural hearing loss and pili torti

branchio-oto-renal syndrome autosomal dominant disorder consisting of branchial clefts, fistulas, and cysts, renal malformation, and conductive, sensorineural, or mixed hearing loss

Carpenter syndrome autosomal recessive craniosynostosis disorder that may include low-set ears, preauricular pits, and associated conductive hearing loss

cervico-oculo-acoustic syndrome congenital branchial arch syndrome, occurring primarily in females, characterized by fusion of two or more cervical vertebrae; similar to Klippel-Feil syndrome, with retraction of eyeballs, lateral gaze weakness, and hearing loss

CHARGE association genetic association featuring *c*oloboma, *h*eart disease, *a*tresia choanae (nasal cavity), *r*etarded growth and development, *g*enital hypoplasia, and *e*ar anomalies and/or hearing loss that can be conductive, sensorineural, or mixed

chondrodystrophia fetalis autosomal dominant disorder characterized by short stature, short limbs, large head, and middle and inner ear anomalies with associated hearing loss; SYN: achondroplasia

chromosome 21-trisomy syndrome congenital genetic abnormality, characterized by mental retardation and characteristic facial features, with high incidence of chronic otitis media and associated conductive, mixed, and sensorineural hearing loss; SYN: Down syndrome

cleidocranial dysostosis autosomal dominant disorder of the skeleton due to retarded bone formation, characterized by absence of clavicles and irregular formation of bones, with associated conductive and sensorineural hearing loss

cochleosaccular aplasia congenital malformation of the membranous portion of the cochlea and saccule, including atrophy of the striae vascularis and abnormalities of the tectorial membrane

Cockayne syndrome rare autosomal recessive disorder characterized by delayed-onset dwarfism, mental and motor retardation, and retinal atrophy, with progressive sensorineural hearing loss

Cogan syndrome any autoimmune disorder characterized by nonsyphilitic interstitial keratitis, associated with Ménière-like symptoms

congenital rubella teratogenic disorder caused by maternal rubella, characterized by cataract or glaucoma, cardiovascular defects, mental retardation, psychomotor retardation, and severe to profound sensorineural hearing loss

Cornelia de Lange syndrome small-stature syndrome characterized by severe mental and growth retardation,

abnormally shaped skull and face, and anomalies of the external ear and auditory meatus, with associated conductive, sensorineural, or mixed hearing loss

Costen syndrome a symptom complex of otalgia, tinnitus, headache, and dizziness associated with temporomandibular joint disorder

craniocervical dysplasia primarily inherited disorder characterized by bony, vascular, and neural malformations of the craniocervical region, with associated unilateral fluctuating progressive sensorineural hearing loss

craniodiaphyseal dysplasia craniotubular disorder with mixed hearing loss as a predominant feature

craniofacial dysostosis SYN: Crouzon syndrome

Crouzon syndrome congenital autosomal dominant disorder with manifestations related to premature fusion of the cranial sutures including ear canal atresia, commonly with sensorineural, conductive, or mixed hearing loss; SYN: craniofacial dysostosis

cryptophthalmia congenital autosomal recessive eye disorder, characterized by absence of eyelids and by skin covering a rudimentary eye, with associated conductive hearing loss

diastrophic dwarfism autosomal dominant craniofacial disorder, characterized by marked shortness of stature, hand deformity, and severe clubfoot, which may include congenital sensorineural hearing loss

DiGeorge syndrome congenital disorder characterized by agenesis of the thymus and parathyroid glands with anomalies of the cardiovascular and renal systems and craniofacial structures, including pinna malformation and atresia of the external auditory meatus

dominant hereditary hearing loss hearing loss due to transmission of a genetic characteristic or mutation in which only one gene of a pair must carry the characteristic in order to be expressed, and both sexes have an equal chance of being affected

dominant progressive hearing loss DPHL; genetic condition in which sensorineural hearing loss gradually worsens over a period of years, caused by dominant inheritance

Down syndrome congenital genetic abnormality, characterized by mental retardation and characteristic facial features, with high incidence of chronic otitis media and associated conductive, mixed, and sensorineural hearing loss

Duane retraction syndrome autosomal dominant eye disorder, characterized by congenital paralysis of Cranial Nerve VI, with congenital sensorineural or conductive hearing loss

dysplasia, Scheibe developmental abnormality of the phylogenetically newer parts of the inner ear, specifically the cochlea and saccule, and sparing of the utricle and semicircular canals, with associated sensorineural hearing loss

ectodermal dysplasia autosomal dominant facial-limb disorder, characterized by peculiar lobster-claw deformity of hands and feet, associated with small or malformed auricles, ossicular malformation, and conductive and sensorineural hearing loss

Edward syndrome chromosomal abnormality, characterized by microcephaly, agenesis of bones of the extremities, congenital heart disease, craniofacial anomalies, and mental retardation, with associated outer, middle, and inner ear anomalies; SYN: trisomy 18 syndrome

endemic cretinism type of congenital hypothyroidism resulting from failure of normal thyroid development during gestation, often accompanied by growth retardation, mental retardation, and mixed hearing loss

Engelmann syndrome autosomal dominant skeletal disorder associated with progressive sensorineural, mixed, or conductive hearing loss

familial goiter form of congenital hypothyroidism caused by defects in thyroid biosynthesis; may be accompanied by sensorineural hearing loss, as in the case of Pendred syndrome

Fehr corneal dystrophy autosomal recessive eye disorder associated with progressive sensorineural hearing loss of delayed onset; SYN: Harboyan syndrome

fetal alcohol syndrome syndrome in children of women who abuse alcohol during pregnancy, characterized by low birthweight, failure to thrive, and mental retardation, associated with recurrent otitis media and sensorineural hearing loss

Friedrich ataxia autosomal recessive nervous system disorder characterized by progressive spinocerebellar ataxia, associated with progressive sensorineural hearing loss of delayed onset

goiter, stippled epiphysis, and high protein-bound iodine congenital metabolic syndrome, characterized by thyroid overactivity, associated with profound sensorineural hearing loss

Goldenhar syndrome congenital musculoskeletal anomalies including microtia and atresia of the external auditory meatus; SYN: oculoauriculovertebral dysplasia

Gradenigo syndrome disorder characterized by the triad of paralysis of the external rectus muscle, pain behind the eye, and persistent otitis media and mastoiditis

Hallgren syndrome recessive genetic disorder characterized by vestibulocerebellar ataxia, pigmentary retinal dystrophy, congenital sensorineural hearing loss, and cataract

hand-hearing syndrome autosomal dominant disorder characterized by congenital hand abnormalities, including contracture of the digits and wasting of finger muscles, and sensorineural hearing loss

Harboyan syndrome autosomal recessive eye disorder associated with progressive sensorineural hearing loss of delayed onset; SYN: Fehr corneal dystrophy

hemifacial microsomia craniofacial disorder, including eye and facial malformation, with preauricular tags, pinna malformation, microtia, and atresia

Herrmann syndrome autosomal dominant nervous system disorder beginning in late childhood or early adolescence, with photomyoclonus and progressive sensorineural hearing loss, followed by diabetes mellitus and progressive dementia

Hunter syndrome mucopolysaccharidosis II; X-linked recessive disorder characterized by early onset and progression of growth failure, mental retardation, and other metabolic disorders, associated with conductive and sensorineural hearing loss

Hurler syndrome mucopolysaccharidosis

I; autosomal recessive disorder characterized by early onset and severe progression of growth failure, mental retardation, and other metabolic disorders, associated with some degree of progressive hearing loss

hyperbilirubinemia abnormally large amount of bilirubin (red bile pigment) in the blood at birth; risk factor for sensorineural hearing loss; SYN: erythroblastosis fetalis

hyperprolinemia II autosomal dominant metabolic disorder with late-onset progressive sensorineural hearing loss

hyperuricemia endocrine-metabolic disorder with late-onset, progressive sensorineural hearing loss

Jervell and Lange-Nielsen syndrome autosomal recessive cardiovascular disorder accompanied by congenital bilateral profound sensorineural hearing loss

Kearns-Sayre syndrome autosomal dominant disorder, characterized by cardiac abnormalities, progressive ophthalmoplegia, myopathies, neuropathies, and hearing loss

keratopachyderma and digital constrictions autosomal dominant disorder characterized by hyperkeratosis, ring-like furrows on fingers and toes, and congenital progressive sensorineural hearing loss

Klippel-Feil syndrome craniofacial disorder, characterized by short neck of limited mobility and eye disorders, including abducens nerve palsy; associated with severe to profound sensorineural hearing loss

knuckle pads and leukonychia autosomal dominant disorder, characterized by calluslike thickening of finger and toe joints and progressive whitening of finger and toenails; associated with conductive or sensorineural hearing loss

Krabbe disease autosomal recessive leukodystrophy with neonatal onset, characterized by progressive loss of muscle control, optic atrophy, tonic spasms, and sensorineural hearing loss

large vestibular aqueduct syndrome congenital disorder, often associated with Mondini dysplasia, resulting from faulty embryogenesis of the endolymphatic duct and sac, leading to endolymphatic hydrops with childhood-onset, bilateral, progressive sensorineural hearing loss

Laurence-Moon-Biedl-Bardet syndrome recessive eye disorder, characterized by retinitis pigmentosa, hypogenitalism, mental retardation, and progressive sensorineural hearing loss

Leri-Weill disease autosomal dominant craniofacial-skeletal disorder, characterized by deformity of the radius and ulna bones, with conductive hearing loss due to outer-ear and middle-ear deformity; SYN: dyschondrosteosis; Madelung deformity

Lermoyez syndrome atypical form of Ménière's disease in which fluctuation of hearing and vertiginous episodes are inversely related, so that hearing improves before, during, and immediately after a vertiginous attack

lobster-claw syndrome autosomal dominant facial-limb disorder, characterized by lobster-claw deformity of hands and feet, associated with small or malformed auricles, ossicular malformation, and conductive and sensorineural hearing loss; SYN: ectodermal dysplasia

long arm 18 deletion syndrome genetic imbalance syndrome involving partial deletion of the long arm of the 18th chromosome, characterized by mental retardation, microcephaly, short stature, retinal changes, and conductive hearing loss due to external and middle ear anomalies

Madelung deformity autosomal dominant craniofacial-skeletal disorder, characterized by deformity of the radius and ulna bones, with conductive hearing loss due to ossicular deformity and microtia; SYN: dyschondrosteosis; Leri-Weill disease

malformed low-set ears syndrome craniofacial disorder, characterized by deformed low-set ears and possible mental retardation, associated with conductive hearing loss commensurate with degree of auricular malformation

malignant sclerosteosis skeletal bone sclerosing disorder present at birth and fatal at an early age, characterized by optic atrophy, retarded growth, fractures, hearing loss, mental retardation, and facial palsy

mandibulofacial dysostosis disorder of embryonic development, resulting in ocular anomalies, defects of the mandible, palate, teeth, and auricle, with associated conductive hearing loss commensurate with the degree of auricular malformation

Marfan syndrome autosomal dominant craniofacial-skeletal disorder, characterized by arachnodactyly, scoliosis, joint hypermobility, and cardiac anomalies, with associated conductive, mixed, or sensorineural hearing loss

Marshall syndrome autosomal dominant disorder, characterized by severe myopia, cataracts, and a malformed nose, with congenital progressive sensorineural hearing loss; SYN: saddle nose and myopia

Melnick-Fraser syndrome autosomal dominant branchial arch syndrome with auricular anomalies and conductive, mixed, or sensorineural hearing loss; SYN: branchio-oto-renal syndrome

Ménière's syndrome constellation of symptoms of episodic vertigo, hearing loss, tinnitus, and aural fullness

mitochondrial disorders abnormalities of mitochondrial DNA that can result in isolated sensorineural hearing loss or hearing loss associated with other features of the disease, including encephalopathy, myopathy, seizure disorder, ataxia, and ophthalmoplegia

Möbius syndrome severe congenital bilateral facial paralysis, associated with neurological, ocular, and musculoskeletal anomalies due to lesions of Cranial Nerves III, V, VI, VII, and XII, with associated middle ear anomalies and sensorineural hearing loss

Mohr syndrome autosomal recessive craniofacial disorder, characterized by deformities of face, mouth, and fingers, associated with conductive hearing loss due to ossicular malformation

Mondini dysplasia congenital anomaly of the osseous and membranous labyrinths, exhibiting a wide range of morphologic and functional abnormality, including severe loss of hearing and vestibular function

Morquio syndrome rare autosomal recessive metabolic disorder, or mucopolysaccharidosis, characterized by dwarfism, major skeletal disorders, corneal clouding, and hearing loss

Muckle-Wells syndrome autosomal dominant endocrine and metabolic disorder of teenage onset characterized by progressive nephropathy and renal failure, with coincident progressive sensorineural hearing loss

multiple lentigines syndrome autosomal dominant integumentary-pigmentary disorder, characterized by small brown spots on the neck and upper trunk and multiple anomalies, including sensorineural hearing loss

muscular dystrophy autosomal recessive disorder characterized by muscle wasting; severe infantile muscular dystrophy is associated with mild-to-moderate sensorineural hearing loss

myoclonic epilepsy autosomal dominant nervous system disorder, characterized by myoclonic jerking and progressive ataxia; associated with late-onset progressive sensorineural hearing loss

myopia and congenital deafness autosomal recessive disorder, characterized by myopia and congenital moderate-to-severe sensorineural hearing loss

myositis ossificans dominant skeletal disorder, characterized by formation of osseous tissue in skeletal muscles, with associated conductive, mixed, or sensorineural hearing loss

Nager syndrome branchial arch disorder characterized by mandibulofacial dysostosis with limb defects, particularly the absence of thumbs, with hearing loss secondary to outer ear and middle ear malformation; SYN: acrofacial dysostosis

nephrosis, urinary tract malformations autosomal recessive renal disorder, characterized by kidney degeneration, digital anomalies, bifurcation of the uvula, and congenital conductive hearing loss

nonsyndromic hearing loss autosomal recessive or dominant genetic condition in which there are no other significant features besides hearing loss; SYN: recessive nonsyndromic hearing loss; ANT: syndromic hearing loss

Norrie syndrome X-linked recessive ocular disorder, characterized by progressive eye degeneration, mental retardation, and late-onset, progressive, bilateral, symmetric sensorineural hearing loss; SYN: oculoacousticocerebral degeneration

oculoacousticocerebral degeneration autosomal recessive ocular disorder, characterized by progressive eye degeneration, mental retardation, and late-onset, progressive, bilateral, symmetric sensorineural hearing loss; SYN: Norrie syndrome

oculoauricovertebral dysplasia congenital disorder characterized by musculoskeletal anomalies, including microtia and atresia of the external auditory meatus; SYN: Goldenhar syndrome

onychodystrophy autosomal recessive skin disorder, characterized by rudimentary fingernails and toenails, triphalangeal thumbs, and congenital, severe sensorineural hearing loss

optic atrophy and diabetes mellitus autosomal recessive disorder, characterized by childhood-onset visual impairment and diabetes mellitus, with associated progressive sensorineural hearing loss

optic atrophy and polyneuropathy autosomal recessive disorder, characterized by progressive bilateral optic atrophy, childhood polyneuropathy, and progressive sensorineural hearing loss

opticocochleodentate degeneration rare autosomal recessive nervous system disorder, characterized by progressive visual loss, progressive spastic quadriplegia, and progressive sensorineural hearing loss

osteogenesis imperfecta autosomal dominant disorder, characterized by symptoms related to having brittle bones; symptoms include multiple fractures at birth, weak joints, bone deformities, nerve-root compression, and temporal bone malformation; SYN: Van Der Hoeve syndrome

osteopetrosis autosomal recessive craniofacial and skeletal disorder characterized by brittle bones; may include disarticulated ossicular chain and progressive sensorineural hearing loss; SYN: Albers-Schönberg disease

oto-spondylo-megaepiphyseal dysplasia autosomal recessive disorder characterized by severe to profound sensorineural hearing loss, short extremities, and abnormally thick joints

otopalatodigital syndrome X-linked recessive disorder characterized by generalized bone dysplasia, resulting in conductive hearing loss, cleft palate, wide spacing of toes, broad thumbs, and other signs of dysplasia

Paget disease autosomal recessive skeletal disorder in which bones progressively soften, thicken, and deform; involves the auditory system when the temporal bone is affected

Patau syndrome chromosomal disorder, trisomy 13, characterized by numerous anomalies, including microcephaly, severe mental retardation, low-set ears, auricular malformation, atresia, and middle- and inner-ear malformation

Pelizaeus-Merzbacher disease X-linked demyelinating disorder, characterized by childhood onset of nystagmus, ataxia, dysarthria, and psychomotor dysfunction, with associated sensorineural hearing loss due to both cochlear and auditory brainstem pathway disorder

Pendred syndrome autosomal recessive endocrine metabolism disorder resulting in goiter and congenital, symmetric, moderate-to-profound sensorineural hearing loss

piebaldness recessive, X-linked, or dominant forms of skin-pigmentary syndromes, characterized by patchy absence of pigment of scalp hair; may include profound congenital sensorineural hearing loss

Pierre Robin syndrome autosomal dominant craniofacial-skeletal disorder, characterized by micrognathia and abnormal smallness of the tongue, often with cleft palate, severe myopia, congenital glaucoma, retinal detachment, and conductive or sensorineural hearing loss

pili torti [L. twisted hair] recessive skin disorder, characterized by dry, brittle twisted hair of the scalp, eyebrows, and eyelashes; often with bilateral sensorineural hearing loss

progressive adult-onset hearing loss autosomal dominant nonsyndromic hearing loss with onset in adulthood, characterized by progressive, symmetric sensorineural hearing loss

Pyle disease autosomal recessive craniofacial-skeletal disorder, which may include nystagmus and progressive mixed or sensorineural hearing loss

Ramsay Hunt syndrome herpes zoster infection that lingers in the ganglia and can be activated by systemic disease, resulting in vesicular eruptions of the auricle, facial nerve palsy, and sensorineural hearing loss; SYN: herpes zoster oticus

recessive hereditary sensorineural hearing loss most common inherited hearing loss, in which both parents are carriers of the gene but only 25% of offspring are affected; occurring in either nonsyndromic or syndromic form

Refsum syndrome autosomal recessive eye disorder, characterized by retinitis pigmentosa, peripheral neuropathy, and cerebellar ataxia, with associated progressive, asymmetric sensorineural hearing loss

renal-genital syndrome autosomal recessive disorder, characterized by renal anomalies and internal genital malformation, with low-set auricles, stenotic ear canals, and malformed middle ears with associated conductive hearing loss

Richards-Rundle syndrome autosomal recessive nervous system disorder, characterized by ataxia, muscle wasting, and severe mental retardation, with early-onset, progressive sensorineural hearing loss; SYN: ataxia-hypogonadism syndrome

rubella, congenital teratogenic disorder caused by maternal rubella, characterized by cataract or glaucoma, cardiovascular defects, mental retardation, psychomotor retardation, and severe to profound sensorineural hearing loss

saddle nose and myopia autosomal dominant disorder, characterized by severe myopia, cataracts, and a malformed nose, with congenital progressive sensorineural hearing loss; SYN: Marshall syndrome

Sanfilippo syndrome a type of mucopolysaccharidosis, characterized by severe mental retardation, minimal skeletal and visceral abnormalities, and hearing loss

Scheibe dysplasia developmental abnormality of the phylogenetically newer parts of the inner ear, specifically the cochlea and saccule, and sparing of the utricle and semicircular canals, with associated sensorineural hearing loss

sclerosteosis subgroup of congenital disorders involving skeletal sclerosis, the autosomal dominant or malignant form of which often results in otic dysplasia and associated hearing loss

sensory radicular neuropathy autosomal dominant nervous system disorder, characterized by young-adult-onset lightning pains in the distal extremities and painless ulcerations of the feet, with progressive sensorineural hearing loss

Stickler syndrome craniofacial disorder characterized by a flat facial profile, cleft palate, ocular changes, and joint disease, with conductive or mixed hearing loss associated with eustachian tube dysfunction secondary to cleft palate

symphalangism autosomal dominant skeletal disorder, characterized by bony ankylosis of the finger and toe joints, with conductive hearing loss associated with stapes fixation

Tietze syndrome autosomal dominant hereditary disorder characterized by generalized pigment loss, absence of eyebrows, blue irises, and profound hearing loss

Townes-Brocks syndrome autosomal dominant disorder characterized by anomalies of the ear, hand, foot, anus, and kidney, with associated mixed or progressive sensorineural hearing loss

Treacher Collins syndrome autosomal dominant disorder of craniofacial morphogenesis, characterized by downward sloping palpebral fissures, depressed cheek bones, malformed pinna, receding chin, and large mouth, with associated atresia and ossicular malformation

trisomy 13-15 syndrome chromosomal abnormality, characterized by microphthalmia, cleft lip and palate, and polydactyly, with associated outer, middle, and inner ear anomalies

trisomy 18 syndrome chromosomal abnormality, characterized by microcephaly, agenesis of bones of the extremities, congenital heart disease, craniofacial anomalies, and mental retardation, with associated outer, middle, and inner ear anomalies; SYN: Edward syndrome

trisomy 21 syndrome congenital genetic abnormality, characterized by mental retardation and characteristic facial features, with high incidence of chronic otitis media and associated conductive, mixed, and sensorineural hearing loss; SYN: Down syndrome

Turner syndrome chromosomal abnormality in females characterized by a missing X chromosome, resulting in small stature, lack of ovarian tissue, and eye, heart, and ear anomalies with associated conductive and sensorineural hearing loss; SYN: XO syndrome

Usher syndrome autosomal recessive disorder characterized by congenital sensorineural hearing loss and progressive loss of vision due to retinitis pigmentosa

Van Buchem syndrome autosomal recessive craniofacial disorder characterized by childhood-onset generalized osteosclerotic narrowing of the skull foramen, resulting in cranial nerve paresis, including sensorineural hearing loss

Van Der Hoeve syndrome autosomal dominant disorder, characterized by symptoms related to having brittle bones, including multiple fractures at birth, weak joints, bone deformities, nerve-root compression, and temporal bone malformation; SYN: osteogenesis imperfecta

Waardenburg syndrome autosomal dominant disorder characterized by lateral displacement of the medial canthi, increased width of the root of the nose, multicolored iris, white forelock, and mild to severe sensorineural hearing loss

Wegener granulomatosis syndrome of necrotizing granulomatous vasculitis of the airway and kidneys, which can result in otitis media with effusion, and occasional secondary sensorineural loss, due to encroachment on the eustachian tube by the granuloma

Wildervanck syndrome congenital branchial arch syndrome, occurring primarily in females, characterized by fusion of two or more cervical vertebrae, similar to Klippel-Feil syndrome, with retraction of eyeballs, lateral gaze weakness, and hearing loss

X-linked hearing disorder hereditary hearing disorder due to a faulty gene located on the X chromosome, such as that found in Alport syndrome and Hunter syndrome

XO syndrome chromosomal abnormality leading to an XO configuration with 45 chromosomes; results in small stature, obesity, low hairline, webbing of digits, narrow palate, and anomalous auricles, with associated conductive and sensorineural hearing loss; SYN: Turner Syndrome

Disorders of the Outer Ear and Tympanic Membrane

accessory auricle craniofacial anomaly characterized by an additional auricle or additional auricular tissue

acute circumscribed external otitis reddened, pustular lesion surrounding a hair follicle, usually due to staphylococci infection during hot, humid weather; SYN: furunculosis

acute diffuse external otitis diffuse reddened, pustular lesions surrounding hair follicles, usually due to gram-negative bacterial infection during hot, humid weather and often initiated by swimming; COL: swimmer's ear

acute tympanitis short-duration inflammation of the tympanic membrane; SYN: acute myringitis

anotia congenital absence of the pinna; SYN: auricular aplasia

aspergillus auricularis fungus that grows in the external ear canal and on the tympanic membrane

atresia, aural absence of the opening to the external auditory meatus

atresia, bilateral congenital absence of the external auditory meatus on both ears

atresia, bony congenital absence of the external auditory meatus due to a wall of bone separating the external auditory meatus from the middle ear space

atresia, congenital absence or pathologic closure at birth of a normal anatomical opening, such as the external auditory meatus

atresia, membranous congenital absence of the external auditory meatus due to a dense soft tissue plug between the external auditory canal and middle ear space

attic perforation perforation of the pars flaccida portion of the tympanic membrane

aural adenoma, benign glandular tumor of the external auditory canal and middle ear, which appears as a painless mass and may be accompanied by conductive hearing loss

aural adenoma, malignant   rare malignant glandular tumor of the external auditory canal and middle ear, which is accompanied by hearing loss, otorrhea, pain, and cranial nerve palsies

aural atresia   absence of the opening to the external auditory meatus

aural myiasis   infection due to invasion of the external, middle, or inner ear by larvae of certain insects

aural polyp   benign lesion in the external auditory meatus, protruding from a perforation of the tympanic membrane

auricle, accessory   craniofacial anomaly characterized by an additional auricle or additional auricular tissue

auricular aplasia   congenital absence of an auricle; SYN: anotia

auricular perichondritis   inflammation of the connective tissue membrane around the cartilage of the auricle

basal-cell carcinoma   slow-growing malignant skin cancer which can occur on the pinna and external auditory meatus as a flat, painless, slightly raised lesion followed by the development of a penetrating bleeding ulcer

benign aural adenoma   glandular tumor of the external auditory canal and middle ear, which appears as a painless mass and may be accompanied by conductive hearing loss

bilateral atresia   congenital absence of the external auditory meatus on both ears

bony atresia   congenital absence of the external auditory meatus due to a wall of bone separating the external auditory meatus from the middle ear space

bullous myringitis   acute painful viral inflammation of the tympanic membrane accompanied by bullae formation between layers of the tympanic membrane, commonly occurring in association with influenza

carcinoma, basal-cell   slow-growing malignant skin cancer which can occur on the pinna and external auditory meatus as a flat, painless, slightly raised lesion followed by the development of a penetrating bleeding ulcer

carcinoma, epidermoid   cancerous neoplasms of the auricle, external auditory canal, middle ear, and/or mastoid

carcinoma, squamous cell   most common malignant tumor of the auricle, charac-

terized by a progression of skin thickening with scaling, painless out-growth, and formation of an ulcer with a raised edge

cauliflower ear   thickening and malformation of the auricle following repeated trauma, commonly related to injury caused by the sport of wrestling

cavernous hemangioma   benign tumor consisting of newly formed blood vessels that may involve the external auditory canal, tympanic membrane, and middle ear, with associated hearing loss and pulsatile tinnitus

cellulitis   inflammatory lesion of the pinna, characterized by redness, warmth to touch, tenderness, and tenseness on palpation

cerumen, impacted   cerumen that causes blockage of the external auditory meatus

ceruminoma   benign tumor of ceruminous glands

ceruminosis   excessive cerumen in the external auditory meatus

chondrodermatitis nodularis chronica helicis   tender, benign, pea-shaped, nodular lesion on the free edge of the pinna

chronic diffuse external otitis   inflammation of the external auditory meatus, characterized by itching and a persistent or recurring scaling or weeping dermatitis, caused by bacterial infection

cleft pinna   congenital fissure of the pinna

collapsed canal   condition in which the cartilaginous portion of the external auditory meatus narrows, usually in response to pressure from a circumaural earphone against the pinna, resulting in apparent high-frequency conductive hearing loss

coloboma lobuli   congenital fissure of the earlobe

congenital atresia   absence or pathologic closure at birth of a normal anatomical opening, such as the external auditory meatus

dermatitis   nonspecific skin condition that may affect the pinna, characterized by dryness, itching, crusting, and weeping

dimeric tympanic membrane   thin area of the tympanic membrane, secondary to the healing of a perforation; consists of epidermis and mucous membrane

ear canal stenosis   narrowed or constricted external auditory meatus

epidermoid carcinoma cancerous neoplasms of the auricle, external auditory canal, middle ear, and/or mastoid

erysipelas acute inflammatory disease of the skin, which can affect the external ear

exostosis rounded hard bony nodule, usually bilateral and multiple, growing from the osseous portion of the external auditory meatus, caused by extended exposure to cold water; often found in divers or surfers

external otitis inflammation of the lining of the external auditory meatus

external otitis, acute circumscribed reddened, pustular lesion surrounding a hair follicle, usually due to staphylococci infection during hot, humid weather; SYN: furunculosis

external otitis, acute diffuse diffuse reddened, pustular lesions surrounding hair follicles, usually due to gram-negative bacterial infection during hot, humid weather and often initiated by swimming; COL: swimmer's ear

external otitis, chronic diffuse inflammation of the external auditory meatus, characterized by itching and a persistent or recurring scaling or weeping dermatitis, caused by bacterial infection

external otitis, malignant severe bacterial inflammation of the temporal bone, beginning as a focal area of ulceration in the external auditory meatus, which may spread through the tympanic membrane to the middle ear and soft tissue of the mastoid space

false fundus membrane formed across the ear canal lateral to the tympanic membrane following chronic inflammation

fibroproliferation, tympanic membrane proliferation of fibrous tissue growth in the submucosal and subcutaneous layers of the tympanic membrane, resulting from chronic inflammation, causing thickening and stiffness

fibroproliferative external otitis chronic diffuse outer ear bacterial inflammation, characterized by narrowing of the lumen of the canal

fibrotic drum tympanic membrane with reduced function due to the formation of fibrous tissue

furunculosis reddened, pustular lesion surrounding a hair follicle, usually due to staphylococci infection during hot, hu-

mid weather; SYN: acute circumscribed external otitis

granular myringitis focal or diffuse replacement of the dermis of the tympanic membrane with granulation tissue

impacted cerumen cerumen that causes blockage of the external auditory meatus

inclusion cyst firm cystic lesion found on the pinna, following incision or trauma

keloid excessive scar tissue formation on the lobule, in the form of a shiny, firm mass, following trauma, surgery, or, often, ear piercing

keratosis obturans rapidly forming keratin-mass tumor, often mixed with cerumen, caused by abnormal migration of the skin in the external auditory meatus

lupus pernio cutaneous epithelioid granulomas on the ears and hands

lupus vulgaris cutaneous tuberculosis characterized by nodular lesions on the nose and ears

macrotia congenital excessive enlargement of the auricle

malignant aural adenoma rare malignant glandular tumor of the external auditory canal and middle ear, which is accompanied by hearing loss, otorrhea, pain, and cranial nerve palsies

malignant external otitis severe bacterial inflammation of the temporal bone, beginning as a focal area of ulceration in the external auditory meatus, which may spread through the tympanic membrane to the middle ear and soft tissue of the mastoid space

marginal perforation hole at the edge or margin of the tympanic membrane

melotia congenital displacement of the auricle

membranous atresia congenital absence of the external auditory meatus due to a dense soft tissue plug between the external auditory canal and middle ear space; COM: bony atresia

microtia abnormal smallness of the auricle

monomeric tympanic membrane eardrum membrane that is missing a portion of the fibrous layer

mycomyringitis fungal inflammation of the tympanic membrane

myringitis inflammation of the tympanic membrane, usually associated with infection of the middle ear or external auditory meatus; SYN: tympanitis

myringitis, bullous acute painful viral inflammation of the tympanic membrane accompanied by bullae formation between layers of the tympanic membrane, commonly occurring in association with influenza

myringitis, granular focal or diffuse replacement of the dermis of the tympanic membrane with granulation tissue

myringomycosis fungal infection of the tympanic membrane and adjoining skin of the external auditory meatus

osteoma benign, slowly growing mass of bony tissue, sometime occurring at the junction of bone and cartilage in the external auditory meatus

otitis externa inflammation of the outer ear, usually the external auditory meatus

otomycosis fungal infection of the external auditory meatus

pachyotia abnormally thick and coarse auricles

perforation, attic perforation of the pars flaccida portion of the tympanic membrane

perforation, marginal hole at the edge or margin of the tympanic membrane

perforation, tympanic membrane abnormal opening in the tympanic membrane

perichondritis, auricular inflammation of the connective tissue membrane around the cartilage of the auricle

pinna, cleft congenital fissure of the pinna

pit, preauricular craniofacial anomaly characterized by a small hole of variable depth lying anterior to the auricle

polychondritis connective tissue disorder, characterized by inflammation and loss of multiple cartilage, including that of the auricle and eustachian tube; SYN: relapsing polychondritis

polyotia presence of an additional auricle on one or both sides of the head

polyp, aural benign lesion in the external auditory meatus, protruding from a perforation of the tympanic membrane

preauricular pits craniofacial anomaly characterized by a small hole of variable depth lying anterior to the auricle

preauricular tag craniofacial anomaly characterized by a small appendage, often containing cartilage, lying anterior to the auricle

prolapsed canal external auditory meatus that is occluded by cartilaginous tissue

that has lost rigidity; SYN: collapsed canal

retraction of the tympanic membrane a drawing back of the eardrum into the middle ear space due to negative pressure formed in the cavity secondary to eustachian tube dysfunction

scroll ear auricular deformity in which the rim is rolled forward and inward

seroma mass caused by a collection of serosanguineous fluid within tissue that can occur on the auricle following trauma

Shrapnell membrane perforation attic perforation of the pars flaccida

squamous cell carcinoma most common malignant tumor of the auricle, characterized by a progression of skin thickening with scaling, painless out-growth, and formation of an ulcer with a raised edge

stenotic ear canal narrowed or constricted external auditory meatus

subcutaneous fibro proliferative external otitischronic diffuse external otitis characterized by stenosis of the lumen of the external auditory meatus

swimmer's ear colloquial term for diffuse red, pustular lesions surrounding hair follicles, usually due to gram-negative bacterial infection during hot, humid weather and often initiated by swimming; SYN: acute diffuse external otitis

tag, preauricular craniofacial anomaly characterized by a small appendage, often containing cartilage, lying anterior to the auricle

tympanic membrane, dimeric thin area of the tympanic membrane, secondary to the healing of a perforation; consists of epidermis and mucous membrane

tympanic membrane, monomeric eardrum membrane that is missing a portion of the fibrous layer

tympanic membrane fibroproliferation proliferation of fibrous tissue growth in the submucosal and subcutaneous layers of the tympanic membrane, resulting from chronic inflammation, causing thickening and stiffness

tympanic membrane retraction a drawing back of the eardrum into the middle ear space due to negative pressure formed in the cavity secondary to eustachian tube dysfunction

tympanitis inflammation of the tympanic membrane; SYN: myringitis

Disorders of the Middle Ear

acute otitis media inflammation of the middle ear having a duration of fewer than 21 days

acute serous otitis media acute inflammation of middle ear mucosa, with serous effusion

acute suppurative otitis mediaa cute inflammation of the middle ear with infected effusion containing pus

adhesive otitis media inflammation of the middle ear caused by prolonged eustachian tube dysfunction resulting in severe retraction of the tympanic membrane and obliteration of the middle ear space

aerotitis media traumatic inflammation disorder of the middle ear caused by sudden changes in air pressure in the pneumatized spaces of the temporal bone on descent from high altitude or ascent from underwater diving; SYN: otitic barotrauma

aspergillosis infectious lung disease caused by aspergillus, often involving the middle ear by direct extension of the infection from the upper respiratory tracts

aviator's ear traumatic inflammation disorder of the middle ear caused by sudden changes in air pressure in the pneumatized spaces of the temporal bone on descent from high altitude; SYN: aerotitis media

barotitis media traumatic inflammation disorder of the middle ear caused by sudden changes in air pressure in the pneumatized spaces of the temporal bone on descent from high altitude or ascent from underwater diving; SYN: aerotitis media

blue eardrum bluish appearance of the tympanic membrane due to a variant of otitis media with effusion, idiopathic hemotympanum, in which the fluid is bluish in color caused by bleeding of granulomas

catarrhal otitis media middle ear inflammation resulting from catarrh of the nasopharynx with congestion of the eustachian tube

cholesteatoma tumorlike mass of squamous epithelium and cholesterol in the middle ear that may invade the mastoid and erode the ossicles, usually secondary to chronic otitis media or marginal tympanic membrane perforation

cholesterol granuloma circumscribed mass, formed in reaction to cholesterol deposits occurring in fluid-filled cells that are usually pneumatized, occurring in either the tympanomastoid compartment or the petrous apex, resulting in conductive or retrocochlear disorder

chronic adhesive otitis media long-standing inflammation of the middle ear caused by prolonged eustachian tube dysfunction resulting in severe retraction of the tympanic membrane and obliteration of the middle ear space

chronic atticoantral suppurative otitis media persistent purulent inflammation of the attic and mastoid antrum of the middle ear

chronic otitis media persistent inflammation of the middle ear having a duration of greater than 8 weeks

chronic otitis media with effusion persistent inflammation of the middle ear, accompanied by fluid in the middle ear space

chronic suppurative otitis media persistent inflammation of the middle ear with infected effusion containing pus

chronic tubotympanic catarrh persistent inflammation of the mucosal membrane of the eustachian tube and middle ear

disarticulation, ossicular detachment or break in the bones of the ossicular chain

effusion, middle ear exudation of fluid from the membranous walls of the middle ear cavity, secondary to inflammation

effusion, mucoid thick, viscid, mucuslike fluid

effusion, purulent fluid containing pus

effusion, serous thin, watery, sterile fluid secreted by a mucous membrane

embryonal rhabdomyosarcoma malignant neoplasm in young children, arising in many parts of the body including the middle ear, associated with bleeding from the ear or otorrhea

epidermoid cyst early term for cholesteatoma, describing a tumorlike mass of squamous epithelium and cholesterol in the middle ear

fracture, longitudinal linear break that courses longitudinally through the temporal bone, often tearing the tympanic membrane and disrupting the ossicles, typically caused by a blow to the parietal or temporal regions of the skull

glomus jugulare glomus tumor arising on the jugular bulb or hypotympanum

glomus tympanicum glomus tumor arising in the mesotympanum, with associated conductive hearing loss and pulsatile tinnitus

glue ear inflammation of the middle ear with thick, viscid, mucuslike effusion; SYN: mucoid otitis media

hemotympanum presence of blood in the middle ear

heterotopia displacement of tissue from its normal location, as in salivary gland tissue in the middle ear

longitudinal fracture linear break that courses longitudinally through the temporal bone, often tearing the tympanic membrane and disrupting the ossicles, typically caused by a blow to the parietal or temporal regions of the skull; ANT: transverse fracture

malleus ankylosis stiffness or fixation of the malleus at its abutment to the tegmen tympani

middle ear effusion exudation of fluid from the membranous walls of the middle ear cavity, secondary to inflammation

mucoid otitis media inflammation of the middle ear, with mucoid effusion

mucosanguinous otitis media inflammation of the middle ear with effusion consisting of blood and mucus

necrotizing otitis media persistent inflammation of the middle ear that results in tissue necrosis

nonsuppurative otitis media inflammation of the middle ear with effusion that is not infected, including serous and mucoid otitis media

ossicular disarticulation detachment or break in the bones of the ossicular chain

otitic barotrauma traumatic inflammation of the middle ear caused by a rapid marked change in atmospheric pressure, during descent from altitude or ascent from diving; results in sudden severe negative air pressure in the middle ear cavity; SYN: aerotitis media

otitis media inflammation of the middle ear, resulting predominantly from eustachian tube dysfunction

otitis media, acute inflammation of the middle ear having a duration of fewer than 21 days

otitis media, acute serous acute inflammation of middle ear mucosa, with serous effusion

otitis media, acute suppurative acute inflammation of the middle ear with infected effusion containing pus

otitis media, adhesive inflammation of the middle ear caused by prolonged eustachian tube dysfunction resulting in severe retraction of the tympanic membrane and obliteration of the middle ear space

otitis media, catarrhal middle ear inflammation resulting from catarrh of the nasopharynx with congestion of the eustachian tube

otitis media, chronic persistent inflammation of the middle ear having a duration of greater than 8 weeks

otitis media, chronic adhesive long-standing inflammation of the middle ear caused by prolonged eustachian tube dysfunction resulting in severe retraction of the tympanic membrane and obliteration of the middle ear space

otitis media, chronic atticoantral suppurative persistent purulent inflammation of the attic and mastoid antrum of the middle ear

otitis media, chronic suppurative persistent inflammation of the middle ear with infected effusion containing pus

otitis media, mucoid inflammation of the middle ear, with mucoid effusion

otitis media, mucosanguinous inflammation of the middle ear with effusion consisting of blood and mucus

otitis media, necrotizing persistent inflammation of the middle ear that results in tissue necrosis

otitis media, nonsuppurative inflammation of the middle ear with effusion that is not infected, including serous and mucoid otitis media

otitis media, persistent middle ear inflammation with effusion for 6 weeks or longer following initiation of antibiotic therapy

otitis media, purulent inflammation of the

middle ear with infected effusion containing pus; SYN: suppurative otitis media

otitis media, recurrent middle ear inflammation that occurs 3 or more times in a 6-month period

otitis media, reflux inflammation of the middle ear mucosa resulting from the passage of nasopharyngeal secretions through the eustachian tube

otitis media, sanguineous inflammation of the middle ear, accompanied by bloody effusion

otitis media, secretory otitis media with effusion, usually referring to serous or mucoid effusion

otitis media, seromucinous inflammation of the middle ear with an accumulation of fluid of varying viscosity in the middle ear cavity and other pneumatized spaces of the temporal bone; SYN: otitis media with effusion

otitis media, serous inflammation of middle ear mucosa, with serous effusion

otitis media, subacute inflammation of the middle ear ranging in duration from 22 days to 8 weeks

otitis media, suppurative inflammation of the middle ear with infected effusion containing pus

otitis media, tuberculous chronic inflammation of the middle ear and mastoid secondary to tuberculosis, resulting in early perforation and suppurative otorrhea

otitis media, unresponsive middle ear inflammation that persists after 48 hours of initial antibiotic therapy, occurring more frequently in children with recurrent otitis media

otitis media with effusion OME; inflammation of the middle ear with an accumulation of fluid of varying viscosity in the middle ear cavity and other pneumatized spaces of the temporal bone; SYN: seromucinous otitis media

otitis media with perforation inflammation of the middle ear, with secondary perforation of the tympanic membrane

otitis media without effusion inflammation of the middle ear

otosclerosis remodeling of bone, by resorption and new spongy formation around the stapes and oval window, resulting in stapes fixation and related conductive hearing loss

patulous eustachian tube abnormally patent eustachian tube, resulting in sensation of stuffiness, autophony, tinnitus, and audible respiratory noises

persistent otitis media middle ear inflammation with effusion for 6 weeks or longer following initiation of antibiotic therapy

purulent otitis media inflammation of the middle ear with infected effusion containing pus; SYN: suppurative otitis media

recurrent otitis media middle ear inflammation that occurs 3 or more times in a 6-month period

reflux otitis media inflammation of the middle ear mucosa resulting from the passage of nasopharyngeal secretions through the eustachian tube

relapsing polychondritis connective tissue disorder, characterized by inflammation and loss of cartilage, usually involving the auricles first; associated with conductive hearing loss secondary to eustachian tube collapse and sensorineural hearing loss

retraction pocket invagination into the middle ear space of a weakened portion of the tympanic membrane

sanguineous otitis media inflammation of the middle ear, accompanied by bloody effusion

secretory otitis media otitis media with effusion, usually referring to serous or mucoid effusion

seromucinous otitis media inflammation of the middle ear with an accumulation of fluid of varying viscosity in the middle ear cavity and other pneumatized spaces of the temporal bone; SYN: otitis media with effusion

serous otitis media SOM; inflammation of middle ear mucosa, with serous effusion

stapes fixation immobilization of the stapes at the oval window, often due to new bony growth resulting from otosclerosis

subacute otitis media inflammation of the middle ear ranging in duration from 22 days to 8 weeks

suppurative otitis media inflammation of the middle ear with infected effusion containing pus

tuberculous otitis media chronic inflammation of the middle ear and mastoid secondary to tuberculosis, resulting in early perforation and suppurative otorrhea

tubotympanitis inflammation of the middle ear cavity and eustachian tube

tympanomastoiditis inflammation of the mucosal linings of the middle ear and mastoid cavities

tympanosclerosis formation of whitish plaques in the tympanic membrane and nodular deposits in the mucosa of the middle ear, secondary to chronic otitis media, that may result in ossicular fixation

unresponsive otitis media middle ear inflammation that persists after 48 hours of initial antibiotic therapy, occurring more frequently in children with recurrent otitis media

Disorders of the Cochlea

acoustic trauma 1. damage to hearing from a transient, high-intensity sound; 2. long-term insult to hearing from excessive noise exposure

acquired syphilis venereal disease, caused by the spirochete Treponema pallidum, which in its secondary and tertiary stages may result in auditory and vestibular disorders due to membranous labyrinthitis

acquired syphilis, secondary secondary stage of a syphilis infection, which can result in membranous labyrinthitis associated with acute meningitis

acquired syphilis, tertiary late stage of development of syphilis infection, occurring within 3 years to 10 years of initial infection, often resulting in otosyphilis

acute labyrinthitis inflammation of the labyrinth resulting in acute vertigo, vegetative symptoms, sensorineural hearing loss, and tinnitus

acute mastoiditis inflammation of the mastoid, secondary to acute suppurative otitis media, that can lead to acute suppurative labyrinthitis, facial nerve paralysis, meningitis, and brain abscess

acute suppurative labyrinthitis acute inflammation of the labyrinth with infected effusion containing pus

autoimmune hearing loss auditory disorder characterized by bilateral, asymmetric, progressive, sensorineural hearing loss in patients who test positively for autoimmune disease

bacterial labyrinthitis inflammation of the membranous labyrinth due to bacterial invasion

cinchonism in hearing, the temporary hearing loss related to ingestion of quinine, an alkaloid derivative of cinchona

circumscribed labyrinthitis inflammation of the labyrinth restricted to a defined, limited area

cochlear Ménière's disease atypical form of Ménière's disease in which only the characteristic auditory symptoms are present without vertiginous episodes; SYN: cochlear hydrops

cochlear otosclerosis disease process involving new formation of spongy bone near the oval window resulting in sensorineural or mixed hearing loss

cochleosaccular degeneration, infantile idiopathic or viral selective degeneration of the cochlea and saccule with preservation of the utricle and cristae, occurring in infancy and resulting in unilateral or bilateral profound sensorineural hearing loss

contralateral delayed endolymphatic hydrops endolymphatic hydrops occurring in two phases—an initial profound hearing loss in one ear followed by development of fluctuating hearing loss and episodic vertigo in the previously normal ear

cryoglobulinemia disorder characterized by markedly increased blood viscosity, with associated progressive hearing loss secondary to cochlear degeneration

cytomegalic inclusion disease condition caused by the introduction of cytomegalovirus into cells and tissues of the body, which may result in progressive, fluctuating sensorineural hearing loss

cytomegalovirus CMV; intrauterine-prenatal or postnatal herpetoviral infection, usually transmitted in utero, which can cause central nervous system disorder, including brain damage, hearing loss, vision loss, and seizures

degeneration, infantile cochleosaccular idiopathic or viral selective degeneration in infancy of the cochlea and saccule with preservation of the utricle and cristae, resulting in unilateral or bilateral profound sensorineural hearing loss

delayed endolymphatic hydrops endolymphatic hydrops occurring in two phases—an initial profound hearing loss in one ear followed by development of episodic vertigo in the ipsilateral ear or fluctuating hearing loss and episodic vertigo in the previously normal hearing ear

endolymphatic fistula unhealed rupture of the cochlear duct

endolymphatic hydrops excessive accumulation of endolymph within the cochlear and vestibular labyrinths, resulting in fluctuating sensorineural hearing loss, vertigo, tinnitus, and a sensation of fullness

endolymphatic hydrops, contralateral delay edendolymphatic hydrops occurring in two phases—an initial profound hearing loss in one ear followed by development of fluctuating hearing loss and episodic vertigo in the previously normal hearing ear

endolymphatic hydrops, ipsilateral delayed endolymphatic hydrops occurring in two phases—an initial profound hearing loss in one ear followed by development of episodic vertigo in the ear with the hearing loss

epidemic parotitis contagious systemic viral disease, characterized by painful enlargement of parotid glands, fever, headache, and malaise, associated with sudden, permanent, profound unilateral sensorineural hearing loss; SYN: mumps, parotiditis

fistula, perilymphatic abnormal passageway between the perilymphatic space and the middle ear, resulting in the leak of perilymph at the oval or round window, caused by congenital defects or trauma

fistula, round window passageway between the perilymphatic space and the middle ear occurring at the round window, caused by congenital defects or trauma, resulting in the leak of perilymph

fracture, transverse a break that traverses the temporal bone perpendicular to the long axis of the petrous pyramid; usually caused by a blow to the occipital region of the skull, resulting in extensive destruction of the membranous labyrinth

herpes zoster oticus HZO; herpes zoster infection that lingers in the ganglia and can be activated by systemic disease, resulting in vesicular eruptions of the auricle, facial nerve palsy, and sensorineural hearing loss; SYN: Ramsey-Hunt syndrome

hydrops, cochlear excessive accumulation of endolymph within the cochlear labyrinth, resulting in fluctuating sensorineural hearing loss, tinnitus, and a sensation of fullness

hydrops, endolymphatic excessive accumulation of endolymph within the cochlear and vestibular labyrinths, resulting in fluctuating sensorineural hearing loss, vertigo, tinnitus, and a sensation of fullness

hydrops, labyrinthine excessive accumulation of endolymph within the membranous labyrinth; SYN: endolymphatic hydrops

icterus malignant jaundice that can result in sensorineural hearing loss

infantile cochleosaccular degeneration idiopathic or viral selective degeneration in infancy of the cochlea and saccule with preservation of the utricle and cristae, resulting in unilateral or bilateral profound sensorineural hearing loss

infantile meningogenic labyrinthitis inflammatory invasion of the labyrinth from the subarachnoid space via the cochlear aqueduct or internal auditory canal, secondary to meningitis, resulting in bilateral profound sensorineural hearing loss and impaired vestibular function

ipsilateral delayed endolymphatic hydrops endolymphatic hydrops occurring in two phases—an initial profound hearing loss in one ear, followed by development of episodic vertigo in the ear with the hearing loss

irradiation injury delayed-onset, progressive atrophy of the membranous labyrinth, particularly the spiral and annular ligaments, secondary to x-ray irradiation

jaundice disorder characterized by yellowish staining of tissue with bile pigments (bilirubin), which are excessive in the serum; in its severe form, it has been associated with sensorineural hearing loss; SYN: icterus

kernicterus form of severe neonatal jaundice associated with sensorineural hearing loss

labyrinthine hydrops excessive accumulation of endolymph within the membranous labyrinth; SYN: endolymphatic hydrops

labyrinthitis inflammation of the labyrinth, affecting hearing, balance, or both

labyrinthitis, acute inflammation of the labyrinth resulting in acute vertigo, vegetative symptoms, sensorineural hearing loss, and tinnitus

labyrinthitis, acute suppurative acute inflammation of the labyrinth with infected effusion containing pus

labyrinthitis, bacterial inflammation of the membranous labyrinth due to bacterial invasion

labyrinthitis, circumscribed inflammation of the labyrinth restricted to a defined, limited area

labyrinthitis, infantile meningogenic inflammatory invasion of the labyrinth from the subarachnoid space via the cochlear aqueduct or internal auditory canal, secondary to meningitis, resulting in bilateral profound sensorineural hearing loss and impaired vestibular function

labyrinthitis, otogenic suppurative inflammation of the labyrinth caused by bacterial invasion from the middle ear into the vestibule, resulting in severe vertigo and hearing loss

labyrinthitis, serous inflammation of the labyrinth caused by otogenic or meningogenic bacterial toxins or contamination during surgery; SYN: toxic labyrinthitis

labyrinthitis, subclinical infantile meningogenic labyrinthitis secondary to subclinical bacterial or viral meningitis in a young infant, resulting in mild to profound loss of auditory and vestibular function

labyrinthitis, suppurative inflammation of the labyrinth caused by bacterial invasion of the cochlea by contiguous areas of the temporal bone, resulting in severe vertigo and hearing loss

labyrinthitis, syphilitic acquired or congenital labyrinthitis, secondary to syphilis, that results in progressive, fluctuating sensorineural hearing loss due to endolymphatic hydrops and degenerative changes in sensory and neural structures

labyrinthitis, toxic inflammation of the labyrinth caused by degradation of the tissue fluid environment in the inner ear due to bacterial toxins or contamination of perilymph during surgery; SYN: serous labyrinthitis

labyrinthitis, viral inflammation of the labyrinth due to viral infections, including mumps, measles, rubella, and herpes zoster oticus

labyrinthitis ossificans ossification within the cochlea, usually most severe in the basal turn of the scala tympani near the round window, often secondary to meningitis

Lermoyez syndrome atypical form of Ménière's disease in which fluctuation of hearing and vertiginous episodes are inversely related, so that hearing improves before, during, and immediately after a vertiginous attack

malignant otosclerosis severe active otosclerosis involving the oval window, round window, and most of the bony labyrinth, resulting in a mixed hearing loss that eventually progresses to severe or profound levels

measles highly contagious viral infection, characterized by fever, cough, conjunctivitis, and cutaneous rash, which can cause purulent labyrinthitis and consequent bilateral severe to profound sensorineural hearing loss

Ménière's disease idiopathic endolymphatic hydrops, characterized by fluctuating vertigo, hearing loss, tinnitus, and aural fullness

Ménière's disease, cochlear atypical form of Ménière's disease in which only the characteristic auditory symptoms are present without vertiginous episodes

Ménière's syndrome constellation of symptoms of episodic vertigo, hearing loss, tinnitus, and aural fullness

meningitis bacterial or viral inflammation of the meninges, which can cause significant auditory disorder due to suppurative labyrinthitis or inflammation of the lining of Cranial Nerve VIII

meningo-neuro-labyrinthitis inflammation of the membranous labyrinth and Cranial Nerve VIII meninges, occurring as a predominant lesion in early congenital syphilis or in acute attacks of secondary and tertiary syphilis

mumps contagious systemic viral disease, characterized by painful enlargement of parotid glands, fever, headache, and malaise; associated with sudden, permanent, profound unilateral sensorineural hearing loss; SYN: parotitis, epidemic parotitis

noise-induced hearing loss permanent sensorineural hearing loss caused by acoustic trauma from exposure to excessive sound levels

otogenic suppurative labyrinthitis inflammation of the labyrinth caused by bacterial invasion from the middle ear into the vestibule, resulting in severe vertigo and hearing loss

otosclerosis, cochlear disease process involving new formation of spongy bone near the oval window resulting in sensorineural or mixed hearing loss

otosclerosis, malignant severe active otosclerosis involving the oval window, round window, and most of the bony labyrinth, resulting in a mixed hearing loss that eventually progresses to severe or profound levels

otosyphilis membranous labyrinthitis secondary to syphilis infection, resulting in sensorineural hearing loss

parotiditis contagious systemic viral disease, characterized by inflammation and enlargement of parotid, associated with sudden, permanent, profound unilateral sensorineural hearing loss; SYN: mumps; parotitis

parotitis parotiditis

perilymphatic fistula abnormal passageway between the perilymphatic space and the middle ear, resulting in the leak of perilymph at the oval or round window, caused by congenital defects or trauma

perilymphatic gusher abnormal spontaneous or surgically induced, profuse, jet-like outflow of perilymphatic fluid from the oval window

pneumolabyrinth abnormal entrance of air into the labyrinth by traumatic or surgical fistulization, resulting in acute vertigo and hearing loss

presbyacusis; presbycusis age-related hearing impairment

presbyacusis, neural loss of cochlear and higher-order neurons associated with the aging process

presbyacusis, sensory age-related hearing loss caused by hair cell loss at the basal end of the cochlea

presbyacusis, strial age-related hearing loss due to patchy atrophy of the stria vascularis in the middle and apical turns of the cochlea

radionecrosis death of tissue due to excessive exposure to radiation, which in the auditory system may occur immediately or have later onset and is characterized by atrophy of the spiral and annular ligaments resulting in degeneration of the organ of Corti

round window fistula passageway between the perilymphatic space and the middle ear occurring at the round window, caused by congenital defects or trauma, resulting in the leak of perilymph

scala communis cochleae inner ear anomaly, characterized by a fissure in the bony partition separating the middle and apical turns of the cochlea, common in Mondini dysplasia

secondary acquired syphilis secondary stage of a syphilis infection, which can result in membranous labyrinthitis associated with acute meningitis

sensory presbyacusis age-related hearing loss caused by hair cell loss at the basal end of the cochlea

serous labyrinthitis inflammation of the labyrinth caused by otogenic or meningogenic bacterial toxins or contamination during surgery; SYN: toxic labyrinthitis

sociocusis loss of hearing sensitivity due to the combined influences of aging, noise exposure, and environmental exposure

strial presbyacusis age-related hearing loss due to patchy atrophy of the stria vascularis in the middle and apical turns of the cochlea

subclinical infantile meningogenic labyrinthitis labyrinthitis secondary to subclinical bacterial or viral meningitis in a young infant, resulting in mild to profound loss of auditory and vestibular function

suppurative labyrinthitis inflammation of the labyrinth caused by bacterial invasion of the cochlea by contiguous areas of the temporal bone, resulting in severe vertigo and hearing loss

syphilis, acquired venereal disease, caused by the spirochete Treponema pallidum, which in its secondary and tertiary stages may result in auditory and vestibular disorders due to membranous labyrinthitis

syphilis, secondary acquired secondary stage of a syphilis infection, which can result in membranous labyrinthitis associated with acute meningitis

syphilis, tertiary acquired late stage of development of syphilis infection, occurring within 3 years to 10 years of initial infection, often resulting in otosyphilis

syphilitic labyrinthitis acquired or congenital labyrinthitis, secondary to syphilis, that results in progressive, fluctuating sensorineural hearing loss due to endolymphatic hydrops and degenerative changes in sensory and neural structures

tertiary acquired syphilis late stage of development of syphilis infection, occurring within 3 years to 10 years of initial infection, often resulting in otosyphilis

TORCH infections congenital perinatal infections grouped as risk factors associated with hearing impairment and other disorders, including *t*oxoplasmosis, *o*ther infections, especially syphilis, *r*ubella, *c*ytomegalovirus infection, and *h*erpes simplex

toxic hearing loss loss in hearing sensitivity due to exposure to ototoxic drugs

toxic labyrinthitis inflammation of the labyrinth caused by degradation of the tissue fluid environment in the inner ear due to bacterial toxins or contamination of perilymph during surgery; SYN: serous labyrinthitis

transverse fracture a break that traverses the temporal bone perpendicular to the long axis of the petrous pyramid; usually caused by a blow to the occipital region of the skull, resulting in extensive destruction of the membranous labyrinth; ANT: longitudinal fracture

trauma, acoustic 1. damage to hearing from a transient, high-intensity sound; 2. long-term insult to hearing from excessive noise exposure

viral labyrinthitis inflammation of the labyrinth due to viral infections, including mumps, measles, rubella, and herpes zoster oticus

Waldenstrom's macroglobulinemia vascular disorder characterized by increased blood viscosity and increased resistance to blood flow, one neurological manifestation of which is sudden, bilateral, progressive sensorineural hearing loss

x-ray irradiation injury atrophy of the membranous labyrinth, particularly the spiral and annular ligaments, secondary to x-ray irradiation, resulting in delayed-onset, progressive, sensorineural hearing loss

Disorders of the Auditory Nervous System

acoustic neurilemoma; neurilemmoma cochleovestibular Schwannoma; benign encapsulated neoplasm composed of Schwann cells arising from the intracranial segment of Cranial Nerve VIII; SYN: acoustic neuroma, acoustic neurinoma, acoustic tumor

acoustic neurinoma cochleovestibular Schwannoma

acoustic neuritis inflammation of the auditory portion of Cranial Nerve VIII, often of a viral nature, resulting in acute retrocochlear disorder; SYN: cochlear neuritis

acoustic neuroma generic term referring to a neoplasm of Cranial Nerve VIII, most often a cochleovestibular Schwannoma; SYN: acoustic tumor

acoustic tumor SYN: acoustic neuroma

acquired immunodeficiency syndrome AIDS; disease compromising the efficacy of the immune system, characterized by opportunistic infectious diseases that can affect the middle ear and mastoid as well as peripheral and central auditory nervous system structures

cerebellopontine angle tumor most often a cochleovestibular Schwannoma located or growing outside the internal auditory canal at the juncture of the cerebellum and pons

cochlear neuritis inflammation of the auditory portion of Cranial Nerve VIII, often of a viral nature, resulting in acute retrocochlear disorder; SYN: acoustic neuritis

cochleovestibular Schwannoma benign encapsulated neoplasm composed of

Schwann cells arising from the intracranial segment of Cranial Nerve VIII, commonly the vestibular portion; SYN: acoustic neuroma, acoustic neurilemoma, Schwannoma

demyelinating disease autoimmune disease process that causes scattered patches of demyelination of white matter throughout the central nervous system, resulting in retrocochlear disorder when the auditory nervous system is affected

diabetes mellitus metabolic disorder caused by a deficiency of insulin, with chronic complications including neuropathy and generalized degenerative changes in blood vessels

eighth nerve tumor generic term referring to a neoplasm of Cranial Nerve VIII, most often a cochleovestibular Schwannoma; SYN: acoustic tumor

focal capillary hyperplasia proliferation of small blood vessels within the trunk of Cranial Nerve VIII in the internal auditory meatus, resulting in an enlargement of the nerve trunk

human immunodeficiency virus cytopathic retrovirus that causes AIDS and can result in infectious diseases of the middle ear and mastoid as well as peripheral and central auditory nervous system disorder; SYN: HTLV-III

inferior pontine syndrome vascular lesion of the pons involving several cranial nerves; symptoms include ipsilateral facial palsy, ipsilateral hearing loss, loss of taste from the anterior two-thirds of the tongue, and paralysis of lateral conjugate gaze movement

lateral inferior pontine syndrome vascular lesion of the inferior pons, with symptoms that include facial palsy, loss of taste from the anterior two-thirds of the tongue, analgesia of the face, paralysis of lateral conjugate gaze movements, and hearing loss

lipoma common form of benign neoplasm composed of mature fat cells, not commonly found in the central nervous system, but reported occasionally as a tumor of the cerebellopontine angle

lymphomatoid granulomatosis necrotizing infiltrative lesion of the blood, occurring in patients with immunodeficiency, that can affect the auditory nervous system in extreme cases

meningioma benign tumor arising from the arachnoid villi of the sigmoid and petrosal sinuses at the posterior aspect of the petrous pyramid, which may encroach on the cerebellopontine angle, resulting in retrocochlear disorder

meningo-neuro-labyrinthitis inflammation of the membranous labyrinth and Cranial Nerve VIII meninges, occurring as a predominant lesion in early congenital syphilis or in acute attacks of secondary and tertiary syphilis

miliary tuberculosis infectious bacterial disease characterized by formation of tubercles of millet-seed size in the central nervous system; involvement of the auditory pathways can result in retrocochlear disorder

multiple sclerosis MS; demyelinating disease in which plaques form throughout the white matter of the brainstem, resulting in diffuse neurologic symptoms, including hearing loss, speech-understanding deficits, and abnormalities of the acoustic reflexes and ABR

neural presbyacusis loss of cochlear and higher-order neurons associated with the aging process

neuritis, acoustic inflammation of the auditory portion of Cranial Nerve VIII, often of a viral nature, resulting in acute retrocochlear disorder

neuritis, cochlear acoustic neuritis

neuritis vestibularis viral inflammation of Cranial Nerve VIII, resulting in acute rotary vertigo, vegetative symptoms, and auditory disorder

neurofibroma benign nonencapsulated tumor resulting from proliferation of Schwann cells in a poorly defined pattern that may include nerve fibers

neurofibromatosis I autosomal dominant disorder, characterized by childhood-onset multiple neurofibromas, located on any nerve, with associated sequelae; SYN: von Recklinghausen's disease

neurofibromatosis II autosomal dominant disorder characterized by bilateral cochleovestibular Schwannomas, which are faster growing and more virulent than the unilateral type; associated with secondary hearing loss and other intracranial tumors

Schwannoma, cochleovestibular benign encapsulated neoplasm composed of

Schwann cells arising from the intracranial segment, commonly the vestibular portion, of Cranial Nerve VIII; SYN: acoustic neuroma; acoustic neurilemoma

sclerosis, multiple   MS; demyelinating disease in which plaques form throughout the white matter of the brainstem, resulting in diffuse neurologic symptoms, including hearing loss, speech-understanding deficits, and abnormalities of the acoustic reflexes and ABR

tuberculosis, miliary   infectious bacterial disease characterized by formation of tubercles of millet-seed size in the central nervous system; involvement of the auditory pathways can result in retrocochlear disorder

tumor, acoustic   generic term referring to a neoplasm of Cranial Nerve VIII, most often a cochleovestibular Schwannoma; SYN: acoustic neuroma

tumor, cerebellopontine angle   most often a cochleovestibular Schwannoma located or growing outside the internal auditory canal at the juncture of the cerebellum and pons

tumor, eighth nerve   generic term referring to a neoplasm of Cranial Nerve VIII, most often a cochleovestibular Schwannoma; SYN: acoustic tumor

tumor, extra-axial   lesion that originates outside the brainstem, e.g., cochleovestibular Schwannoma

tumor, glomus   small neoplasm of paraganglionic tissue with a rich vascular supply located near or within the jugular bulb

tumor, intra-axial   tumor that originates within the brainstem

von Recklinghausen's disease   autosomal dominant disease characterized by café-au-lait spots and multiple cutaneous tumors, with associated optic gliomas, peripheral and spinal neurofibromas, and, rarely, acoustic neuromas; SYN: neurofibromatosis I

REPORT WRITING GLOSSARY

Use of standard terminology is important in the efficient and effective communication of audiometric test results to referral sources. Over the years, the following terminology has proven to be valuable in describing the majority of outcomes of audiometric testing. A typical report might include a description of the audiometric configuration, immittance measurement results, and, if abnormal, speech audiometric results for each ear individually, followed by a recommendation. Codes are used as entries in a word-processing glossary for generation of the outcome descriptors.

Description of Audiometric Configuration

Code	Descriptor
NH	Normal hearing.
NHS	Normal hearing sensitivity.
CMI	Mild conductive hearing loss.
CMIR	Mild, rising conductive hearing loss.
CMIL	Mild, low-frequency conductive hearing loss.
CMO	Moderate conductive hearing loss.
CMOR	Moderate, rising conductive hearing loss.
CMOL	Moderate, low-frequency conductive hearing loss.
CS	Severe conductive hearing loss.
MMI	Mild mixed hearing loss.
MMIR	Mild, rising mixed hearing loss.
MMIS	Mild, sloping mixed hearing loss.
MMO	Moderate mixed hearing loss.
MMOR	Moderate, rising mixed hearing loss.
MMOS	Moderate, sloping mixed hearing loss.
MS	Severe mixed hearing loss.
MSR	Severe, rising mixed hearing loss.
MSS	Severe, sloping mixed hearing loss.
MP	Profound mixed hearing loss.
SNMI	Mild sensorineural hearing loss.
SNMIR	Mild, rising sensorineural hearing loss.
SNMIL	Mild, low-frequency sensorineural hearing loss.
SNMIS	Mild, sloping sensorineural hearing loss.
SNMIH	Mild, high-frequency sensorineural hearing loss.
SNMO	Moderate sensorineural hearing loss.
SNMOR	Moderate, rising sensorineural hearing loss.
SNMOL	Moderate, low-frequency sensorineural hearing loss.
SNMOS	Moderate, sloping sensorineural hearing loss.
SNMOH	Moderate, high-frequency sensorineural hearing loss.
SNS	Severe sensorineural hearing loss.
SNSR	Severe, rising sensorineural hearing loss.
SNSL	Severe, low-frequency sensorineural hearing loss.
SNSS	Severe, sloping sensorineural hearing loss.
SNSH	Severe, high-frequency sensorineural hearing loss.
SNP	Profound sensorineural hearing loss.

SUNCH	Sensitivity is essentially unchanged since the previous evaluation on *.
SDEC	Sensitivity is decreased since the previous evaluation on *.
SIMP	Sensitivity is improved since the previous evaluation on *.

Description of Immittance Measurement Results

Code	*Descriptor*
IMPNORM	Acoustic immittance measures are consistent with normal middle ear function.
TYMPNORM	Acoustic immittance measures yield a normal, Type A, tympanogram.
IMPABN	Acoustic immittance measures indicate middle ear disorder.
IMPDIS	Acoustic immittance measures indicate middle ear disorder. The combination of a deep, Type A tympanogram and abnormal acoustic reflex thresholds is consistent with discontinuity of the ossicular chain.
IMPFIX	Acoustic immittance measures indicate middle ear disorder. The combination of a shallow, Type A tympanogram and abnormal acoustic reflex thresholds is consistent with fixation of the ossicular chain.
IMPNEGB	Acoustic immittance measures indicate middle ear disorder. The tympanogram is Type C, with the compliance peak at -*** daPa, indicating significant negative pressure in the middle ear space.
IMPOM	Acoustic immittance measures indicate middle ear disorder. The combination of a Type B tympanogram, low static compliance, and absent acoustic reflexes indicates significant increase in the mass of the middle ear mechanism.
IMPERF	Acoustic immittance measures are consistent with a perforation of the tympanic membrane.
IMPPE	Acoustic immittance measures are consistent with a patent pressure equalization tube.
IMPWAX	Acoustic immittance measures are consistent with excessive cerumen in the ear canal.
ARTABN	Acoustic immittance measures indicate middle ear disorder. The tympanogram is normal, but acoustic reflex thresholds are abnormally elevated.
IMPCONS	Acoustic immittance measures are consistent with a history of otologic surgery.
IMPCHL	Acoustic immittance measures yield a Type A tympanogram. Acoustic reflexes are absent consistent with the severity of the hearing loss.
IMPFLUC	Acoustic immittance measures yield a Type A tympanogram and high static compliance. Acoustic reflexes could not be measured due to excessive compliance fluctuation.
IMPMOVE	Acoustic immittance measures yield a Type A tympanogram. Acoustic reflexes could not be measured due to patient movement during the test.
IMPSEAL	Acoustic immittance measure could not be completed due to an inability to maintain an air-tight seal.
IMPSURG	Acoustic immittance measures were not carried out due to history of otologic surgery.
IMPNO	Acoustic immittance measures were not carried out at the referring physician's request.
TARABN	Acoustic immittance measures yield a Type A tympanogram, but acoustic reflex thresholds are abnormally elevated.

Description of Speech Audiometric Results

Code   *Descriptor*

SPAGE   Decreased speech understanding performance is consistent with the patient's age.

SPPBROL   Speech audiometric results show significant rollover of the PI-PB function.

SSIROL   Speech audiometric results show significant rollover of the PI-SSI function.

PBSSIROL   Speech audiometric results show significant rollover of the PI-PB and PI-SSI functions.

PBSSIDIS   Speech audiometric results show significant discrepancy in performance for words (PB) versus performance for sentences (SSI).

SPDEP   Speech audiometric results are significantly depressed for both PI-PB and PI-SSI functions.

SSIDEP   Speech audiometric results are significantly depressed for the PI-SSI function.

Description of Auditory Electrophysiologic Results

Code   *Descriptor*

ABRNORM1   Auditory brainstem response (ABR) audiometry shows well-formed responses to click stimuli at normal absolute latencies and interwave intervals. There is no evidence of eighth nerve or auditory brainstem pathway disorder.

ABRNORM2   Auditory brainstem response (ABR) audiometry shows well-formed responses to click stimuli at normal absolute latencies and interwave intervals.

ABRNORM3   Auditory brainstem response (ABR) audiometry shows well-formed responses to click stimuli at intensity levels consistent with normal hearing sensitivity in the 1000 Hz to 4000 Hz frequency range. In addition, absolute and interwave latencies are age-appropriate.

ABRHL   Auditory brainstem response (ABR) audiometry shows responses to click stimuli down to **** dB nHL. This is consistent with a **** hearing loss in the 1000 Hz to 4000 Hz frequency range. In addition, interwave latencies are age-appropriate.

ABRCL   Auditory brainstem response (ABR) audiometry shows responses to click stimuli down to **** dB nHL by air conduction, and down to **** dB nHL by bone conduction. This is consistent with a **** hearing loss in the 1000 Hz to 4000 Hz frequency range. In addition, interwave latencies are age-appropriate.

ABRABN   Auditory brainstem response (ABR) audiometry shows abnormal responses to click stimuli. Both the absolute latency of Wave V and the I to V interwave interval are significantly prolonged.

ABRCHL   Auditory brainstem response (ABR) audiometry shows responses to click stimuli at absolute latencies consistent with peripheral sensitivity loss. There is no evidence of Eighth Nerve or auditory brainstem disorder.

ECOG   Electrocochleography shows an SP/AP ratio of ***%, which is within the limits of normal.

MLRNORM   In addition, middle latency and late latency responses are normal.

LLRNORM	Late latency response is normal.
TOAENORM	Transient-evoked otoacoustic emissions are present, suggesting normal cochlear function.
TOAEABN	Transient-evoked otoacoustic emissions are absent.
DPNORM	Distortion-product otoacoustic emissions are present, suggesting normal cochlear function.
DPABN	Distortion-product otoacoustic emissions are absent.

Description of Site of Auditory Disorder

Code	*Descriptor*
SITECOCH	The overall pattern of results is most consistent with cochlear site.
NOTCOCH	Speech audiometric results cannot be explained on the basis of age or degree of hearing sensitivity loss.
SITEVIII	The overall pattern of results is most consistent with retrocochlear site.
SITECAPD	The overall pattern of results is consistent with central auditory processing disorder.
SITEWIMP	These results, while not definitive, suggest the possibility of central auditory pathway disorder.
SITENEG	There is no evidence of central auditory disorder.

Recommendations

Code	*Descriptor*
HANR	Hearing aid use is not recommended.
HAENEG	In view of the relatively mild sensitivity loss, hearing aid use is not recommended.
HAEQ	In view of the audiometric configuration, the prognosis for successful hearing aid use is only marginal.
HAENO	In view of the audiometric configuration, the prognosis for successful hearing aid use is unfavorable. Therefore, a hearing aid evaluation is not recommended.
HAEPOS	In view of the significant sensitivity loss, we recommend a hearing aid evaluation to assess the potential for successful use of amplification.
HAEPEND	In view of the significant sensitivity loss, we recommend a hearing aid evaluation to assess the potential for successful use of amplification, pending medical clearance.
CIREC	In view of the significant sensitivity loss, we recommend a cochlear implant evaluation.
RECALD	We recommend the use of an assistive listening device.
DEFER	Rehabilitative recommendations are deferred pending otologic consultation.
NOTINT	The patient is not interested in pursuing amplification at this time.
EMHAE	Ear impressions were made, and a hearing aid evaluation has been scheduled.
HASUC	The patient reports successful hearing aid use.
HAOK	Electroacoustic analysis of the patient's hearing aid shows it to be functioning properly and providing adequate gain for the degree of hearing loss.
HASOK	Electroacoustic analysis of the patient's hearing aids show them to be functioning properly and providing adequate gain for the degree of hearing loss.

RECUSE	We recommend continued use of current amplification
NOISPRO	We recommend the use of ear protection in noisy environments.
OTOCON	We recommend otologic consultation for evaluation of middle ear disorder.
MEDCON	We recommend medical consultation for evaluation of middle ear disorder.
RECRE	We recommend audiologic re-evaluation following completion of medical management.
RECMON	We recommend continued monitoring of hearing.
RECABR	This pattern of test results suggests retrocochlear disorder. We recommend further evaluation by auditory evoked potentials.
RECAEP	We recommend evoked potential audiometry to further assess hearing sensitivity.
NOREC	No audiologic recommendations are indicated at this time.
PASSSCREEN	This child passed our hearing screening measures. No further audiologic recommendations are indicated at this time.
FAILSCREEN	This child failed our hearing screening measures. We recommend further assessment by evoked potential audiometry.
PEDINORM	Although results are limited on a child of this young age, the overall pattern suggests normal hearing sensitivity and normal middle ear function bilaterally.

ASSOCIATIONS AND OTHER ORGANIZATIONS

Academy of Dispensing Audiologists [ADA]
3008 Millwood Ave.
Columbia, SC 29205
803/252–5646, (800) 445–8629
FAX: 803/765–0860
ada@audiologist.org
http://www.audiologist.org

Academy of Rehabilitative Audiology [ARA]
Box 26532
Minneapolis, MN 55426
612/920–6095

Acoustic Neuroma Association
P.O. Box 12402
Atlanta, GA 30355
404/237–8023
FAX: 404/237–2704

Acoustical Society of America [ASA]
500 Sunnyside Boulevard
Woodbury, NY 11797
516/576–2360
FAX: 516/349–7669
516/576–2360 (TDD)

Alexander Graham Bell Association for the Deaf
3417 Volta Pl. NW
Washington, DC 20007
202/337–5220 (Voice/TDD)
agbell2@aol.com
http://www.agbell.org

American Academy of Audiology [AAA]
8201 Greensboro Dr., Suite 300
McLean, VA 22102
703/610–9022, 800/222–2336
FAX: 703/610–9005
deh@audiology.org
http://www.audiology.org

American Academy of Otolaryngology— Head and Neck Surgery [AAO—HNS]
1 Prince St.
Alexandria, VA 22314
703/836–4444
FAX: 703/683–5100
http://www.entnet.org

American Auditory Society [AAS]
512 E. Canterbury Lane.
Phoenix, AZ 85022
602/942–4939
FAX: 602/942–1486
wstaab@aol.com
http://www.boystown.org/aas

American Neurotology Society [ANS]
950 York Road, #102
Hinsdale, IL 60521–8608
708/789–3110
FAX: 708/789–3137

American Speech-Language-Hearing Association [ASHA]
10801 Rockville Pike
Rockville, MD 20852
301/897–5700
301/897–0157 (TTY)
FAX: 301/571–0457,
HELPLINE 800/638–8255
http://www.asha.org

American Speech-Language-Hearing Foundation
10801 Rockville Pike
Rockville, MD 20852
301/897–5700
FAX: 301/571–0457

American Tinnitus Association [ATA]
1618 SW 1st, #417, Box 5
Portland, OR 97207
503/248–9985
FAX: 503/248–0024
tinnitus@ata.org
http://www.teleport.com/~ata

Association for Research in Otolaryngology [ARO]
431 E. Locust St., Ste 202
Des Moines, IA 50309
515/243–1558
FAX: 515/243–2049
msjohnson@aro.org
http://www.aro.org/showcase/aco

288

Audiological Resource Association
6802 Lee Highway
Chattanooga, TN 37421
615/894–1133
FAX: 615/894–0292

Audiology Foundation of America [AFA]
207 North St., Ste 103B
West Lafayette, IN 47906
317/743–6283
FAX: 317/743–6283
audfound@holli.com

Auditory-Verbal International, Inc. [AVI]
2121 Eisenhower Ave., Ste. 402
Alexandria, VA 22314–4688
703/739–1049, 703/739–0874 (TDD)
FAX: 703/739–0395
avi@csgi.com
http://www.digitalmation.com/aui

Better Hearing Institute [BHI]
5021-B Backlick Road
Annandale, VA 22003
703/642–0580
800/EAR-WELL
FAX: 703/750–9302
betterhearing @juno.com
http://www.betterhearing.org

Canadian Auditory Equipment Association
500 Trillium Dr., Unit 15
Kitchener, ON N2R 1A7
Canada
519/748–6669
FAX: 519/748–9158

Canadian Hearing Society
271 Spadina Road
Toronto, ON M5R 2V3
Canada
416/964–9595
416/964–0023 (TDD)
FAX: 416/928–2506
info@chs.ca
http://www.chs.ca

Cochlear Implant Club International, Inc. [CICI]
P.O. Box 464
Buffalo, NY 14223–0464
716/838–4662 (Voice/TDD)

Committee on Hearing, Bioacoustics, and Biomechanics
National Academy of Sciences
National Research Council
2101 Constitution Ave., HA178
Washington, DC 20418
202/334–3026
FAX: 202/334–3584

Council for Accreditation in Occupational Hearing Conservation [CAOHC]
611 E. Wells St.
Milwaukee, WI 53202
414/276–5338
FAX: 414/276–3349
caottc@globaldialog.com
http://www.globaldialog.com/~cooke

Deafness Research Foundation [DRF]
15 W. 39th St., 6th Fl.
New York, NY 10018
212/768–1181
FAX: 212/768–1906

Educational Audiology Association [EAA]
4319 Ehrlich Road
Tampa, FL 33624
800/460 7322
FAX: 813/968–3597
ltgraye@ix.netcom.com

European Hearing Instrument Manufacturers Association (EHIMA)
Bosch 135
1780 Wemmel
Belgium
32 2 460 22 84
FAX: 32 2 460 42 49

Friends of NIDCD
515 King Street, Suite 420
Alexandria, VA 22314
703/684–9055
FAX: 703/684–6048

Hear Now
9745 E. Hampden Ave., #300
Denver, CO 80231
303/695–7797
800/648–4327
FAX: 303/695–7789
http://www.leisureian.com/~hearnow

Hearing Education and Awareness for Rockers [HEAR]
P.O. Box 460847
San Francisco, CA 94146
415/441–9081
FAX: 415/576–7113
415/476–7600 (TDD)

Hearing Industries Association (HIA)
515 King St., Ste. 420
Alexandria, VA 22314
703/684–5744
FAX: 703/684–6048
hiallears@aol.com

Hearing Research Foundation
55 E. Washington St., Ste. 2022
Chicago, IL 60602
312/726–9670
FAX: 312/726–9695

HIMSA AIS
Lyngbyvej 24, Ground Floor
2100 Copenhagen
Denmark
45 3916 2203
FAX: 45 3916 2216
himsa@inet.uni-c.dk, 100533.3527@compuserve.com
http://www.himsa.dk/

International Hearing Society (IHS)
20361 Middlebelt Road
Livonia, MI 48152
810/478–2610
FAX: 810/478–4520

Military Audiology Association
3600 West Tulare Avenue
Tulare, CA 93274.

National Association of Special Equipment Distributors [NASED]
Box 870923
Stone Mountain, GA 30087–0024
610/325–7600
FAX: 610/325–0369

National Association of Earmold Laboratories [NAEL]
c/o Earmold Design
3424 E. Lake St.
Minneapolis, MN 55406
800/334–6466
FAX: 612/721–1116

National Association of the Deaf [NAD]
814 Thayer Ave.
Silver Spring, MD 20910
301/587–1788 (V)
301/587–1789 (TDD)

National Board For Certification In Hearing Instrument Sciences [NBC-HIS]
20361 Middlebelt Road
Livonia, MI 48152
810/478–5712
FAX: 810/478–9668

National Captioning Institute [NCI]
1900 Gallows Road, Ste. 3000
Vienna, VA 22182
703/917–7600
FAX: 703/917–9878
ncicap.org
http://www.ncicap.org/nci

National Hearing Conservation Association [NHCA]
611 E. Wells St.
Milwaukee, WI 53202
414/276–6045
FAX: 414/276–3349

National Institute on Deafness and Other Communication Disorders [NIDCD]
U.S. Dept. of Health and Human Services
Building 31, Room 3C35
Bethesda, MD 20892
301/402–0900
FAX: 301/402–1590

National Institute for Hearing Instrument Studies [NIHIS]
20361 Middlebelt Road
Livonia, MI 48152
810/478–2610
FAX: 810/478–4520

Self Help For Hard of Hearing People, Inc. [SHHH]
7910 Woodmont Ave., Ste. 1200
Bethesda, MD 20814
301/657–2248 (Voice)
FAX: 301/913–9413,
TTY 301/657–2249
71162.634@compuserve.com
http://www.ourworld.compuserve.com/home-pages/shhh

Sertoma International
1912 E. Meyer Blvd.
Kansas City, MO 64132
816/333–8300
FAX: 816/333–4320
infosertoma@sertoma.org
http://www.sertoma.org

Society of Certified Audioprosthologists
212 W. California
El Paso, TX 79902
915/532–4768